CLINICAL CASES
Gynecologic Surgery

Eugene C. Toy, MD
The John S. Dunn Senior Academic Chair and Program Director
Obstetrics and Gynecology Residency Program
Vice Chair of Academic Affairs
Department of Obstetrics and Gynecology
The Methodist Hospital-Houston Clerkship Director and Clinical Professor
Department of Obstetrics and Gynecology
University of Texas Medical School at Houston
Houston, Texas

Konrad P. Harms, MD
Assistant Professor of Obstetrics and Gynecology
Weill Cornell Medical College
Associate Program Director, The Methodist Hospital Ob/Gyn Residency Program
Houston, Texas

Keith O. Reeves, MD
Clinical Professor of Obstetrics and Gynecology
Weill Medical College of Cornell University
Medical Director, Methodist Center for Restorative Pelvic Medicine
Houston, Texas

Cristo Papasakelariou, MD, FACOG
Clinical Professor Department of Obstetrics/Gynecology
University of Texas Medical Branch
Galveston, Texas
Director of Gynecologic Surgery
St Joseph Medical Center
Houston, Texas

McGraw Hill Education (India) Private Limited
NEW DELHI

McGraw Hill Education Offices
New Delhi New York St Louis San Francisco Auckland Bogotá Caracas
Kuala Lumpur Lisbon London Madrid Mexico City Milan Montreal
San Juan Santiago Singapore Sydney Tokyo Toronto

McGraw Hill Education (India) Private Limited

Clinical Cases: Gynecologic Surgery

Notice

Medicine is an ever-changing science. As new research and clinical experience broaden our knowledge, changes in treatment and drug therapy are required. The authors and the publisher of this work have checked with sources believed to be reliable in their efforts to provide information that is complete and generally in accord with the standards accepted at the time of publication. However, in view of the possibility of human error or changes in medical sciences, neither the authors nor the publisher nor any other party who has been involved in the preparation or publication of this work warrants that the information contained herein is in every respect accurate or complete, and they disclaim all responsibility for any errors or omissions or for the results obtained from use of the information contained in this work. Readers are encouraged to confirm the information contained herein with other sources. For example and in particular, readers are advised to check the product information sheet included in the package of each drug they plan to administer to be certain that the information contained in this work is accurate and that changes have not been made in the recommended dose or in the contraindications for administration. This recommendation is of particular importance in connection with new or infrequently used drugs.

McGraw Hill Education (India) Edition 2013

RZZYCDRORBQRR

Reprinted in India by arrangement with The McGraw Hill Companies, Inc., New York

Sales territories: India, Pakistan, Nepal, Bangladesh, Sri Lanka and Bhutan

Library of Congress Cataloging-in-Publication Data

Clinical Case: Gynecologic surgery / Eugene C. Toy …[et al.].
p. ; cm
Other title: Gynecologic surgery
Includes bibliographical references and index.
ISBN 978-0-07-159280-2 (pbk. : alk. paper)
ISBN 0-07-159280-6 (pbk. : alk. paper)
I Generative organs, Female—Surgery—Case studies. I. Toy, Eugene C.
II. Title: Gynecologic surgery.
[DNLM: 1. Gynecologic Surgical Procedures—Case Reports. 2. Gynecologic Surgical Procedures—Problems and Exercises. 3. Genital Diseases, Female—surgery—Case Reports. 4. Genital Diseases, Female—surgery—Problems and Exercises. 5. Genitalia, Female—surgery—Case Reports. 6. Genitalia, Female—surgery—Problems and Exercises. WP 18.2 C3372010]
RG104.C37 2010
618.1'059—dc22 2010015378

ISBN-13: 978-93-5134-339-4
ISBN-10: 93-5134-339-1

Published by McGraw Hill Education (India) Private Limited, P-24, Green Park Extension, New Delhi 110 016, and printed at Rajkamal Electric Press, Kundli-131028, Haryana

DEDICATION

To the aspiring gynecologic surgeons everywhere; to those who dedicate themselves to scholarly discernment of who needs medicines or the scalpel; and to those who are committed to obtaining manual dexterity, may those hands be graced with divine guidance and unlimited compassion.

— ECT

CONTENTS

CONTRIBUTORS

Barrett Blaue, MD
Central Texas Medical Center
San Marcos, Texas
16. Ectopic Pregnancy-Laparotomy
22. Surgical Management of Postpartum Hemorrhage
37. Ovarian Cystectomy

Tri A. Dinh, MD
Assistant Professor
Department of Obstetrics and Gynecology
Weill Cornell Medical College
Chief, Division of Gynecologic Oncology
The Methodist Hospital
Houston, Texas
18. Ovarian Cancer Surgery
19. Radical Hysterectomy

Jonathan M. Espana, MD
Fellow, Minimally Invasive Gynecological Surgery
Department of Obstetrics and Gynecology
The Methodist Hospital
Houston, Texas
4. Laparoscopic Diagnostic
5. Robotic Surgery

Tametra Johnson Garnier, MD
Obstetrics and Gynecology Specialist for Women
Memorial Hermann Hospital
The Woodlands, Texas
40. Treatment of Cervical Dysplasia
41. Cold Knife Conization

R. Moss Hampton, MD
Associate Professor
Department of Obstetrics and Gynecology
Texas Tech University Health Sciences Center of the Permi Basin
Odessa, Texas
6. Electrocautery with Laparoscopy (bowel injury)
17. Total Abdominal Hysterectomy

Jeané Simmons Holmes, MD, FACOG
Assistant Professor
Weill Cornell Medical College
The Methodist Hospital
Obstetrics and Gynecology Residency Program
Houston, Texas
34. Surgical Indications for DUB
35. Surgical Indications for Chronic Pelvic Pain
36. Hysteroscopic Complications

Eric A. Hurtado, MD
Urogynecology and Reconstructive Pelvic Surgery
Mid-Atlantic Pelvic Surgery Associates
Assistant Clinical Professor of Obstetrics and Gynecology
The George Washington University School of Medicine
Fairfax, Virginia
27. Sling Procedures
28. Cystoscopy

Alan L. Kaplan, MD
Professor, Obstetrics and Gynecology
Weill Medical College of Cornell University
Chairman, Department of Obstetrics and Gynecology
The Methodist Hospital
Houston, Texas
18. Ovarian Cancer Surgery

George A. Pados, MD, PhD
Assistant Professor, Obstetrics and Gynecology
Department of Obstetrics and Gynceology
Aristotle University
Papageorgiou General Hospital
Thessaloniki, Greece
11. Laparoscopic Myomectomy
13. Laparoscopic Endometriosis

Harry Reich, MD, FACOG
Emeritus Staff
Wilkes-Barre General Hospital
Wilkes-Barre, Pennsylvania
9. Total Laparoscopic Hysterectomy

Gwyn Richardson, MD, JD
Assistant Professor
Department of Obstetrics and Gyneoclogy
University of Texas Medical Branch
Division of Gynecologic Oncology
Galverston, Texas
18. Ovarian Cancer Surgery
19. Radical Hysterectomy

Priti P. Schachel, MD, FACOG
Faculty, The Methodist Hospital-Houston
Obstetrics and Gynecology Residency Program
Assistant Professor, Obstetrics and Gynecology
Weill Cornell Medical College
Houston, Texas
8. Laparoscopic Complication
14. Laparoscopic Appendectomy
20. Myomectomy
33. Surgical Therapy for Fibroids

Dimitris Tsolakidis, MD, PhD
Scientific Fellow
Department of Obstetrics and Gynceology
Aristotle University
Papageorgiou General Hospital
Thessaloniki, Greece
11. Laparoscopic Myomectomy
13. Laparoscopic Endometriosis

David E. Zepeda, MD
Clinical Associate Professor
Baylor College of Medicine
Director of Gynecologic Minimally Invasive Surgery
The Methodist Hospital
Houston, Texas
4. Laparoscopic Diagnostic
5. Robotic Surgery

ACKNOWLEDGMENTS

The curriculum that evolved into the ideas for this series was inspired by Larry C. Gilstrap III, MD, when he was chairman of obstetrics and gynecology at the University of Texas Medical School at Houston. Dr. Gilstrap is a man of such a myriad of talents and is my personal inspiration for much of the teaching that I do today. It has been a tremendous joy to work with my excellent coauthors: Konrad Harms, who is a loyal and talented associate program director and excellent surgeon; Dr. Keith O. Reeves who as codirector of the Methodist Hospital Pelvic and Reconstructive Surgical Program is an outstanding scientist, vaginal surgeon, and leader; and to my dear friend and colleague, Dr. Cristo Papasakelariou, whose expertise in minimally invasive surgery is known worldwide. I am greatly indebted to my editor, Catherine Johnson, whose exuberance, experience, and vision helped to shape this series. I appreciate McGraw-Hill's believing in the concept of teaching through clinical cases, and I would like to especially acknowledge Cindy Yoo for her editing expertise and Catherine Saggese and Rajni Pisharody for the excellent production. I appreciate Linda Bergstrom for her sage advice and support. At Methodist, I appreciate Drs. Alan Kaplan, Judy Paukert, Dirk Sostman, Marc Boom, and Karin Larson-Pollock; Ayse McCracken, and David Campbell for their leadership; and Barbara Hagemeister and Tyler Kinney, who hold the department together. Without my dear colleagues, Drs. Jeane Holmes and Priti Schachel, this book could not have been written. Most of all, I appreciate my ever-loving wife Terri, and our four wonderful children, Andy, Michael, Allison, and Christina, for their patience and understanding.

Eugene C. Toy

HOW TO USE THIS BOOK

Mastering the surgical approaches to clinical problems within a field as broad such as obstetrics and gynecology is a formidable task. It requires drawing on a knowledge base, to procure and filter through the clinical and laboratory data, to develop a differential diagnosis, and finally to make a rational treatment plan. To gain these skills, the clinician is best guided and instructed by experienced teachers and accomplished surgeons, and inspired toward self-directed, diligent reading and practicing one's craft. Clearly, there is no replacement for experience at the bedside and the surgical suite. Unfortunately, younger physicians will not have encountered the diversity of clinical situations, or dealt with the more unusual surgical complications. Perhaps the best alternative is a carefully crafted patient case designed to stimulate the clinical and surgical approach and decision making. In an attempt to achieve that goal, we have constructed a collection of clinical vignettes to teach diagnostic, therapeutic, and surgical approaches relevant to obstetrics and gynecology. Most importantly, the explanations for the cases emphasize the underlying principles, rather than merely rote questions and answers.

This book is organized for versatility: It allows the physician "in a rush" to go quickly through the scenarios and check the corresponding answers, and it provides more detailed information for the clinician who wants thought-provoking explanations. The answers are arranged from simple to complex: a summary of the pertinent points, the bare answers, an analysis of the case, an approach to the topic, a comprehension test at the end for reinforcement and emphasis, and a list of resources for further reading. The clinical vignettes are purposely placed in random order to simulate the way that real patients present to the practitioner. A listing of cases is included in Section III. The information is presented with the degree of evidence of support. Several multiple-choice questions (MCQs) are included at the end of each case discussion (comprehension questions) to reinforce concepts or introduce related topics.

Each case is designed to simulate a patient encounter with open-ended questions. At times, the patient's complaint is different from the most concerning issue, and sometimes extraneous information is given. The answers are organized into four different parts:

PART I

1. **Summary:** The salient aspects of the case are identified, filtering out the extraneous information to identify the key issues(s).
2. A **straightforward answer** is given to each open-ended question, often with a differential diagnosis.
3. The analysis consists of two parts:
   a. **Objectives:** A listing of the two or three main principles that are crucial for a practitioner to manage the patient. Again, the students are challenged to make educated "guesses" about the objectives of the case upon initial review of the case scenario, which helps to sharpen their clinical and analytical skills.
   b. **Considerations:** A discussion of the relevant points and brief approach to the specific patient.

PART II

Approach to the Disease Process: It consists of two distinct parts:

a. **Definitions:** Terminology pertinent to the disease process.
b. **Clinical Approach:** A discussion of the approach to the clinical problem in general, including tables, figures, and algorithms.

PART III

Comprehension Questions: Each case contains several MCQs, which reinforce the material, or which introduce new and related concepts. Questions about material not found in the text will have explanations in the answers.

PART IV

Clinical Pearls: Several clinically important points are reiterated as a summation of the text. This allows for easy review, such as before an examination.

SECTION I

How to Approach Clinical Problems

- Part 1. Approach to the Patient
- Part 2. Approach to Clinical Problem Solving
- Part 3. Approach to Surgical Therapy

Part 1. Approach to the Patient

As delineated in nearly every clinical book and guide, the first step in the approach to the patient is gathering information and establishing the database. This includes taking the history, performing the physical examination, and obtaining selective laboratory examinations or special evaluations, such as urodynamic testing and/or imaging tests. Of these, the historical examination is most important and useful. The gynecologist should be unbiased and balanced in the approach to the patient; discipline should be exercised to refrain from being influenced by preconceived ideas of the patient's findings or best therapy. The practitioner should use an appropriate balance of open-ended and directive questioning to efficiently determine the diagnosis without ignoring other patient concerns, or overeagerly focusing on one diagnosis too early.

Clinical Pearl

➤ The history is usually the single most important tool in obtaining a diagnosis. The art of seeking the information in a nonjudgmental, sensitive, and thorough manner cannot be overemphasized.

HISTORY

1. Basic information:
   a. Age must be recorded because some conditions are more common at certain ages; for instance, women younger than 30 years with an adnexal mass are more likely to have a benign cystic teratoma or other germ cell tumors, whereas women older than 30 years with an adnexal mass are more likely to have epithelial tumors.
   b. Gravidity: Number of pregnancies, including current pregnancy (includes miscarriages, ectopic pregnancies, and stillbirths).
   c. Parity: Number of pregnancies that have ended at gestational age(s) greater than 20 weeks.
   d. Abortuses: Number of pregnancies that have ended at gestational age(s) less than 20 weeks (includes ectopic pregnancies, induced abortions, and spontaneous abortions).
2. Last menstrual period (LMP): The first day of the LMP. In obstetric patients, the certainty of the LMP is important in determining the gestational age in pregnancy. Because of delay in ovulation in some cycles, this is not always accurate. The LMP and menstrual history is also important in assessing dysfunctional uterine bleeding, or the menorrhagia associated with uterine leiomyomata.

3. Chief complaint: What is it that brought the patient into the hospital or office? Is it a scheduled appointment, or an unexpected symptom, such as abdominal pain or vaginal bleeding in pregnancy? The duration and character of the complaint, associated symptoms, and exacerbating and relieving factors should be recorded. The chief complaint engenders a differential diagnosis, and the possible etiologies should be explored by further inquiry. For example, if the chief complaint is postmenopausal bleeding, the concern is endometrial cancer. Thus, some of the questions should be related to the risk factors for endometrial cancer, such as hypertension, diabetes, anovulation, early age of menarche, late age of menopause, obesity, infertility, nulliparity, and so forth.

Clinical Pearl

- The chief complaint, as voiced by the patient or identified by the physician as most urgent, is probed through the clinical database, engendering a differential diagnosis.

4. Past gynecologic history:
   a. Menstrual history:
      i. Age of menarche (should normally be > 9 years and < 16 years).
      ii. Character of menstrual cycles: Interval from the first day of one menses to the first day of the next menses (normal is 28 +/− 7 days, or between 21 and 35 days).
      iii. Quantity of menses: Menstrual flow should last less than 7 days (or be < 80 mL in total volume). Menstrual flow that is excessive, that is, menorrhagia, should be further characterized as associated with clots, pain, or pressure. The number of pads used and degree that they are saturated are helpful.
      iv. Menometrorrhagia, which involves both excessive and irregular bleeding, should be distinguished from menorrhagia, and usually involves anovulatory cycles or genital lesions such as endometrial or cervical cancer.
   b. Contraceptive history: Duration, type, and last use of contraception, and any side effects. Some agents such as the intrauterine contraceptive device may be associated with ectopic pregnancy in a pregnant woman, or pelvic inflammatory disease.
   c. Sexually transmitted diseases: A positive or negative history of herpes simplex virus, syphilis, gonorrhea, *Chlamydia*, human immunodeficiency virus (HIV), pelvic inflammatory disease, or human papillomavirus (HPV). Number of sexual partners, whether a recent change in partners, and use of barrier contraception.

5. Obstetric history: Date and gestational age of each pregnancy at termination, and outcome; if induced abortion, then gestational age and method. If delivered, then whether the delivery was vaginal or cesarean; if applicable, vacuum or forceps delivery, or type of cesarean (low-transverse vs classical). All complications of pregnancies should be listed.
6. Past medical history: Any illnesses, such as hypertension, hepatitis, diabetes mellitus, cancer, heart disease, pulmonary disease, and thyroid disease, should be elicited. Duration, severity, and therapies should be included. Any hospitalizations should be listed with reason for admission, intervention, and location of hospital.
7. Past surgical history: Year and type of surgery should be elucidated and any complications documented. Type of incision (laparoscopy vs laparotomy) should be recorded. The operative report is useful particularly with attention to the intra-abdominal findings, surgery performed, and possible complications.
8. Allergies: Reactions to medications should be recorded, including severity and temporal relationship to medication. Nonmedicine allergies such as to latex or iodine are also important to note. Immediate hypersensitivity should be distinguished from an adverse reaction.
9. Medications: A list of medications, dosage, route of administration and frequency, and duration of use should be obtained. Prescription, over-the-counter, and herbal remedies are all relevant. The patient's symptoms and whether there is improvement or change with the use of medications are important to record. Use or abuse of illicit drugs, tobacco, or alcohol should also be recorded.
10. Review of systems: A systematic review should be performed but focused on the more common diseases. For example, in pregnant women, the presence of symptoms referable to preeclampsia, such as headache, visual disturbances, epigastric pain, or facial swelling should be queried. In an elderly woman, symptoms suggestive of cardiac disease, such as chest pain, shortness of breath, fatigue, weakness, or palpitations should be elicited.

PHYSICAL EXAMINATION

1. General appearance: Cachectic versus well-nourished, anxious versus calm, alert versus obtunded.
2. Vital signs: Temperature, blood pressure, heart rate, and respiratory rate. Height and weight are often placed here, including body mass index (weight in kg/height in m^2).
3. Head and neck examination: Evidence of trauma, tumors, facial edema, goiter, and carotid bruits should be sought. Cervical and supraclavicular nodes should be palpated.
4. Breast examination: Inspection for symmetry, skin or nipple retraction with the patient's hands on her hips (to accentuate the pectoral muscles), and with arms raised. With the patient supine, the breasts should then be

palpated systematically to assess for masses. The nipple should be assessed for discharge, and the axillary and supraclavicular regions should be examined for adenopathy.

5. Cardiac examination: The point of maximal impulse (PMI) should be ascertained, and the heart auscultated at the apex of the heart as well as base. Heart sounds, murmurs, and clicks should be characterized. Systolic flow murmurs are fairly common due to the increased cardiac output, but prolonged or louder systolic or significant diastolic murmurs are unusual.
6. Pulmonary examination: The lung fields should be examined systematically and thoroughly. Wheezes, rales, rhonchi, and bronchial breath sounds should be recorded.
7. Abdominal examination: The abdomen should be inspected for scars, distension, masses or organomegaly (ie, spleen or liver), and discoloration. For instance, the Grey Turner sign of discoloration at the flank areas may indicate intra-abdominal or retroperitoneal hemorrhage. Auscultation of bowel sounds should be accomplished to identify normal versus high-pitched and hyperactive versus hypoactive sounds. The abdomen should be percussed for the presence of shifting dullness (indicating ascites). Careful palpation should begin initially away from the area of pain, involving one hand on top of the other to assess for masses, tenderness, and peritoneal signs. Tenderness should be recorded on a scale (eg, 1 to 4, where 4 is the most severe pain). Guarding, whether it is voluntary or involuntary, should be noted.
8. Back and spine examination: The back should be assessed for symmetry, tenderness, or masses. In particular, the flank regions are important to assess for pain on percussion since that may indicate renal disease.
9. Pelvic examination (adequate preparation of the patient is crucial, including counseling about what to expect, adequate lubrication, and sensitivity to pain and discomfort):
   a. The external genitalia should be observed for masses or lesions, discoloration, redness, or tenderness. Ulcers in this area may indicate herpes simplex virus, vulvar carcinoma, or syphilis; a vulvar mass at the 5:00 or 7:00 o'clock positions can suggest a Bartholin gland cyst or abscess. Pigmented lesions may require biopsy since malignant melanoma is not uncommon in the vulvar region. The level of estrogen effect should also be characterized, such as vaginal rugae and vaginal pH.

Clinical Pearl

- The vaginal pH of less than 4.5 correlates with estrogen effect, whereas a vaginal pH greater than 4.5 can indicate a hypoestrogenic state or various microbial infections.

b. Speculum examination: The vagina should be inspected for lesions, discharge, estrogen effect (well-rugated vs atrophic), and presence of a cystocele or a rectocele. The appearance of the cervix should be described, and masses, vesicles, or other lesions should be noted.
c. Bimanual examination: Initially, the index and middle finger of the one gloved hand should be inserted into the patient's vagina, systematically probing the urethra, bladder, vagina, and finally, underneath the cervix, while the clinician's other hand is placed on the abdomen at the uterine fundus. With the uterus trapped between the two hands, the examiner should identify whether there is cervical motion tenderness, and evaluate the size, shape, and directional axis of the uterus. The adnexa should then be assessed with the vaginal hand in the lateral vaginal fornices. The normal ovary is approximately the size of a walnut.
d. Rectal examination: A rectal examination will reveal masses in the posterior pelvis, and may identify occult blood in the stool. Nodularity and tenderness in the uterosacral ligament can be signs of endometriosis. The posterior uterus and palpable masses in the cul-de-sac can be identified by rectal examination. Occult blood should not be assessed through digital examination since false positives may occur.

10. Extremities and skin: The presence of joint effusions, tenderness, skin edema, and cyanosis should be recorded.
11. Neurologic examination: Patients who present with neurologic complaints usually require a thorough assessment, including evaluation of the cranial nerves, strength, sensation, and reflexes.
12. Laboratory assessment for obstetric patients:
    a. Screening laboratory tests usually include
        i. Complete blood count, to assess for anemia and thrombocytopenia.
        ii. Basic or comprehensive metabolic panel to assess for electrolytes and renal and liver function tests.
        iii. Hepatitis B surface antigen: Indicates that the patient is infectious. Further testing will determine whether this is a chronic carrier status (normal liver function tests) or active hepatitis (elevated liver function tests).
        iv. Syphilis nontreponemal test (rapid plasma reagin [RPR] or Venereal Disease Research Laboratories [VDRL]): A positive test necessitates confirmation with a treponemal test, such as microhemagglutination-*Treponema pallidum* (MHA-TP) or fluorescent treponemal antibody absorbed (FTA-ABS).
        v. HIV test: The screening test is usually the enzyme-linked immunosorbent assay (ELISA) and, when positive, will necessitate the Western blot or other confirmatory test.
        vi. Urine culture or urinalysis: To assess for asymptomatic bacteriuria.
        vii. Cytological examination: To assess for cervical dysplasia or cervical cancer; involves both ectocervical component and endocervical sampling. Evidence points toward the liquid-based media as being superior cellular sampling and allows for HPV subtyping.

viii. Endocervical assays for gonorrhea and/or *Chlamydia trachomatis* for high-risk patients.

ix. Pregnancy test: Urine pregnancy assays are both sensitive and specific, and quantitative serum human chorionic gonadotropin (hCG) assays can be used to follow the progress of a pregnancy.

x. Endometrial sampling: Sampling the endometrium is useful to assess for endometrial hyperplasia or malignancy as well as to assess for hormonal alterations.

13. Other tests are dependent on age, presence of coexisting disease, and chief complaint.
    a. Common scenarios:
        i. Threatened abortion: Serum quantitative hCG and/or progesterone levels may help to establish the viability of a pregnancy and risk of ectopic pregnancy.
        ii. Menorrhagia due to uterine fibroids: Complete blood cell count (CBC), endometrial biopsy, and Papanicolaou (Pap) smear. The endometrial biopsy is performed to assess for endometrial cancer and the Pap smear for cervical dysplasia or cancer.
        iii. A woman 55 years or older with an adnexal mass: CA-125, carcinoembryonic antigen (CEA), and/or CA 19-9 tumor markers for epithelial ovarian tumors.
        iv. A woman aged 25 with a complex adnexal mass: hCG level, α-fetoprotein level, and lactic acid dehydrogenase (LDH) level for germ cell tumor markers.
14. Imaging procedures:
    a. Ultrasound examination:
        i. Adnexal masses evaluated by sonography are assessed for size and echogenic texture; simple (fluid-filled) versus complex (fluid and solid components) versus solid. Various scoring systems are used to assess for malignancy, taking into account septations and the thickness of the septa, papillations, and solid components. Doppler flow may help to distinguish benign versus malignant processes, usually with high flow, low resistance being consistent with malignancy.
        ii. The uterus can be characterized for presence of masses, such as uterine fibroids, and the endometrial stripe can be measured. In postmenopausal women, a thickened endometrial stripe exceeding 5 mm may indicate malignancy. Fluid in the cul-de-sac may indicate ascites.
        iii. The gynecologic ultrasound examination usually also includes investigation of the kidneys, because hydronephrosis may suggest a pelvic process (ureteral obstruction).
        iv. Saline infusion into the uterine cavity via a transcervical catheter can enhance the ultrasound examination of intrauterine growths such as polyps. Emerging frontiers include the use of ultrasonic contrast agents to assess for tubal patency.

Clinical Pearl

> ➤ Sonohysterography is a special ultrasound examination of the uterus that involves injecting a small amount of sterile saline into the endometrial cavity to better define the intrauterine cavity. It can help to identify endometrial polyps or submucous myomata.

b. Computed tomography (CT) scan:
   i. Because of radiation concerns, this procedure is usually not performed on pregnant women unless sonography is not helpful and it is deemed necessary.
   ii. The CT scan is useful in women with possible abdominal and/or pelvic masses, and may help to delineate the lymph nodes and retroperitoneal disorders.

c. Magnetic resonance imaging (MRI):
   i. Identifies soft tissue planes very well and may assist in defining müllerian defects, such as vaginal agenesis or uterine didelphys (condition of double uterus and double cervix), and in selected circumstances may also aid in the evaluation of uterine pathology.
   ii. May be helpful in establishing the location of a pregnancy, such as in differentiating a normal pregnancy from a cervical pregnancy.

d. Intravenous pyelogram (IVP):
   i. Intravenous dye is used to assess the concentrating ability of the kidneys, the patency of the ureters, and the integrity of the bladder.
   ii. It is also useful in detecting hydronephrosis, ureteral stone, or ureteral obstruction.

e. Hysterosalpingogram (HSG):
   i. A small amount of radiopaque dye is introduced through a transcervical cannula and radiographs are taken.
   ii. It is useful for the detection of intrauterine abnormalities (submucous fibroids or intrauterine adhesions) and patency of the fallopian tubes (tubal obstruction or hydrosalpinx).

Part 2. Approach to Clinical Diagnosis and Staging

There are typically six distinct steps that a clinician undertakes to solve most clinical problems systematically:

1. Identifying the most important clinical condition
2. Developing a differential diagnosis
3. Making the diagnosis
4. Assessing the severity and/or stage of the disease
5. Rendering a treatment based on the stage of the disease
6. Following the patient's response to the treatment

IDENTIFYING THE MOST IMPORTANT CONDITION

The patient's chief complaint is generally the problem to be evaluated and worked up; however, at times, the physician may identify an issue that is more concerning than the patient's reason for seeking care. The practitioner should clearly define and communicate that key clinical condition to the patient. If the clinical problem is different from the patient's chief complaint, then the reason for its priority should also be explained so as not to alienate the patient. Patients or family members often feel as though their concerns are not addressed if this step is not taken. Other clinical problems should likewise be listed and noted, but the primary condition should be given first attention.

DEVELOPING A DIFFERENTIAL DIAGNOSIS

After the key issue or issues have been identified and prioritized, the next step is to develop a differential diagnosis. The differential diagnosis is usually between three and five disease processes, based on clinical presentation, risk factors, disease prevalence, and potential danger of the disease. A seasoned clinician will "key in" on the most important possibilities. A good clinician also knows how to ask the same question in several different ways, and use different terminology. For example, patients at times may deny having been treated for "pelvic inflammatory disease," but will answer affirmatively to being hospitalized for "a tubal infection." Reaching a diagnosis may be achieved by systematically reading about each possible cause and disease. The patient's presentation is then matched against each of these possibilities, and each is either placed high up on the list as a potential etiology or moved lower down because of disease prevalence, the patient's presentation, or other clues. A patient's risk factors may influence the probability of a diagnosis.

Usually, a long list of possible diagnoses can be pared down to two to three most likely ones, based on selective laboratory or imaging tests. For example, a woman who complains of lower abdominal pain *and* has a history of a prior sexually transmitted disease may have salpingitis; another patient who has abdominal pain, amenorrhea, *and* a history of prior tubal surgery may have an ectopic pregnancy. Furthermore, yet another woman with a 1-day history of periumbilical pain localizing to the right lower quadrant may have acute appendicitis.

MAKING THE DIAGNOSIS

The diagnosis is made by a careful evaluation strategy. An efficient, cost-effective, and evidence-based approach is best. The clinician should be careful not to have "blinders" to only focus on one diagnosis, such as a 25-year-old woman with a pelvic mass has uterine fibroids, but rather keep an "open mind" to various diagnoses and be on the alert for "red flags" that may indicate inconsistencies with the primary diagnosis. Patients are conscious of the time, convenience, and number of visits required to reach a diagnosis, and these factors should also be taken into account in formulating the diagnostic plan. Finally, the diagnostic plan should be individualized for the particular patient, since a preconceived algorithm is rarely "one size fits all." Surgery is sometimes performed for diagnostic purposes to establish the diagnosis. In general, surgery should be reserved for those instances when noninvasive methods are unrevealing, or when urgent conditions exist.

Clinical Pearl

- The first three steps in clinical problem solving include identifying the key issue(s), developing a differential diagnosis, and making the diagnosis.

ASSESSING THE SEVERITY OF THE DISEASE

After ascertaining the diagnosis, the next step is to characterize the severity of the disease process; in other words, describe "how bad" a disease is. With malignancy, this is done formally by staging the cancer. Most cancers are categorized from stage I (least severe) to stage IV (most severe). Some diseases, such as preeclampsia, may be designated as mild or severe. With other ailments, there is a moderate category. With some infections, such as syphilis, the staging depends on the duration and extent of the infection and follows the natural history of the infection (ie, primary syphilis, secondary, latent period, and tertiary/neurosyphilis).

Clinical Pearl

- The fourth step is to establish the severity or stage of disease. There is usually prognostic or treatment significance based on the stage.

TREATING BASED ON STAGE

Many illnesses are stratified according to severity because prognosis and treatment often vary based on the severity. If neither the prognosis nor the treatment was influenced by the stage of the disease process, there would not be a reason to subcategorize a disease as mild or severe. As another example, urinary tract infections may be subdivided into lower tract infections (cystitis) that are treated by oral antibiotics on an outpatient basis and upper tract infections (pyelonephritis) that generally require hospitalization and intravenous antibiotics.

Bacterial vaginosis (BV), which has been associated with preterm delivery, endometritis, and vaginal cuff cellulitis (following hysterectomy), does not have a severe or mild substaging. The presence of BV may slightly increase the risk of problems, but neither the prognosis nor the treatment is affected by "more" BV or "less" BV. Hence, the student should approach a new disease by learning the mechanism, clinical presentation, staging, and the treatment based on stage.

Treatment is broadly divided into medical therapy and surgical therapy. The astute clinician will be aware of the various types of medical therapy available and the indications for surgery. Often, there will be various types of surgical approaches and possible associated or prophylactic procedures considered with the primary operation. For instance, in a 44-year-old woman undergoing a hysterectomy for symptomatic uterine fibroids that have failed medical management, should the ovaries be removed? Current review of the literature, assessment of the risks and benefits of each alternative, and a careful discussion with the patient and her family are paramount.

Clinical Pearl

- The treatment, whether medical or surgical, is tailored to the extent or "stage" of the disease.

FOLLOWING THE RESPONSE TO TREATMENT

The final step in the approach to disease is to follow the patient's response to the therapy. The "measure" of response should be recorded and monitored. Some responses are clinical, such as improvement (or lack of improvement) in a patient's abdominal pain, temperature, or pulmonary examination. Obviously, the physician must work on being more skilled in eliciting the data in an unbiased and standardized manner. Subjective complaints such as chronic pelvic pain due to endometriosis may be followed by an analogue pain scale and validated questionnaires. Other responses may be followed by imaging tests, such as a CT scan, to establish retroperitoneal node size in a patient receiving chemotherapy, or a tumor marker, such as the CA-125 level in a woman receiving chemotherapy for ovarian cancer. When the patient's condition does not improve, it may be time to reconsider the diagnosis, or to repeat the metastatic workup, or to follow up with another more specific test. Because different physicians may follow the same patient, the methodology and plan for follow-up should be clearly documented so that the clinical assessment is reproducible.

Clinical Pearl

- The final step is to monitor treatment response or efficacy, which may be measured in different ways. It may be symptomatic (patient feels better), or based on physical examination (fever), a laboratory test (CA-125 level), or an imaging test (ultrasound size of ovarian cyst).

Part 3. Approach to the Surgical Therapy

When surgery is contemplated in treating a patient, the timing, operative approach, optimization of comorbidities, risk-benefit analysis, and alternatives should be explored.

1. Timing: When the patient presents with an urgent clinical finding, urgent surgical intervention is warranted. For instance, when a woman has abdominal pain and hypotension consistent with a ruptured ectopic pregnancy, expeditious surgery is indicated. Nevertheless, even with emergency situations, patient stabilization is critical. For instance, it may be prudent to initiate intravenous fluid hydration, and perhaps ensure the availability of cross-matched blood. In most conditions, the patient should be treated with medical therapy first, and the symptoms monitored. Nevertheless, with some diseases, surgery is the best initial treatment, such as the postmenopausal woman with a 10 cm ovarian mass, due to the concern of ovarian neoplasm/malignancy.
2. Operative approach: Once surgery is decided as the best treatment alternative, the surgeon should consider the best operative approach. In women with a vaginal vault prolapse, should the approach be vaginal and a sacrospinous ligament fixation, or a uterosacral ligament fixation, or should it be an abdominal route such as an sacrocolpopexy. Although physicians will naturally have preferences for their favorite method, the patient should not be counseled toward one approach due to the surgeon's limitations. In other words, if the best technique is not within the scope of the physician's expertise, then the patient should be referred to a colleague who can perform that procedure. The patient's underlying pathophysiology should be sought, so that not just the "tip of the iceberg" symptom is addressed, but also the etiologies under the waterline. For instance, in women with vaginal vault prolapse, an enterocele is almost always present, and needs to be repaired to prevent recurrence.
3. Optimization of comorbidities: The patient's medical conditions, such as cardiovascular disease, pulmonary disease, diabetes, hypothyroidism, and other processes, need to be explored and optimized to reduce the perioperative complications. An understanding of the patient's anesthesia risk is

also important. Thus, a history of snoring and uneasy sleep may indicate sleep apnea. Consultants' recommendations are vitally important; yet, blindly following recommendations is unwise, as the consummate surgeon should be aware of the important complications of the more common diseases. For instance, the gynecologist should assess for end-organ involvement from processes such as diabetes mellitus or hypertension.

4. Risk-benefit analysis: Each individual patient should be assessed for the benefits of the proposed procedure and the risks of doing nothing, an alternative, or the surgery contemplated. An evidence-based approach is best—literature should be used rather than speculation or impression of the past experience. A clear idea of the indication for the surgery should be documented, and the realistic incidence of complications associated with the procedure. Although patients are counseled every day on the possibility of complications, most surgeons and patients do not believe that those complications will happen to them. Thus, it is an important discipline to "fast forward" to the possibility of complications, and ask oneself the question: "If this patient develops a serious complication from the surgery, will the indication and surgery still be viewed as appropriate?"
5. Alternatives: Before embarking on surgery, the gynecologist should review the alternative therapies one last time before proceeding to the operative approach. The clinician is best served by taking a dispassionate view, trying to look objectively at the patient's condition from an "outsider's view." This exercise allows for the patient to have the best treatment. The short- and long-term clinical course should be projected for the recommended surgery as well as the alternatives, including doing nothing.

REFERENCES

Rock JA, Jones HW. *TeLinde's Operative Gynecology*. 10th ed. Philadelphia, PA: Lippincott Williams and Wilkins; 2008.

Baggish MS, Karram MM. *Atlas of Pelvic Anatomy and Gynecologic Surgery*. 2nd ed. New York, NY: Saunders; 2006.

SECTION II

Clinical Cases

Case 1

A 43-year-old G3P2002 woman presents to the emergency department (ED) complaining of nausea, vomiting, abdominal distention, and vaginal bleeding of 2-day duration. Her last normal LMP (last menstrual period) was 9 weeks ago. She has no known medical problems and two previously normal-term vaginal deliveries. She has not been using any contraception. On examination, she is in no acute distress. Her blood pressure (BP) is 110/90 mm Hg and heart rate (HR) 100 beats/min. The pelvic examination reveals an enlarged uterus, closed cervix, and minimal vaginal bleeding. Her serum quantitative β human chorionic gonadotropin (β-hCG) level is 120,000 mIU/mL, and a transvaginal ultrasound reveals an 18-cm uterus with a "snowstorm" pattern within the uterine cavity consistent with a hydatidiform mole.

- ➤ What is your management plan?
- ➤ What are some risk factors for the development of a hydatidiform mole?
- ➤ What are some differences between complete and partial hydatidiform moles?

ANSWERS TO CASE 1:
D&C Indications (Molar Pregnancy)

Summary: This is a 43-year-old G3P2002 woman at 9 weeks' gestation by LMP, who has nausea and vomiting, and ultrasound findings consistent with a molar pregnancy.

- **Management plan:** Metastatic workup including chest radiograph, CBC, liver function tests, and then suction dilation and curettage (D&C) or possible total abdominal hysterectomy.
- **Risk factors:** History of molar pregnancy, ethnicity, maternal age.
- **Differences between complete and partial hydatidiform moles:** Complete moles are genetically composed of only paternal genetic material after a process of androgenesis. There are a total of 46 chromosomes with a complete mole (nearly always 46, XX) as compared to a partial mole which has 69 chromosomes and is derived from both maternal and paternal genotypes. Gestational trophoblastic tumors are more likely to be associated with complete moles rather than partial ones. Unlike a complete mole, partial moles may contain fetal tissue and may present similar to a missed abortion.

ANALYSIS

Objectives

1. Understand the different indications for a D&C.
2. Review the surgical technique of D&C.
3. Familiarize yourself with the differences between an obstetrical versus gynecologic D&C.

Considerations

The case described is typical of a patient with a molar pregnancy. She presents with vaginal bleeding, elevated hCG level, enlarged uterus, and ultrasound findings of "snowstorm" appearance. Her only risk factor for the development of a molar pregnancy was her age. The most important risk factor in general is history of previous molar pregnancy. Clinical symptoms of a molar pregnancy include abnormal bleeding/passage of villi, development of preeclampsia in less than 20 weeks' gestation, hyperemesis, enlarged uterus for gestational age, abdominal pain, hyperthyroidism, and theca luteal cysts. Confirmation of a molar pregnancy is usually established with ultrasound.

One of the important goals of the gynecologist is to determine if this is an uncomplicated molar pregnancy situation or a complicated gestational trophoblastic disease. Uncomplicated molar pregnancy is treated by evacuation of the uterus or possible hysterectomy (if childbearing is completed). In contrast, gestational trophoblastic disease should be referred to the specialist, such as the gynecologic oncologist or special referral centers, if feasible. Complications include high-risk metastases (brain or liver) or high risk for choriocarcinoma. Although fertility plans were not mentioned in this case scenario, at age 43, she would be a good candidate for an abdominal hysterectomy. Approximately 80% of molar pregnancies will resolve with D&C, and the remainder develop persistent disease or other malignant features. Even though a hysterectomy does not eliminate the risk of gestational trophoblastic tumor (GTT), it reduces its risk as compared to that of D&C alone. In addition, patients older than 40 years with a molar pregnancy have at least a 33% chance of the development of GTT, making hysterectomy a good treatment option for this patient. Prior to the treatment, the patient should be assessed for some potential medical problems which may occur with molar pregnancies such as preeclampsia, anemia, hyperthyroidism, hyperemesis, and possibly pulmonary insufficiency.

After uterine evacuation, the patient should be followed closely for the development of GTT. To evaluate for the presence of possible GTT, serum β-hCG values are monitored for normal regression. Weekly β-hCG values are followed until a negative value is obtained. After the β-hCG value has reached a negative level, it may then be measured monthly for the next 6 to 12 months. Patients are usually started on some form of reliable birth control as to not become pregnant while β-hCG values are being followed. If normal regression of the β-hCG does not occur, or if the β-hCG value increases after reaching normal levels, the patient should be evaluated for the presence of GTT.[1-5]

APPROACH TO D&C

There are numerous indications for the performance of a D&C. Table 1–1 lists both obstetrical and gynecologic indications for D&C.

Table 1–1 INDICATIONS FOR D&C

OBSTETRICAL	GYNECOLOGIC
Spontaneous abortion	Evaluation of dysfunctional bleeding
Elective abortion	Treatment of acute excessive bleeding
Molar pregnancy	Treatment of cervical stenosis
Ectopic pregnancy evaluation	

With the exception of ectopic pregnancy evaluation, all other obstetrically indicated D&Cs are therapeutic in nature. Because of the risks associated with surgical management of miscarriages, numerous other management options are now available for the management of abortion and include expectant management and medical therapy. It has been reported that the overall success rate with expectant management is approximately 39%.[6] The efficacy of expectant management is inversely proportional to the gestational age. Medical management success rates have been reported between 62% and 85%, depending on the agent used.[7] Common medical regimens include the use of misoprostol (orally or vaginally) with or without mifepristone. American College of Obstetricians and Gynecologists (ACOG) literature states that, "Medical abortion should be considered a medically acceptable alternative to surgical abortion in selected, carefully counseled, and informed women."[8] However, patients being treated medically need to have a 24-hour availability for emergent curettage as fewer than 1% of women undergoing medical abortion will have excessive bleeding.[8] When comparing all three management strategies for abortions, surgical management was most likely to induce complete evacuation of uterus and is the preferred method of management for gestations of longer than 11 weeks. The appropriate management strategy should be determined by both clinical factors and patient preference. A diagnostic D&C can be used in the evaluation of a possible ectopic pregnancy. If no chorionic villi are seen on frozen section, an ectopic pregnancy can be assumed. It has been reported that a frozen section was accurate in identifying chorionic villi 93% of the time.[9,10]

Gynecologic D&Cs are most often diagnostic, in other words, assessing for a disease process such as abnormal uterine bleeding or postmenopausal bleeding. However, because D&Cs are blind procedures and may miss focal areas of abnormalities, some experts recommend that a hysteroscopy be performed at the same time to evaluate the entire uterine cavity. **Studies have shown that when comparing endometrial biopsy, D&C, and hysteroscopy, 17% of patients who underwent hysteroscopy had additional pathology picked up that was not detected with either blind procedure.**[11] Studies have also demonstrated that ultrasound and sonohysterogram are also effective in evaluating the uterine cavity.[12]

D&C TECHNIQUE

When performing a D&C for obstetrical indications, a suction device is often used. Suction curettage is the surgical management of choice for abortions at less than 12 weeks' gestation or for molar pregnancies. Either local or general anesthesia may be used. The patient is then placed in dorsal lithotomy position. After a pelvic examination is performed to determine the axis of the uterus, a tenaculum or Allis clamp can be placed on the anterior lip of the cervix for traction during the D&C. A uterine sound may be used by some physicians as a means to assess uterine size and direction of cervical canal.

The cervix is then gently dilated with cervical dilators (ie, Pratt, Hank, Hegar); see Figure 1–1. Care must be taken to not "force" cervical dilation and risk perforation. During the preoperative phase, the gynecologist should determine whether dilation is anticipated to be difficult; if dilation is thought to be difficult, osmotic dilators and vaginal administration of misoprostol may be considered. After adequate cervical dilation has been achieved, the appropriate suction cannula should be inserted into the uterine cavity until the fundus is felt. Suction is only applied after reaching the fundus and with curette moving in a downward direction (Figure 1–2). Evacuation is usually complete when bubbles appear in the cannula and a gritty sensation of the cavity is felt. The appropriate cannula is usually 1 mm smaller than the weeks' gestation (although one must be aware that the smaller the diameter of the cannula, the higher the risk of uterine perforation). After suctioning contents from uterus, some physicians use a sharp curette to confirm evacuation. Oxytocic agents are given at the discretion of the physician as studies are conflicting.

Because of the significant risk of hemorrhage and uterine perforation, a suction D&C performed for a molar pregnancy is different from that of an abortion. The procedure should be performed in a fully staffed and equipped operating room (OR) under general anesthesia. Intravenous access must be

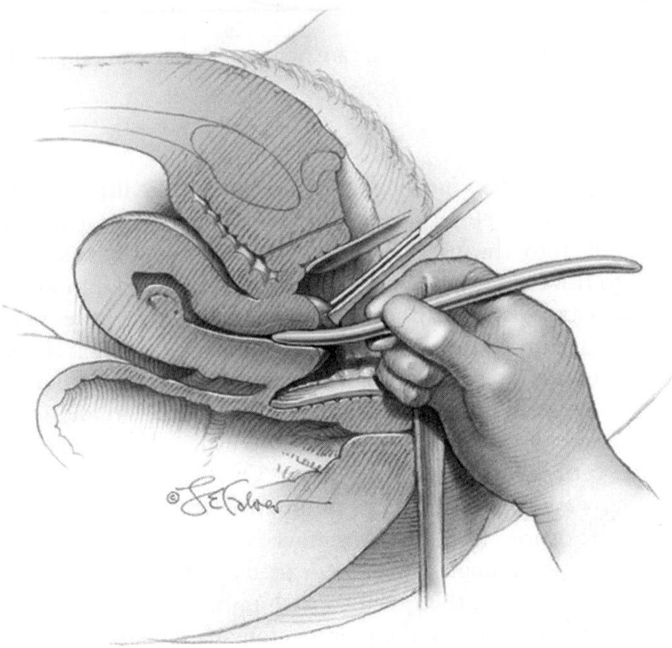

Figure 1–1. Dilation of the cervix with care to introduce the dilator in the direction of the endocervical canal. (*Reproduced, with permission, from Schorge JO, Schaffer JI, Halvorson LM, et al.* Williams Gynecology. *New York: McGraw-Hill, 2008:899.*)

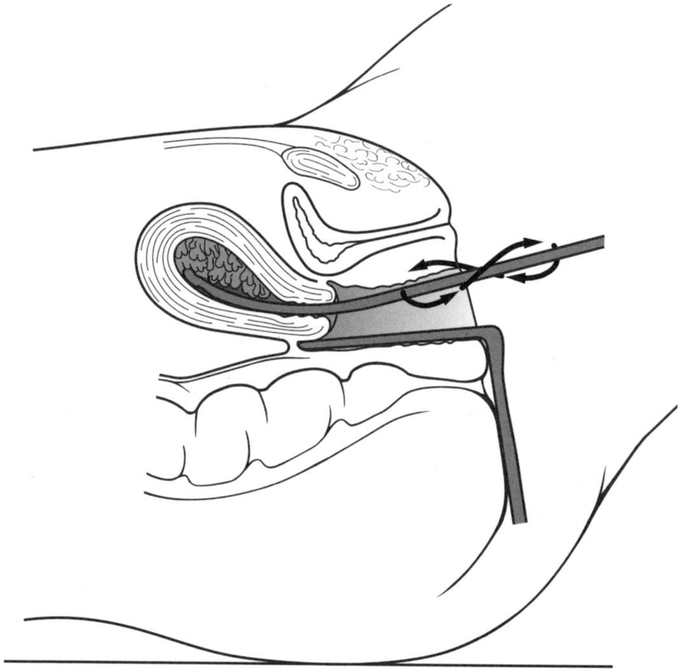

Figure 1–2. Suction curettage taking care not to perforate through the fundus of the uterus.

secured and blood products available. As compared to traditional D&Cs, cervical dilation should be performed gently and enough to get a 10- to 12-mm suction cannula into the uterine cavity. Uterine sounding is not recommended due to risk of inciting hemorrhage and uterine perforation. Once the cervix is dilated and suction cannula is introduced into the lower uterine segment, oxytocin is infused to help reduce blood loss. Evacuation should begin in the lower uterine segment and proceed toward the fundus carefully. Simultaneous use of an ultrasound can aid with evacuation and the prevention of uterine perforation. After contents are evacuated, a sharp curette is used to gently verify evacuation of the uterus. Oxytocic agents should then be continued following the procedure to minimize blood loss. If a hysterectomy is performed, the ovaries need not be removed unless other pathology is present. The ovarian blood supply is usually secured prior to uterine manipulation and the uterine vessels are then secured with minimal uterine manipulation. By securing the blood supply to the uterus before manipulation, the chance of molar villous transportation is diminished.[13,14]

As compared to obstetrical D&Cs, most gynecologic-indicated D&Cs do not require the use of a suction curette. Some practitioners choose to perform a fractional D&C (curetting the endocervical area before the uterine cavity) to better assess uterine pathology. In this setting, the cervical canal should be curetted before the cervix is dilated. Because many of the patients are being evaluated for postmenopausal bleeding, dilation of the cervix is often more difficult, and the hazards include making a false tract or perforating the cervix or uterus. Uterine contracting agents are not necessary for gynecologic D&Cs. Rare does a therapeutic D&C need to be performed for gynecologic reasons. However, a D&C is the treatment of choice in patients with acute excessive vaginal bleeding and hypovolemia.

Comprehension Questions

1.1 A 56-year-old woman with chronic obstructive pulmonary disease (COPD) and congestive heart failure (CHF) presents to your clinic with postmenopausal bleeding. An endometrial biopsy (EMB) is attempted in the clinic but unsuccessful secondary to a stenotic cervix. What is the best next step in managing this patient?

A. Wait for another episode of bleeding and, when present, take the patient to the OR for a D&C.
B. Hysteroscopy with D&C in OR.
C. Office hysteroscopy.
D. Transvaginal ultrasound.

1.2 A 48-year-old woman with vaginal bleeding and a positive pregnancy test is noted to have a molar pregnancy on sonography. A search for metastasis reveals no disease. Which of the following is the best reason for hysterectomy in this patient?

A. Lower incidence of metastasis with hysterectomy
B. Less need for chemotherapy with hysterectomy
C. Improved survival with hysterectomy
D. More cost-effective management with hysterectomy

1.3 A 54-year-old woman is taken to the OR for a fractional D&C for postmenopausal bleeding. During sounding the uterus, the fundus of the uterus is perforated. The patient's vital signs are normal. Which of the following is the best management at this stage?

A. Abandon the procedure and observe the patient in the hospital overnight.
B. Continue the procedure as long as the vital signs are normal.
C. Continue the procedure under laparoscopic guidance.
D. Perform a hysterectomy.

1.4 Which of the following describes the appropriate technique for performing a fractional D&C?
   A. The curette should be held tightly in palm.
   B. Pressure with tip of curette should be applied as it is advanced to the fundus.
   C. The curette should be advanced to fundus and then pressure exerted on uterine wall as it is withdrawn.
   D. The cervix should be dilated before attempting the endocervical curetting.

ANSWERS

1.1 **D.** Although a diagnostic hysteroscopy with D&C could be considered in this patient, her significant medical conditions (COPD and CHF) place her at higher risk for intraoperative surgical complications. A less invasive way to evaluate the uterus would be a transvaginal ultrasound to evaluate the endometrial stripe. If the stripe is less than 4 mm, no further workup is needed unless the patient continues to have bleeding. Numerous studies have validated the use of the endometrial stripe and postmenopausal bleeding.[11]

1.2 **B.** Hysterectomy may be considered in the treatment of a nonmetastatic gestational trophoblastic disease in women who do not desire future fertility. The primary reason for early hysterectomy is the decreased need and shorter duration of chemotherapy needed.

1.3 **C.** Perforation of the uterus usually occurs at the fundus, and is usually asymptomatic. Perforation with a blunt sound typically does not injure any structures; conversely, suction D&C with perforation can lead to bowel injury. Laparoscopic guidance can allow for investigation of injuries or bleeding, and also allows for uterine curettage without fear of further damage.

1.4 **C.** To minimize the risk of uterine perforation, the curette should be held loosely, as with holding a pencil, with pressure on uterine wall only when curetting away from the fundus. The endocervical sample of the fractional D&C should be obtained before cervical dilation and endometrial sampling.

Table 1–2 LEVELS OF EVIDENCE AND STRENGTH OF RECOMMENDATION

- **Level A (randomized controlled trial/meta-analysis):** High-quality randomized controlled trial (RCT) that considers all important outcomes. High-quality meta-analysis (quantitative systematic review) using comprehensive search strategies.
- **Level B (other evidence):** A well-designed, nonrandomized clinical trial. A nonquantitative systematic review with appropriate search strategies and well-substantiated conclusions. Includes lower quality RCTs, clinical cohort studies, and case-controlled studies with nonbiased selection of study participants and consistent findings. Other evidence, such as high-quality, historical, uncontrolled studies or well-designed epidemiological studies with compelling findings, is also included.
- **Level C (consensus/expert opinion):** Consensus viewpoint or expert opinion.

Clinical Pearls

See Table 1-2 for definition of level of evidence and strength of recommendation

- Suction D&C is the treatment of choice for molar pregnancies in patients desiring future fertility (Level A).
- A medically managed abortion is an acceptable alternative to surgical management (Level A).
- Transvaginal ultrasound is an effective screening tool for uterine pathology (Level A).
- The addition of hysteroscopy to a D&C increases diagnostic yield (Level A).

REFERENCES

1. Katz VL, Lentz GM, Lobo RA, Gershenson DM. Gestational trophoblastic disease and abnormal uterine bleeding. In: *Comprehensive Gynecology*. 5th ed. Philadelphia, PA: Mosby; 2007:889-900, 915-929.
2. Gilstrap III LC, Cunningham FG, Vandorsten JP. Gestational trophoblastic disease. In: *Operative Obstetrics*. 2nd ed. New York, NY: McGraw-Hill; 2002:615-628.
3. Goldstein DP, Berkowitz RS, Berstein MR. Reproductive performance after molar pregnancy and gestational trophoblastic tumor. *Clin Obstet Gynecol*. 1984;27:221.
4. Cunningham FG, Leveno KJ, Bloom SL, Gilstrap III LC, Wenstrum KD. Abortion and gestational trophoblastic disease and abortion. In: *Williams Obstetrics*. 22nd ed. New York, NY: McGraw-Hill; 2005:241-247, 273-283.
5. American College of Obstetricians and Gynecologists. *Diagnosis and Treatment of Gestational Trophoblastic Disease*. *ACOG Practice Bulletin*, 53. Washington, DC; 2004.
6. Sotiriadis A, Makrydimas G, Papatheodorou S, Ioannidis JP. Expectant, medical, or surgical management of first trimester miscarriage: a meta-analysis. *Obstet Gynecol*. 2005;105:1104-1113.

7. Chen BA, Creinin MD. Contemporary management of early pregnancy failure. *Clin Obstet Gynecol*. 2007;50:67-88.
8. American College of Obstetricians and Gynecologists. *Medical Management of Abortion*. ACOG *Practice Bulletin*, 67. Washington, DC; 2005.
9. Spandorfer SD, Menzin A, Barnhart KT, et al. Efficacy of frozen section evaluation of uterine curettings in the diagnosis of pregnancy. *Am J Obstet Gynecol*. 1996; 175:603.
10. American College of Obstetricians and Gynecologists. *Management of Anovulatory Bleeding*. ACOG *Practice Bulletin*, 14. Washington, DC; 2000.
11. Gimpelson RJ, Rappold HO. A comparative study between panoramic hysteroscopy with directed biopsies and dilation and curettage. *Am J Obstet Gynecol*. 1988;158:489.
12. Goldstein SR. The role of transvaginal ultrasound or endometrial biopsy in the evaluation of the menopausal endometrium. *Am J Obstet Gynecol*. 2009;201:5-11.
13. Baggish M, Karram M. Trophoblastic disease. *Atlas of Pelvic Anatomy and Gynecologic Surgery*. 2nd ed. Philadelphia, PA: Elsevier Saunders; 2006:1150-1159.
14. Rock J, Jones H. Normal and abnormal bleeding. In: *Te Linde's Operative Gynecology*. 10th ed. Philadelphia, PA: Lippincott Williams & Wilkins; 2008:595-605.

Case 2

A 23-year-old G3P2002 woman at 11 weeks' gestation by last menstrual period presents to the ER with a 4-day history of abdominal pain, vaginal bleeding, and fever. Upon further questioning, she reports possible passage of tissue with the blood clots. She had been seen in the same ER 1 week earlier and diagnosed with an embryonic demise. She was discharged with expectant management of the miscarriage. On examination, she is febrile to 101°F, has HR 100 beats/min, and BP 100/60 mm Hg. She appears ill. Her uterus is extremely tender on examination and cervix dilated 1 cm with "tissue" just inside the cervical os. Minimal bleeding is noted from the cervix. Her white blood cell count is 21,000/mm^3, hemoglobin is 9 g/dL, and blood type is O positive. A transvaginal ultrasound demonstrates "debris" in the uterus but normal ovaries, no adnexal masses, and no free fluid. After beginning intravenous (IV) antibiotics for a septic abortion, she is taken to the OR for a suction D&C. During the D&C, the uterus is suspected to be perforated by the suction curette since there is a sudden loss of resistance and the catheter advances much farther into the cervix than previously.

- ➤ What is your management plan?
- ➤ What are some risk factors for uterine perforation during a D&C?

ANSWERS TO CASE 2: D&C Complications

Summary: This is a 23-year-old G3 P2002 woman has a septic incomplete abortion at 11 weeks' gestation. She experiences a uterine perforation while undergoing a suction D&C procedure.

- **Management plan:** Laparoscopy/laparotomy to determine the extent of injury to intra-abdominal organs/vessels and completion of the evacuation of the uterus under direct visualization.
- **Risk factors:** Enlarged uterus (advanced gestational age), stenotic cervix, uterine infection, multiparity.

ANALYSIS

Objectives

1. Become familiar with the different management strategies for first-trimester abortions (surgical, medical, and expectant management).
2. Understand potential complications of a D&C: immediate, delayed, and late.
3. Become familiar with ways to minimize complication risks.

Considerations

This is a 23-year-old G3P2002 woman at 11 weeks' gestation with septic incomplete abortion. The patient had been diagnosed with an embryonic demise at 10 weeks' gestation and was undergoing expectant management of the abortion. Given her presentation to the ER, she is no longer a candidate from expectant management. Once the products of conception have become infected, evacuation of the contents is critical. The standard surgical management in this case would be suction D&C. Although many D&Cs can be performed as an outpatient under a local anesthetic, this patient is best treated with hospitalization and D&C in the OR. She is at greater risk for surgical complications (perforation, bleeding) than other routine D&Cs performed as an outpatient. Hospital admission is required to monitor for signs of sepsis, bacterial shock, disseminated intravascular coagulopathy, and acute renal failure. Prior to beginning the D&C, it is necessary to begin broad-spectrum antibiotics intravenously. The cause of the infection is usually polymicrobial, including anaerobic organisms. Up to 25% of septic abortions have been reported to be associated with positive blood cultures. This is one of the reasons that antibiotics should be administered prior to D&C. Tissue levels of antibiotics are usually reached about 1 hour after administration intravenously and the patient can then be taken to the OR. After evacuation, a bacterial culture (aerobic and anaerobic) may be obtained from the curetted specimen. Postoperatively, the patient should be continued on antibiotics and observed closely for signs/symptoms of septic shock. Uterine perforation is a known complication of a suction D&C.

APPROACH TO
Complications of a D&C

Early pregnancy failure is clinically recognized in 15% to 20% of pregnancies and can be managed surgically, medically, and expectantly. Many studies have compared the various treatment options, but differences in terminology, medical management, and definitions of failed treatment make comparison difficult. However, medical management seems to be a possible and effective acceptable alternative to surgical curettage. The use of vaginal misoprostol 400 to 800 micrograms has been found to be 80% to 88% successful in achieving a complete miscarriage as compared to 96% to 100% of surgically managed pregnancy failures.[1] The primary side effects of medical therapy include nausea, vomiting, and diarrhea, and those with failed complete miscarriage often require suction D&C. As with any surgery, the risks and benefits of the surgery must be weighted. The benefits of surgical management include high success rate and prompt treatment of pregnancy failure. As the gestational age of the abortion increases, so does the risk of complications. However, not all D&Cs performed are for obstetrical indications. Gynecologic indications for D&C include evaluation of dysfunctional bleeding, treatment of excessive bleeding, and treatment of cervical stenosis.[2-5]

Surgical complications of D&Cs are rare and can be categorized as occurring in the immediate or delayed/late period (Table 2–1). D&Cs performed for obstetrical indications carry a slightly higher risk than nonobstetrical indications due to the increased risk of perforation/bleeding from the gravid uterus. Ben-Baruch et al[6] reported that the risk for nonobstetrical D&Cs varies between 0.5% and 1.8%, depending on the indication. A recent retrospective study confirmed this low complication risk for nonobstetrical D&Cs.[7]

Table 2–1 COMPLICATIONS ASSOCIATED WITH D&C

IMMEDIATE COMPLICATIONS	DELAYED/LATE COMPLICATIONS
Hemorrhage	Infection
Cervical injury	Retained tissue
Acute hematometra	Intrauterine adhesions
Uterine perforation	
Anesthesia complications	

IMMEDIATE COMPLICATIONS

Patients with anatomic distortion from previous operations, cervical stenosis, atrophic conditions of the vagina, congenital anomalies, and distortion from benign or malignant tumors are often the most at risk for complications of hemorrhage/perforation. A recent study by Hefler et al[7] also demonstrated that a retroverted uterus, postmenopausal status, and nulliparity were independent risk factors for intraoperative complications (Figure 2–1). When a patient with one of these conditions is encountered, the intraoperative use of pelvic sonography has been demonstrated to decrease risk of complications.[8] The risk of hemorrhage is also higher for obstetrically indicated D&Cs, increasing further with the greater size of the uterus. If hemorrhage occurs, uterotonic agents and manual compression may be initially used. The use of a Foley catheter within the uterus and uterine packing has also been described if initial management of hemorrhage fails. Delayed hemorrhage can occur with a hematometra (distention of the uterus with blood). Cervical lacerations can occur from the tenaculum or from the dilation process and can be repaired in the OR.[9,10]

The incidence of perforation has been reported to be approximately 0.63%.[11] When a uterine perforation occurs, one important factor is to discern to the best of one's ability the **location** of the perforation (midline vs lateral) and the **instrument** that perforated the uterus (for instance, the uterine sound, because of its blunt design, is less likely to cause abdominal or bowel injury, whereas the suction curette by virtue of its vacuum can cause trauma).

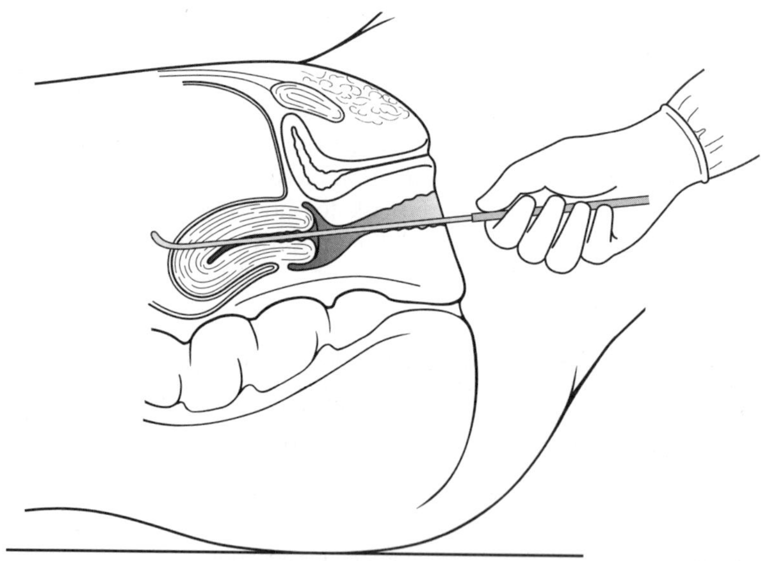

Figure 2–1. Perforation of the uterus due to retroflexion of the uterus, and the operator advances the dilator unaware of the uterine position.

Because the vacuum curette can injure intra-abdominal contents, it is imperative that the suction vacuum not be activated unless the surgeon is certain of the location in the uterine cavity. Risk factors for uterine perforation include an inexperienced operator, advanced gestational age, infection, stenotic cervix, and nulliparity. The primary concerns for uterine perforation are hemorrhage and injury to abdominal contents. Lateral perforations, near the uterine vessels, are much more likely to result in hemorrhage than midline lacerations. When perforation is suspected, the patient needs to be assessed for hemorrhage and hemodynamic stability and the procedure stopped. If patient becomes unstable or experiences unmanageable hemorrhage, an immediate laparotomy is indicated. If the patient is stable, there is no clear consensus on whether the extent of injury is required if a blunt instrument is used in the midline. Laparoscopy can be performed to assess perforation and intra-abdominal injury, and should be employed if there is a possibility of injury. If the D&C has not been completed, the procedure should be completed under direct visualization (either through laparotomy or laparoscopy). Patients who experience severe abdominal/pelvic pain after a D&C should be evaluated for possible perforation.[9,10,12,13]

Anesthesia complications are present with any surgery and depend on the type used. These complications can be minimized by performing the D&C under local anesthesia with/without sedation in the outpatient setting if clinically indicated. Early pregnancy loss may also be managed with manual vacuum aspiration under local anesthesia.[14] Patients undergoing a D&C with general anesthesia carry the highest anesthesia complication rate.

DELAYED/LATE COMPLICATIONS

Delayed complications include infection, retained tissue, and intrauterine adhesions. Patients with retained tissue usually present with cramping and bleeding several days after completion of the D&C. Infection may result from retained products of conception or even a preexisting gonorrhea/chlamydial infection. A meta-analysis performed by Sawaya and colleagues[15] demonstrated that antibiotic prophylaxis is indicated for elective abortion to reduce risk of infection. Although data are lacking, antibiotic prophylaxis may also be considered for missed abortion.[16] Late complications primarily focus on adverse pregnancy outcomes: intrauterine adhesions, stenotic/incompetent cervix, Rh sensitization, and placenta previa/accreta to name a few. In a large study by Schenker and Margalioth,[17] patients who were found to have Asherman syndrome were screened for possible risk factors. Of those who had Asherman syndrome, 90% had a curettage performed for a pregnancy-related problem (67% after curettage for postabortion/miscarriage). Other risk factors for Asherman syndrome include curettage of uterus, infection (especially endometrial tuberculosis), and congenital anomalies of the uterus. Postpartum and lactating patients who undergo a D&C are thought to be at increased risk for intrauterine adhesions secondary to the relative hypoestrogenic state.[18]

If a D&C is necessary, the risk of intrauterine adhesions can be minimized by using the vacuum curette only or gentle and superficial sharp curettage trying to not extend into the myometrium. In addition, suspected intrauterine infections should be treated to decrease risk of intrauterine adhesions. Multiple sharp curettage procedures have been shown to increase the risk of developing placenta accreta (risk not seen with suction curettage).[17,19] Rh sensitization can be minimized with knowledge of the patient's blood type and administration of anti-D immunoglobulin.

Comprehension Questions

2.1 A 23-year-old woman undergoes an uncomplicated suction D&C for a missed abortion at 12 weeks' gestation. About 2 hours after the procedure, the nurse notices the patient to have weakness/diaphoresis. Her uterus is noted to be enlarged and scant minimal bleeding is noted. What is the most likely etiology?

A. Acute hematometra
B. Uterine perforation
C. Uterine infection
D. Intrauterine adhesions

2.2 A 78-year-old postmenopausal woman is being evaluated for postmenopausal bleeding. Her cervix is noted to be stenotic and she is taken to the OR for a diagnostic D&C. Which of the following statements is most accurate?

A. The risk of uterine perforation is no greater than other diagnostic D&C.
B. To minimize the intraoperative and anesthesia risks, this patient is a good candidate for an outpatient D&C.
C. Intraoperative use of pelvic sonography would be beneficial in decreasing surgical risks.
D. A D&C is the only way to evaluate this patient's endometrium.

2.3 Which of the following is the major predisposing factor to the development of intrauterine adhesions?

A. Infection
B. Trauma to nonpregnant uterus
C. Trauma to pregnant uterus
D. Congenital anomalies

ANSWERS

2.1 **A.** Acute hematometra, "postabortal syndrome," occurs about 2 hours after surgery and the patient presents with scant vaginal bleeding, diaphoresis/weakness, and an enlarged/tender uterus. The etiology is unknown and treatment is prompt repeat curettage.

2.2 **C.** The use of intraoperative ultrasound has been found to be useful in the prevention of surgical complications such as uterine perforation in difficult D&Cs. In this case, the patient has three risk factors (postmenopausal state, atrophic vagina, and stenotic cervix) for increased surgical complications. Other risk factors include distortion of anatomy from previous surgery, congenital anomalies, or tumors. The endometrial cavity in a patient with postmenopausal bleeding can be assessed with measurement of the endometrial stripe using pelvic ultrasonography.

2.3 **C.** Trauma to the pregnant uterus is the major predisposing factor for the development of intrauterine adhesions. Two theories for this development are the low level of estrogen at the time of the procedure (or immediately after) doesn't allow for proper endometrial regeneration and that the uterus may be in a vulnerable state after pregnancy (basal layer more easily damaged).[20]

Clinical Pearls

See Table 1-2 for definition of level of evidence and strength of recommendation

- Medical management of an early pregnancy failure has success rate of approximately 80% (Level A).
- Antibiotic prophylaxis is indicated for elective suction curettage abortion (Level A).
- Patients at greatest risk for intraoperative complications are postmenopausal state, vaginal atrophy, cervical stenosis, retroverted uterus, and distorted anatomy from previous surgery/tumors (Level B).
- Patients who have a D&C after a pregnancy have higher risk of developing Asherman syndrome as compared to a nonpregnant uterus (Level B).
- Complications after a D&C can be classified as immediate and delayed/late (Level C).
- The risk of developing intrauterine adhesions in an obstetrically indicated D&C can be minimized by using the suction curette rather than sharp curettage and curetting gently and not deep into the myometrium (Level C).
- The morbidity after a uterine perforation depends on the location of the perforation and the instrument used (Level C).

REFERENCES

1. Chen BA, Creinin MD. Contemporary management of early pregnancy failure. *Clin Obstet Gynecol.* 2007;50:67-88.
2. Graziosi GC, Mol BW, Ankum WM, Bruinse HW. Management of early pregnancy loss. *Int J Gynaecol Obstet.* 2004;86:337-346.
3. Sotiriadis A, Makrydimas G, Papatheodorou S, Ioannidis J. Expectant, medical, or surgical management of first-trimester miscarriage: a meta-analysis. *Obstet Gynecol.* 2005;105:1104-1113.
4. Stubblefield PG, Carr-Ellis S, Borgatta L. Methods for induced abortion. *Obstet Gynecol.* 2004;104:174-184.
5. Trinder J, Brocklehurst P, Porter R, Read M, Vyas S, Smith L. Management of miscarriage: expectant, medical, or surgical? Results of a randomized controlled trial (miscarriage treatment (MIST) trial). *BMJ.* 2006 May;332:1235-1240.
6. Ben-Baruch G, Menczer J, Shalev J, Romen Y, Serr DM. Uterine perforation during curettage: perforation rates and postperforation management. *Isr J Med Sci.* 1980;16:821-824.
7. Hefler L, Lemach A, Seebacher V, Polterauer S, Tempfer C, Reinthaller A. The intraoperative complication rate of nonobstetrical dilation and curettage. *Obstet Gynecol.* 2009;113:1268-1271.
8. Hunter RE, Reuter K, Kopin E. Use of ultrasonography in the difficult postmenopausal dilation and curettage. *Obstet Gynecol.* 1989;73:813-816.
9. Gilstrap III LC, Cunningham FG, Vandorsten JP. Pregnancy termination: first and second trimesters. In: *Operative Obstetrics.* 2nd ed. New York, NY: McGraw-Hill; 2002:543-546.
10. Rock J, Jones H. Normal and abnormal bleeding. In: *TeLinde's Operative Gynecology.* 10th ed. Philadelphia, PA: Lippincott Williams & Wilkins; 2008:595-605.
11. McElin TW, Burd CC, Reeves BE, et al. Diagnostic dilation and curettage. *Obstet Gynecol.* 1969;33:807.
12. Cunningham FG, Leveno KJ, Bloom SL, Gilstrap III LC, Wenstrum KD. Abortion. In: *Williams Obstetrics.* 22nd ed. New York, NY: McGraw-Hill; 2005:241-247.
13. Katz VL, Lentz GM, Lobo RA, Gershenson DM. Spontaneous and recurrent abortion. In: *Comprehensive Gynecology.* 5th ed. Philadelphia, PA: Mosby; 2007:368-369.
14. Milingos DS, Mathur M, Smith NC, Ashok PW. Manual vacuum aspiration: a safe alternative for the surgical management of early pregnancy loss. *BJOG.* 2009; 116:1268-1271.
15. Sawaya GF, Grady D, Kerlikowske K, Grimes DA. Antibiotics at the time of induced abortion: the case for universal prophylaxis based on a meta-analysis. *Obstet Gynecol.* 1996 May; 87:884-890.
16. American College of Obstetricians and Gynecologists. *Antibiotic Prophylaxis for Gynecologic Procedures. ACOG Practice Bulletin No.104.* Washington, DC; 2009.
17. Schenker JG, Margalioth EJ. Intrauterine adhesions: an updated appraisal. *Fertil Steril.* 1982;37:593-610.
18. Westendorp IC, Ankum WM, Mol BW, Vonk J. Prevalence of Asherman's syndrome after secondary removal of placental remnants or a repeat curettage for incomplete abortion. *Hum Reprod.* 1998;13:3347-3350.
19. Johnson LG, Mueller BA, Daling JR. The relationship of placenta previa and history of induced abortion. *Int J Gynaecol Obstet* 2003;81:191.
20. Yu D, Wong Y, Cheong Y, Xia E, Li T. Asherman syndrome-one century later. *Fertil Steril.* 2008;89:759-779.

Case 3

A 25-year-old G2P1001 woman at 19 weeks' gestation presented to the clinic for routine prenatal care. On examination, she was found to have a uterus which was consistent with 18 weeks' gestation, but no fetal heart tones were heard. An ultrasound was performed and a fetal demise was found with the estimated gestational age of 16 weeks. She denies any vaginal bleeding or uterine cramping. Her cervix is closed on pelvic digital examination. She has no known medical problems and her first pregnancy was a term spontaneous vaginal delivery.

- What are your management options?
- How might the management affect future pregnancies?

ANSWERS TO CASE 3: Dilation and Evacuation

Summary: A 25-year-old G2P1001 at 19 weeks' gestation has an intrauterine demise.

- **Management options:** Dilation and evacuation (D&E) or medical evacuation of the uterus (misoprostol).
- **Risks for future pregnancies:** No increase in clinically significant complications in subsequent pregnancies is anticipated.

ANALYSIS

Objectives

1. Become familiar with management options of second-trimester fetal demise.
2. Review options for cervical dilation.
3. Understand some basic surgical principles of D&E.
4. Understand complications which can occur with a D&E.

Considerations

The management of a second-trimester fetal demise depends on both the clinical expertise of the physician as well as the patient's desires after counseling. Options for management include medical induction of labor, D&E, hysterotomy, and hysterectomy. Because of the safety, efficiency, and cost-effectiveness of D&E, it has become the most common surgical management of second-trimester abortions (> 98% of all second-trimester abortions in 2003). A suction D&C is no longer an option after the first trimester, when fetal skeletal parts have begun to calcify, due to a greater risk of complications (uterine perforation, hemorrhage, cervical laceration, and incomplete removal of products). After 15 to 16 weeks' gestation, a D&E is the preferred method of surgical evacuation of the uterus. Given this patient's gestation age, she is no longer a candidate for a simple suction D&C. Her management options include either a D&E or medical management (misoprostol). In order to perform a D&E safely, a physician must have specialized training and adequate experience to even offer this treatment plan. The expertise of her physician will dictate which management plan can be performed safely.[1]

APPROACH TO
Dilation and Evacuation

The technique of a D&E was introduced in the 1970s and is now the preferred surgical technique for second-trimester abortions. After 16 weeks' gestation, the difference in morbidity and mortality between a D&E and medical management becomes less clear. D&E is more complicated than D&C due to the need for increased cervical dilation, the use of special instruments to remove the fetal parts, assurance that all fetal parts are removed, and the requirement for additional anesthesia. Accurate determination of gestational age is essential as the needed cervical dilation increases with advancing gestational ages. Most forceps require a minimal dilation of 14 to 19 mm. A D&E usually requires either general anesthesia or a paracervical block with conscious sedation. In order to perform a D&E safely, specialized training is a requirement. For physicians with less experience with a D&E, medical management will be their primary treatment option. In a recent *Cochrane Database of Systematic Review*,[2] D&E appears to be associated with fewer overall adverse events, side effects, and pain than induction with medical management. However, medical management (misoprostol and mifepristone) appears to be effective and acceptable. The ideal regimen of misoprostol has not been determined.[3,4]

Studies have produced conflicting results as to whether the method of cervical dilation is associated with complications of future pregnancy complications such as preterm labor, miscarriage, and cervical incompetence. Cervical trauma from rapid dilation is thought to be the cause of these potential pregnancy complications. Preoperative osmotic dilators are often needed to achieve adequate dilation prior to the D&E. As the gestational age increases, so does the need for cervical dilation. The cervix can be prepared with either osmotic dilators, prostaglandin analogues (misoprostol), or a combination of the two. Osmotic dilators (Figure 3–1) can be made either from natural sources (laminaria made from the stems of seaweed which are dehydrated and made into cervical tents) or synthetic substances (Lamicel or Dilapan). Because laminaria are made from natural sources, the dilation is unpredictable, anaphylaxis has been reported, and it requires time for dilation (often overnight). Each synthetic agent has its own unique properties but, in general, requires less time for dilation as compared to laminaria. Other potential risks of osmotic dilators include vasovagal symptoms with insertion (5%-20%), allergies/anaphylaxis to laminaria, creation of false passage and perforation if placed with force, and theoretic risk of infection (literature does not support an increased risk).[5-9]

The **use of osmotic dilators has been shown to significantly reduce the risk of cervical laceration and trauma to the cervix and reduction in the induction-to-delivery interval.**[10] In addition, repeated laminaria applications

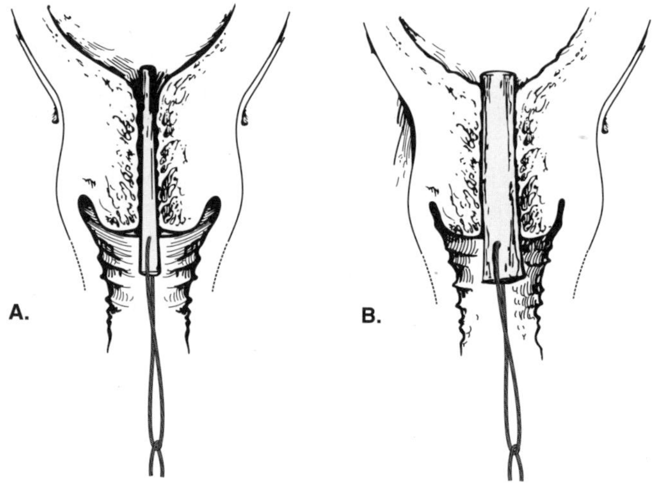

Figure 3–1. Osmotic dilators are introduced into the cervical canal, and slowly enlarge as they absorb water. The tip of the dilator should be placed just above the level of the internal os. (*Reproduced, with permission, from Schorge JO, Schaffer JI, Halvorson LM, et al.* Williams Gynecology. *New York: McGraw-Hill, 2008:898.*)

have been shown to increase cervical dilation when compared to single application.[11] Compared to laminaria, misoprostol alone has been shown to be inferior for cervical dilation. The combination of misoprostol and concurrent placement laminaria often requires only one laminaria application, and thus a shorter time period before procedure can be performed. The **combination of laminaria placement with misoprostol has not been shown to increase induction efficiency**.[12] Proper placement of the laminaria is crucial. The cervix should be cleaned with an antiseptic solution before the laminaria tents are placed through the internal os. After the laminaria have been placed, the use of several saline-soaked gauze sponges in the vagina helps prevent expulsion. Although most practitioners choose to remove the laminaria after 12 hours, laminaria have been noted to continue to expand for up to 24 hours.[13] When a patient's membranes have been ruptured, laminaria should be removed in less than 12 hours and procedure completed. The placement of multiple laminaria is preferred over just one and the number inserted should be recorded in the patient's record. Care should be taken in placement to not break the dilators, since a fragment in the uterus is problematic and may even require hysterotomy for retrieval.

Between 13 and 16 weeks' gestation, vacuum extraction with a 14-mm cannula is probably sufficient after adequate cervical dilation. Beyond 16 weeks' gestation, forcep (Sopher and Bierer) extraction is necessary. These specialized forceps have been found to be superior to standard ring forceps. To minimize perforation risk, the extraction should begin in the lower uterus rather than fundus and continuous ultrasound guidance may aid in the removal of fetal parts. After the cervix is adequately dilated, the large suction cannula is introduced into the uterus and amniotic fluid removed. The surgeon will then extract the fetal parts. At the conclusion of the procedure, the physician must inspect the products and identify all major fetal parts (skull, spine, four extremities) and evaluate the quantity of the placenta.[14]

Reported complications of D&E include cervical trauma, hemorrhage, perforation of the uterus, infection, and retained products. Intracervical vasopressin (as component of cervical block) has been demonstrated to decrease intraoperative blood loss.[15] Intraoperative administration of uterotonic agents (oxytocin or methylergonovine) has been used by some practitioners to minimize blood loss. However, some practitioners prefer not to use these agents because a contracted uterus can make the evacuation more difficult. Recently, there have been case reports published on the use of uterine artery embolization (UAE) to treat hemorrhage from D&E with some success.[16] However, it should be noted that UAE should be considered only when the etiology of the bleeding is from an intracervical injury, abnormal placentation, or presence of submucosal fibroids.[16] Studies show that very few hysterectomies (11/10,000 or 0.11%) are required due to hemorrhage or other complications in those patients who undergo D&E.[4,15,17]

Comprehension Questions

3.1 A 23-year-old woman undergoes a D&E after she was found to have an 18-week fetal demise. Which of the following fetal structures is most likely to be left behind in the uterus after a D&E?

A. Calvarium
B. Extremities
C. Abdomen
D. Spine

3.2 Which type of osmotic dilator requires the longest time before maximum cervical dilation?

A. Lamicel
B. Dilapan
C. Laminaria
D. Misoprostol

3.3 A 32-year-old female patient undergoes a D&E for a fetal demise at 16 weeks. Despite adequate dilation of the cervix, all the fetal parts are not able to be removed. What is the most appropriate next step?

A. Give a uterine relaxing agent and proceed with D&E.
B. Proceed with hysterotomy and removal of remaining fetal parts.
C. Expectant management for spontaneous delivery of fetal parts.
D. Administer oxytocin for 2 to 3 hours and attempt repeat D&E.

ANSWERS

3.1 **A.** The calvarium is the most likely fetal part to be left behind. The use of ultrasound often will help to identify remaining fetal parts. It is imperative for the surgeon to identify all four major body parts prior to concluding the procedure. If the fetal part (most often the calvarium) cannot be removed even under direct ultrasound visualization, oxytocin can be infused for several hours. The remaining fetal part is often closer to the internal os and much easier to remove.

3.2 **C.** The natural product, laminaria, require a longer period of time before the cervix is maximally dilated (usually overnight). Lamicel, a synthetic agent, works within 2 to 6 hours; however, it does not achieve as much dilation as other osmotic agents. Dilapan, also a synthetic agent, works within 4 to 6 hours and achieves the greatest cervical dilation within the shortest time frame. The original Dilapan product was removed from the market between 1995 and 2002 due to its increased risk of retained fragments with removal. The newer product has stronger core to decrease this risk. Misoprostol is not an osmotic dilator.

3.3 **D.** Oxytocin, given intravenously aids in the expulsion of products if D&E is not successful initially. With the combination of ruptured membranes and oxytocin, the remaining fetal parts are often found closer to the cervix and much easier to remove. D&E do not have to be completed in one step. The use of uterine relaxing agent would significantly increase the risk of uterine perforation and hemorrhage and would not be a good option for this patient. Although expectant management would be a possible alternative management strategy, the uncertain time from rupture to delivery of products could possibly increase the risk of infection and therefore is not the best choice. Hysterotomy should only be considered when both surgical and medical managements have failed.

Clinical Pearls

See Table 1-2 for definition of level of evidence and strength of recommendation

- The use of osmotic dilators decreases the induction-to-delivery time (Level A).
- A D&E has been found to be superior to intrauterine injection with prostaglandin $F_{2\alpha}$ (Level B).
- Medical management of second-trimester abortions is as efficacious as a D&E but often with increased pain and side effects (Level B).
- The use of osmotic dilators minimizes cervical trauma and decreases the incidence of cervical lacerations and possibly future pregnancy complications (Level B).
- In experienced hands, D&E is a more effective and safer treatment compared to medical management, hysterotomy, and hysterectomy (Level C).
- Because of the complexity of the procedure and its difficulty as compared to D&C, a D&E procedure should only be performed by practitioners with specialized training (Level C).

REFERENCES

1. Autry AM, Hayes EC, Jacobson GF, Kirby RS. A comparison of medical induction and dilation and evacuation for second-trimester abortion. *Am J Obstet Gynecol.* 2002;187:393-397.
2. Lohr PA, Hayes JL, Gemzell-Danielsson K. Surgical versus medical methods for second trimester induced abortion. *Cochrane Database Syst Rev.* 2008;(1): CD006714.
3. Cunningham FG, Leveno KJ, Bloom SL, Gilstrap III LC, Wenstrum KD. Abortion. In: *Williams Obstetrics*. 22nd ed. New York, NY: McGraw-Hill; 2005:241-243.
4. Gilstrap III LC, Cunningham FG, Vandorsten JP. Pregnancy termination: first and second trimesters. In: *Operative Obstetrics*. 2nd ed. New York, NY: McGraw-Hill; 2002:540-546.
5. Turok DK, Curtcheff SE, Esplin MS, et al. Second trimester termination of pregnancy: a review by site and procedure type. *Contraception*. 2008;77:155-161.
6. Jackson JE, Grobman WA, Haney E, Casele H. Mid-trimester dilation and evacuation with laminaria does not increase the risk for severe subsequent pregnancy complications. *Int J Gynaecol Obstet*. 2007;96:12-15.
7. Kalish RB, Chasen ST, Rosenzweig LB, Rashbaum WK, Chervenak FA. Impact of midtrimester dilation and evacuation on subsequent pregnancy outcome. *Am J Obstet Gynecol*. 2002;187:613-614.
8. Lichtenberg ES. Complications of osmotic dilators. *Obstet Gynecol Surv.* 2004;59:528-535.
9. Society of Family Planning. Cervical preparation for second-trimester surgical abortion prior to 20 weeks of gestation. *Contraception*. 2007;76:486-495.

10. Atlas RO, Lemus J, Reed J, Atkins D, Alger LS. Second trimester abortion using prostaglandin E_2 suppositories with or without intracervical laminaria japonica: a randomized study. *Obstet Gynecol.* 1998;92:398.
11. Stubblefield PG, Altman AM, Goldstein SP. A randomized trial of one versus two days of laminaria treatment prior to late midtrimester abortion by uterine evacuation: a pilot study. *Am J Obstet Gynecol.* 1982;143:481.
12. Jain JK, Mishell DR. A comparison of misoprostol with and without laminaria tents for induction of second trimester abortion. *Am J Obstet Gynecol.* 1996; 175:173.
13. Wheeler RG, Scheider K. Properties and safety of cervical dilators. *Am J Obstet Gynecol.* 1983;146:597.
14. Chasen ST, Kalish RB, Gupta M, Kaufman JE, Rashbaum WK, Chervenak FA. Dilation and evacuation at ≥ 20 weeks: comparison of operative techniques. *Am J Obstet Gynecol.* 2004;190:1180-1183.
15. Peterson WF, Berry FN, Grace MR, Bulbranson CL. Second-trimester abortion by dilation and evacuation: an analysis of 11,747 cases. *Obstet Gynecol.* 1983;62:185-190.
16. Haddad L, Delli-Bovi L. Uterine artery embolization to treat hemorrhage following second-trimester abortion by dilatation and surgical evacuation. *Contraception.* 2009;79:452-455.
17. Rock J, Jones H. Management of abortion. In: *Te Linde's Operative Gynecology.* 10th ed. Philadelphia, PA: Lippincott Williams & Wilkins; 2008:788-791.

Case 4

A 28-year-old G2P2 woman complains of lower abdominal and pelvic pain for 2 years which seems to be worsening. She states that the pain is exacerbated by menses and is located in the lower abdomen in the midline. She describes it as cramping with radiation to the back. She has tried nonsteroidal anti-inflammatory drugs (NSAIDs) with no relief. She denies gastrointestinal symptoms. The patient denies a history of sexually transmitted infections, and has menses every month. She was on the oral contraceptive agent last year without affecting the pelvic pain. On examination, she is 5 ft 5 in tall and weighs 120 lb (54.43 kg). Her abdomen is without surgical scars. She has mild tenderness of the lower abdominal quadrants with normal bowel sounds. On pelvic examination, the external genitalia appear normal. The cervix and vagina are normal. The uterus is retroverted and fixed and tender. The adnexa are bilaterally tender. There are no nodules or barbs noted. The rectovaginal examination reveals some tenderness of the posterior uterus.

- ➤ What is your diagnostic plan?
- ➤ What is your differential diagnosis?
- ➤ What are options for establishing a gynecologic diagnosis?

ANSWERS TO CASE 4: Diagnostic Laparoscopy

Summary: A 28-year-old G2P2 woman has *chronic pelvic pain, consistent with dysmenorrhea, which is not amenable to medical therapy. The examination shows a retroverted uterus that is fixed.*

➤ **Diagnostic plan:** *Assays for gonorrhea, Chlamydia, pregnancy test, and pelvic ultrasound; consider a pain diary.*

➤ **Differential diagnosis:** *Gynecologic conditions*: endometriosis, pelvic adhesions, chronic pelvic inflammatory disease (PID), adenomyosis; *Urologic*: interstitial cystitis; *Gastrointestinal*: irritable bowel syndrome, diverticulitis; *Psychological*: anxiety disorder, depression, somatization, sexual abuse, marital discord, drug abuse; *Neurologic*: pudendal neuralgia, vulvodynia; *Musculoskeletal*: pelvic floor disorder, fibromyalgia.

➤ **Establishing a gynecologic diagnosis:** Diagnostic laparoscopy. The history, physical examination, and limited tests are the key to determining which etiology is most likely. With a gynecologic likelihood, diagnostic laparoscopy is indicated to help to establish the diagnosis.

ANALYSIS

Objectives

1. Describe the role of diagnostic laparoscopy in gynecological conditions.
2. Describe the major surgical approach in minimizing injuries associated with diagnostic laparoscopy.
3. List the most common complications associated with diagnostic laparoscopy.

Considerations

Chronic pelvic pain is one of the most difficult diagnostic challenges that a gynecologist faces. The history is essential in trying to establish the body system etiology. The pain in this patient has been present for 2 years and is worsening. The factors that lean toward a gynecologic cause include the location of the lower abdomen, worsening with menses, and midline in nature. There is no mention of pain with intercourse, dyspareunia, but this is also very important in the investigation process. After establishing a good idea of the location, character, duration, and radiation of the pain, the physician must look for associated conditions. For instance, if the patient has dysuria or urinary urgency or frequency, then a urinary disorder may be considered.

Psychological issues are very common, and the physician should spend time inquiring about depression, anxiety, and the patient's relationship with her partner. Past history of sexual or physical abuse is also relevant. Gastrointestinal symptoms should be sought such as bloating, constipation and diarrhea, or upper abdominal discomfort. When a reasonable etiology belonging to a nongynecologic system exists, the patient should be referred to the appropriate consultant. When a gynecologic disorder is likely, further testing or imaging and, if needed, diagnostic laparoscopy can help to establish the diagnosis.

APPROACH TO Diagnostic Laparoscopy

The advantages of laparoscopy are well known when compared to laparotomy. Advantages include faster recovery to normal activities, decreased cost, decreased adhesion formation, smaller incisions and therefore decreased postoperative pain, and shorter operative times (although this may not hold true for some procedures).[1] Large meta-analysis published in 2002 comparing laparoscopy to laparotomy for benign gynecologic disease found that the overall risk of minor complications such as fever, urinary tract infection, or wound infection was lower in woman undergoing laparoscopic procedures, but both groups had the same risk for major complication such as pulmonary embolism, major bleeding, fistula formation, or damage to surrounding organs.[1] Laparoscopic procedures in gynecology are standard for many conditions, and its widespread use has made the transition to the minimally invasive procedures as standard of care in many respects.

Laparoscopy is the best diagnostic/treatment tool in endometriosis because it allows the gynecologist to assess the extent of the disease and at the same time treat lesions with fulguration and resection. The accuracy of laparoscopic diagnosis depends on location and type of lesion, as well as surgeon experience (see Figure 4–1). Direct biopsies of suspicious lesions are necessary when direct visualization can lead to errors in certain cases.[2] Most common anatomical sites where endometriotic implants are located include the ovaries and the posterior cul-de-sac, although it is not uncommon to see them at the broad ligament, uterosacral ligament, posterior uterine wall, fallopian tubes, sigmoid colon, and appendix. Multiple extra-abdominal organs can be affected as well.

Basic elements for any gynecologic laparoscopic procedure start with positioning the patient in dorsal lithotomy with padded candy cane–type stirrups or Allen stirrups; knees and legs should be in a resting nonflexed position in order to avoid nerve injury. Entry into the peritoneal cavity can be by open or closed technique, although no major differences have been found in the avoidance of major complications among laparoscopic entry techniques.[3]

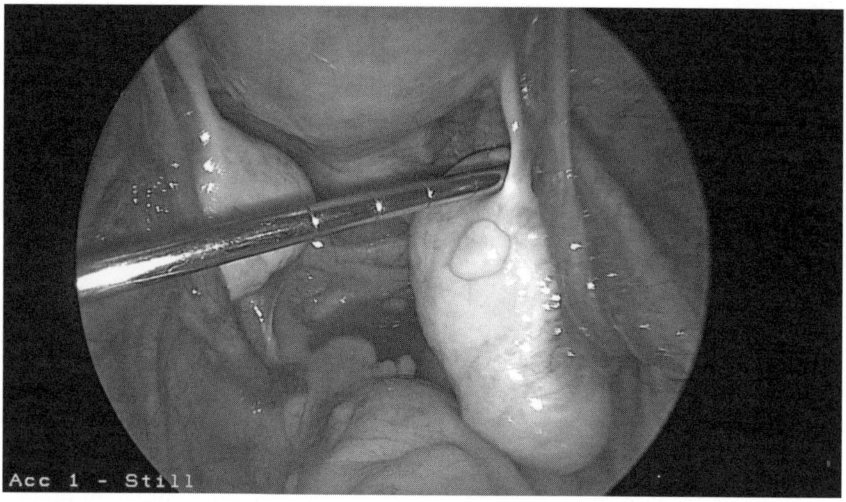

Figure 4–1. Right endometrioma noted, with right ovary significantly larger than the left ovary. (*Courtesy of Dr. Cristo Papasakelariou*.)

Different locations can be used for both techniques, although the periumbilical area is the most widely used. Other locations utilized are the transfundal area, posterior cul-de-sac, left upper quadrant, and the lateral border of the rectus muscle at either left or right McBurney point.

The abdominal cavity is then insufflated with CO_2 (typically with 2-4 L), and insufflation is confirmed once the liver dullness disappears and overall expansion of the abdominal wall appears symmetrical in all quadrants. The entry pressure should not be higher than 10 mm Hg; if in doubt of correct placement, a 10-mL open syringe with saline may be utilized to test for proper placement of the Veress needle. The saline should evacuate the syringe in the peritoneal cavity by gravity if properly placed. Multiple devices have been designed to be used in laparoscopic gynecologic procedures, including graspers, scissors, cutting and coagulating tools, tools for intra- and extracorporeal suturing techniques, and, lately, high-quality sealing and coagulation devices such as the argon beam coagulator (ABC), the LigaSure (Valleylab, Colorado, USA), the harmonic scalpel, and stapler devices.

Removal of tissue from the pelvic cavity can be achieved by morcellation technique and/or retrieval bags. Many companies have developed these tools for such occasions. Potential complications with laparoscopic procedures include bowel injury, vascular injuries, urinary tract injury (bladder or ureteral injuries), nerve damage, hematomas, postoperative incisional hernias, and gas embolism. But almost half of these complications are related to the initial entry to the peritoneal cavity.[4,5]

Comprehension Questions

Match the single best diagnosis (A-F) with the clinical scenario (4.1-4.4).

A. Endometriosis
B. Vaginismus
C. Pelvic inflammatory disease
D. Interstitial cystitis
E. Diverticulitis
F. Hydrosalpinx

4.1 A 35-year-old woman with cyclic pelvic pain related to menses has tried multiple medications, including birth control pills, without success. Occasionally, she experiences rectal bleeding with bloating, and bimanual examination reveals a fixed retroverted uterus.

4.2 A 26-year-old nulligravida woman with pelvic pain mainly on the left side states she has had some malodorous vaginal discharge for the previous 2 days, which she has not had before. She has multiple sexual partners, states she is very careful, and is taking oral contraceptives. Urine pregnancy test is negative.

4.3 A 28-year-old woman with infertility, despite two rounds of treatment with clomiphene citrate, has been unsuccessful in attempts at pregnancy. Otherwise asymptomatic, she has a history of *Chlamydia* 5 years prior.

4.4 A 57-year-old woman presents with left lower quadrant pain and fever; at physical examination, rebound tenderness was noticed. She has a history of ovarian cysts and a surgery for torsion of a left necrotic ovary.

ANSWERS

4.1 **A.** Cyclic pain associated with rectal bleeding and a fixed uterus should lead one toward the diagnosis of endometriosis.

4.2 **C.** A nulliparous woman with multiple sexual partners and unprotected intercourse associated with pelvic pain is very suggestive of pelvic inflammatory disease. Other possibilities would include the presence of a hydrosalpinx, although this condition is not usually associated with malodorous vaginal discharge.

4.3 **F.** Hydrosalpinx would be the best explanation for this reproductive age woman after two rounds of ovulation induction drugs. Hydrosalpinx is almost always bilateral in the presence of infertility.

4.4 **E.** Diverticulitis is the most likely diagnosis, given that the patient had previously had a left salpingo-oophorectomy and was experiencing left lower quadrant pain and fever.

Clinical Pearls

See Table 1-2 for definition of level of evidence and strength of recommendation

- Overall risk of minor complications is lower in woman undergoing operative laparoscopic procedures when compared to laparotomy; however, major complication risks are the same in both groups (Level B).
- The diagnosis of endometriosis is by direct visualization, but confirmatory biopsy of lesions is recommended in cases of suspicious lesions (Level B).
- No major differences have been found in major complications among laparoscopic entry techniques (Level A).
- Roughly half of the complications related to laparoscopic procedures are related to initial entry into peritoneal cavity (Level B).

REFERENCES

1. Chapron C, Fauconnier A, Goffinet F, et al. Laparoscopic surgery is not inherently dangerous presenting with benign gynaecologic pathology. Result of a meta-analysis. *Hum Reprod.* 2002;17:1334.
2. Wykes CB, Clark TJ, Khan KS. Accuracy of laparoscopy in the diagnosis of endometriosis: a systematic quantitative review. *BJOG*. 2004;111:1204.
3. Ahmad G, Duffy JM, Phillips K, Watson A. Laparoscopic entry techniques. *Cochrane Database Syst Rev.* 2008;16:CD006583.
4. Jansen FW, Kolkman W, Bakkum EA, de Kroon CD, Trimbos-Kemper TC, Trimbos JB. Complications of laparoscopy: an inquiry about closed- versus open-entry technique. *Am J Obstet Gynecol.* 2004;190:634.
5. Shirk GJ, Johns A, Redwine DB. Complications of laparoscopic surgery: how to avoid them and how to repair them. *J Minim Invasive Gynecol.* 2006;13:352.

Case 5

A 35-year-old woman is noted to have severe menorrhagia over the past 2 years that is worsening and is associated with severe anemia. She has tried various medical therapies, including oral contraceptives and NSAIDs, which do not help. The patient has been diagnosed with uterine fibroids. She desires more children. On examination, her abdomen is normal with the exception of an irregularly shaped nontender uterus that is approximately 14-week size. She denies having previous surgeries. In counseling her, you review various surgical options. She has heard about robotic surgery and desires more information about this technique.

- ➤ What are your management options?
- ➤ What are the advantages and disadvantages of robotic surgery versus other techniques?

ANSWERS TO CASE 5: Robotic Surgery

Summary: This is a 35-year-old woman with significant menorrhagia and anemia associated with uterine fibroids. Her symptoms have failed medical therapy. Her uterus is 14-week size.

➤ **Management options:** Myomectomy with options of open technique versus laparoscopy versus robotic surgery. She desires to preserve fertility; therefore, less invasive treatment should be at the top of the treatment plan list. Nonsurgical option, such as magnetic resonance–guided focused ultrasound (MRgFUS), is an option that must be considered, but few patients qualify as candidates. Normally, the procedure is reserved for premenopausal women who have completed childbearing[1]; therefore, myomectomy will provide the most benefit in this patient, with the laparoscopic approach providing faster recovery and similar pregnancy rates as the open approach.[2]

➤ **Robotic surgery advantages:**
1. Less postoperative pain as compared to open laparotomy.
2. Shorter hospitalizations.
3. Better visualization (three-dimensional [3D] vision) versus open surgery and conventional laparoscopy.
4. Improved dexterity and precision given the 3D visualization and replication of full range of motion of a surgeon's hand.
5. Reduction in surgeon's fatigue.
6. Decreased blood loss.
7. Correction of tremor amplification.
8. New concept in minimally invasive surgery (remotely performed surgery or telesurgery).

➤ **Robotic surgery disadvantages:**
1. Expensive initial investment.
2. Bulky equipment, therefore large-size ORs are required.
3. Lack of haptics or tactile feedback.
4. Limited uterine manipulation is less when compared with conventional laparoscopy.

ANALYSIS

Objectives

1. Describe the advantages and disadvantages of robotic surgery versus laparoscopy and laparotomy.
2. Describe the robotic manual dexterity capabilities.
3. Describe the 3D visual capability of robotic surgery.
4. Be aware of the limitations of robotic surgery.

Considerations

This 35-year-old woman with severe menorrhagia and anemia has failed medical management with oral control pills and NSAIDs. She has been diagnosed with uterine fibroids, and she desires future fertility. Therefore, procedures like endometrial ablation, uterine artery embolization, or hysterectomy are not options for treatment. Myomectomy is still considered the procedure of choice in women with severe symptoms due to fibroids who desire to preserve fertility. The aforementioned MRgFUS uses focused ultrasound directed into the substance of the large fibroid masses, leading to their degeneration. Unfortunately, many third-party carriers do not pay for this procedure, and many patients fail as candidates due to the nature, location, and size of the myomatous tumors. Management of the leiomyomas endoscopically is one of the major advances in minimally invasive gynecologic surgery, especially in a 35-year-old female patient with no previous abdominal surgery, although currently in the United States the majority of the cases are still performed using laparotomy.[2,3]

When comparing open myomectomy versus robotic approach, the robotic group had showed longer operative times and increased cost, but decreased blood loss and shorter length of stay.[2] Also, comparison between conventional laparoscopy versus robotic myomectomy seems to raise some concerns about the level of difficulty encountered in order to enucleate fibroids and perform multilayer closure in the conventional group. Pregnancy rates after myomectomy are similar whether managed endoscopically (either conventional or robotic) or via laparotomy.[2] Given these facts, usually the less invasive approach is indicated, especially in a 35-year-old patient with history of no previous surgeries.

APPROACH TO Robotic Surgery

Surgical robotics were first used in 1985 in neurosurgery; applications soon followed in the fields of urology and orthopedics, but it was not until 1998 when the first robotic gynecologic surgery in a human patient was performed.[4-6]

Subsequently, the da Vinci Surgical System (Intuitive Surgical, Inc., Sunnyvale, California), the only system available in the market, received Food and Drug Administration (FDA) approval for gynecologic procedures in 2005, resulting in a steady increase in the number of surgical gynecologic procedures performed robotically (Figure 5–1). Multiple specialties in medicine

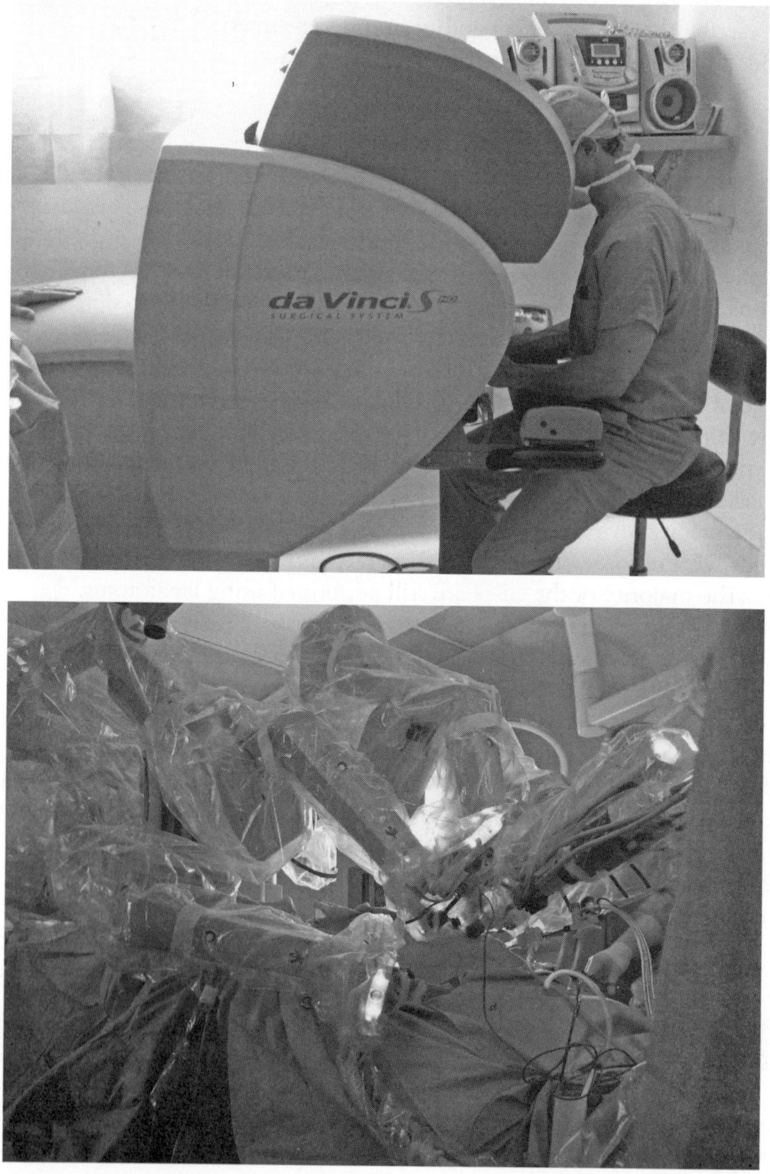

Figure 5–1. The da Vinci Surgical Robotic System. *(Courtesy of Intuitive Surgical Inc.)*

currently utilize robotics, and, in most centers, urologic surgeons are leading the way with radical prostatectomies.[2] Other specialties such as general surgery, gynecology, cardiovascular surgery, orthopedics, and ENT (ear, nose, and throat) are rapidly incorporating robotics into their surgical procedures.

The applications of robotic surgery in gynecology are very broad, including benign gynecology (robotic-assisted hysterectomy, tubal anastomosis, myomectomy, sacrocolpopexy, oophorectomy, ovarian cystectomy, major lysis of adhesions and tuboplasty), gynecologic oncology (radical hysterectomy, lymph node dissections), and even obstetrics (robotic-assisted abdominal cerclage). Traditionally, robotic-assisted gynecologic procedures have been associated with longer OR times, secondary to the learning curve associated with new technology, but generally similar clinical outcomes when compared to open and conventional laparoscopy.[7] This likely will not be an issue as more and more gynecologists receive training across the country. The main, widely agreed upon advantages of robotics in gynecologic procedures include decreased blood loss, shorter hospitalization time, improved surgeon's dexterity, 3D vision, and precision.[3,7-9]

As of today, there is only one FDA-approved robotic surgical system, known as the da Vinci Surgical System (Intuitive Surgical, Inc., Sunnyvale, California). This system basically consists of four components that are standard for all the available different models. These are the following: (1) Surgeon console which is essentially from where the surgeon operates. (2) Patient side cart that executes all the commands and movements performed by the surgeon that is achieved through four robotics arms, camera, and up to three EndoWrist instruments. (3) Vision system which is a high-resolution 3D endoscopic camera that provides the true-to-life 3D images of the operative field. (4) EndoWrist instrument (Figure 5–2) that attaches to the patient side cart and mimics the dexterity of the human hand and wrist. Besides all the aforementioned instruments, the operative assistant provides instrument exchanges, suction and irrigation, suture introduction and retrieval, and additional retraction.[7]

USE IN BENIGN GYNECOLOGY

Robotic-Assisted Hysterectomy

Vaginal hysterectomy continues to be the route of choice for benign pathology whenever technically possible, as morbidity appears to be lower than that of any other method.[10] Hysterectomy by laparotomy remains the most common route in gynecology at the present day.[11] As an alternative, endoscopic surgical approaches have made inroads into the laparotomy percentages and effectively decreased the number of open cases. Robotic laparoscopic technology appears to offer the surgeon a feasible method of surgery that allows for more difficult cases that otherwise may not be challenged by conventional laparoscopic techniques. Robotic surgeons speak of the increasing difficulty in

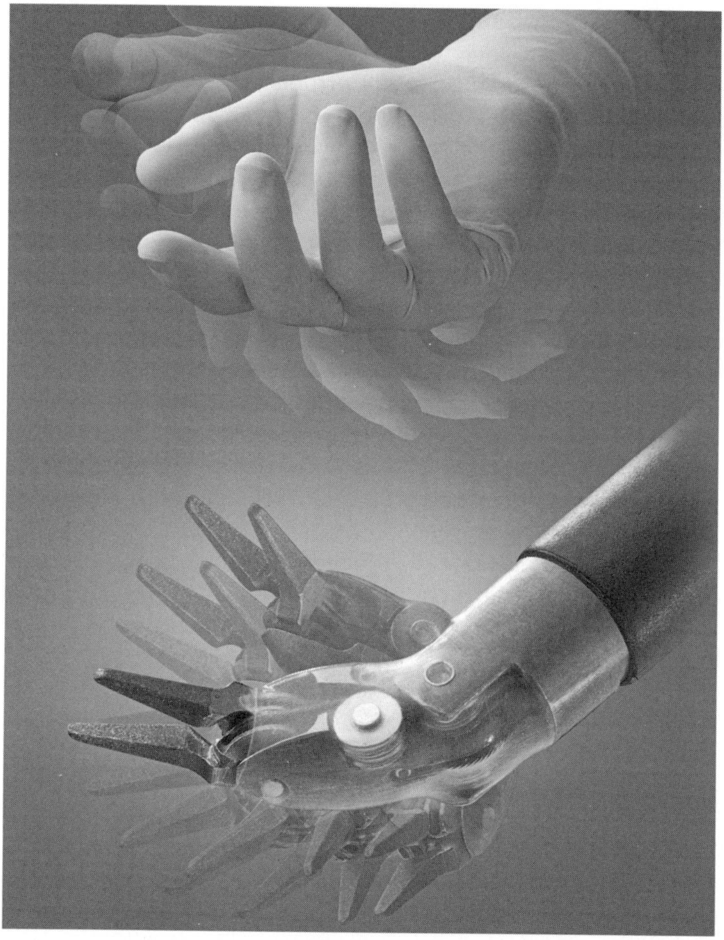

Figure 5–2. EndoWrist instrument allows for the reproduction of the human hand dexterity. *(Courtesy of Intuitive Surgical Inc.)*

certain cases being handled much more easily and precisely than with conventional laparoscopic technology.

Myomectomy

The majority of these procedures are performed by laparotomy because of the complexity encountered during enucleation and multilayer closure with confidence when approached by laparoscopy. Robotic closure allows for confidence in dissection as well as multilayer closure of the myoma bed.[12,13] The EndoWrist instruments allow for the technical aspects of the procedure that only a few

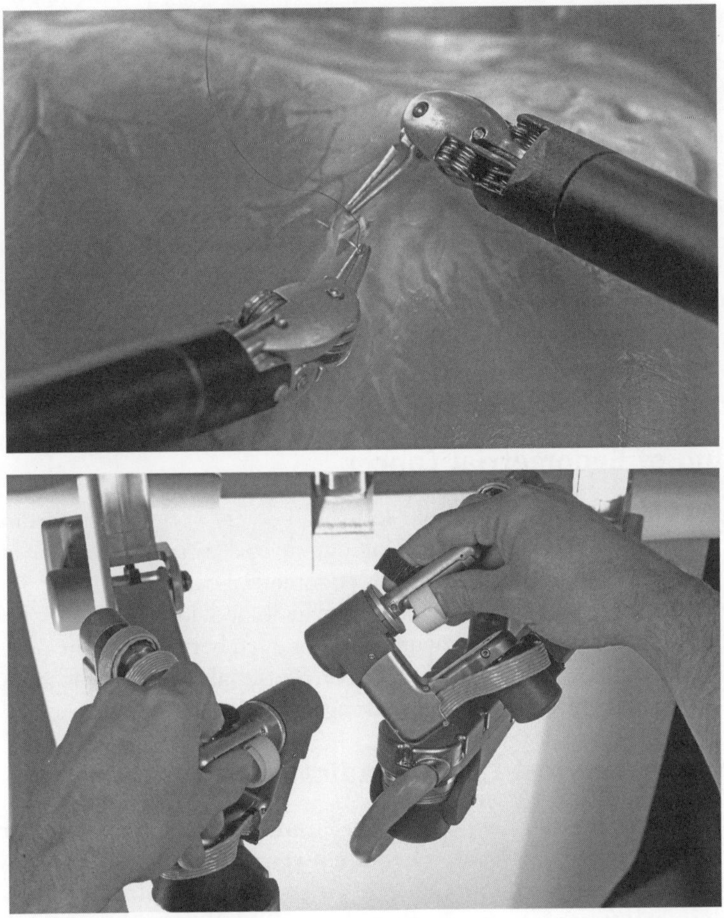

Figure 5–2. (*Continued*)

laparoscopic surgeons possess. Cost-benefit ratios remain to be seen regarding this approach when taking into account time away from regular activity.

Sacrocolpopexy

Robotic-assisted sacrocolpopexy (RAS) offers a reproducible, minimally invasive technique for vaginal vault prolapse with similar short-term durability compared with open sacrocolpopexies.[7] RAS is associated with longer operative time but decreased blood loss and decreased hospital stay. The robotic approach does not rival those surgeons who are capable of performing this procedure by conventional laparoscopy, but it does introduce EndoWrist movement which can facilitate the procedure.

Tubal Anastomosis

When compared to conventional laparoscopy and minilaparotomy, robotic-assisted tubal anastomosis appears to have similar success rate and shorter recovery time, but longer operative time and higher cost.[14,15] Only few comparative studies have been done.

USE IN GYNECOLOGY ONCOLOGY

The use of robotics in gynecology oncology has been limited to basically two main procedures that involve staging of endometrial cancer and radical hysterectomy for cervical cancer. Other procedures that lack sufficient data include the staging of ovarian cancer and radical trachelectomy.

Staging of Endometrial Cancer

All literature available in this field seems to be very optimistic regarding the use of robotics in uterine cancer. When compared to laparoscopy or laparotomy, robotic-assisted hysterectomy for endometrial cancer staging yields similar outcomes such as lymph node retrieval, blood loss, and complication rates. Robotic outcomes are comparable to, or even better than, the other two surgical techniques.[16,17] Robotic and conventional laparoscopic operative times are comparable and are slightly longer than open approaches.

Staging of Cervical Cancer/Radical Hysterectomy

Robotic-assisted radical hysterectomy has been shown to have shorter or similar operative times than laparotomy or conventional laparoscopy.[18,19] Major advantages of robotics in this procedure are shorter hospitalization, decreased blood loss, and faster recovery to normal activities. Robotic laparoscopic surgery applies to a very broad scope of applicability, and more and more gynecologic surgeons seem to be incorporating robotics in their practices.[20,21] Although there is not a national consent about the development and training of this innovative technology, it is definitely here to stay.

Comprehension Questions

5.1 A 50-year-old woman has a history of menorrhagia refractory to medical treatment. She has been diagnosed with uterine polyps by hysteroscopy. Her endometrial biopsy is negative for malignancy. She requests a hysterectomy with salpingo-oophorectomy. Her past surgical history includes three prior cesarean sections, an appendectomy secondary to ruptured appendix, and an exploratory laparoscopy for the evaluation of chronic pelvic pain. The pelvic examination reveals a large 14-week-size uterus, which is fixed and not very mobile and somewhat tender. Which of the following would be the best surgical approach for this patient?

A. Vaginal hysterectomy with bilateral salpingo-oophorectomy
B. Laparoscopic-assisted vaginal hysterectomy with sacrocolpopexy
C. Total abdominal hysterectomy with bilateral salpingo-oophorectomy
D. Robotic-assisted supracervical hysterectomy

5.2 With regard to robotic-assisted gynecologic procedures, which of the following statements *is true*?

A. As compared to the open technique, robotic-assisted myomectomy has better outcomes.
B. Robotic-assisted radical hysterectomy for early stages of cervical cancer has the same operative time as open procedure and shorter times than conventional laparoscopy.
C. Robotic-assisted sacrocolpopexy has better outcomes and less blood loss than open sacrocolpopexy.
D. When adhesive disease is suspected in a patient, laparoscopic approach is preferred over robotic.

5.3 Which of the following statements is most accurate?

A. Robotic machinery is more precise than conventional laparoscopy because of the bulkiness and initial investment.
B. If vaginal hysterectomy is feasible, this approach should be offered first rather than robotics.
C. Robotic-assisted sacrocolpopexy has longer operative time than laparoscopy sacrocolpopexy.
D. Disadvantages to the robotic technology include the lack of the option of morcellation.

ANSWERS

5.1 **C.** Total abdominal hysterectomy with bilateral salpingo-oophorectomy would be the safest choice in this patient, given her extensive past surgical history that includes possible endometriosis and extensive postoperative adhesions. Laparoscopic-assisted vaginal hysterectomy could be considered, except for the fact that this patient has an enlarged uterus which would be less likely to be amenable to vaginal approach; sacrocolpopexy is not indicated in this patient. Robotic-assisted supracervical hysterectomy would be a substandard treatment since the patient desires total hysterectomy that includes cervix, tubes, and ovaries.

5.2 **B.** Data available today suggest that robotic-assisted radical hysterectomy for early cervical cancer stages has similar operative times as the open approach and shorter operative times than conventional laparoscopy. Considering that this procedure is minimally invasive, faster recovery and less blood loss are major advantages. Option A robotic myomectomy has similar short-term outcomes when compared to open approach. Option C robotic-assisted sacrocolpopexy has similar outcomes when compared to open and also less blood loss. Finally, when postoperative or postinflammatory adhesions are suspected, option D, that is, the use of robotics, would be a better option, given the improved dexterity, precision, and improved visualization (3D).

5.3 **B.** Whenever technically feasible and medically appropriate, patients requiring hysterectomy should be offered the vaginal approach because morbidity appears to be lower than any other method.[12]

Clinical Pearls

See Table 1-2 for definition of level of evidence and strength of recommendation

- Robotic sacrocolpopexy has demonstrated similar short-term vaginal vault support compared with abdominal sacrocolpopexy, although with longer operative time, less blood loss, and shorter length of stay (Level B).
- Vaginal hysterectomy has the lower morbidity than any other method (Level A).
- Some advantages of robotic technology over conventional laparoscopy are better dexterity, precision, and 3D imaging (Level C).

REFERENCES

1. Stewart EA, Gedroyc WM, Regan L, et al. Focused ultrasound treatment of uterine fibroid tumors: safety and feasibility of a noninvasive thermoablative technique. *Am J Obstet Gynecol.* 2003;189:48.
2. Mohamed N, Akl MD, Javier Magrina MD. Will robots transform gynecologic surgery? *Contemporary Ob/Gyn.* 2009 Sep;54(9):26-32.
3. Senapati S, Advincula AP. Surgical techniques: robot-assisted laparoscopic myomectomy with the Da Vinci surgical system. *J Robotic Surg.* 2007;1:69-74.
4. Dharia SP, Falcone T. Robotics in reproductive medicine. *Fertil Steril.* 2005;84:1.
5. Satava RM. Robotic surgery: from the past to future- a personal journey. *Surg Clin North Am.* 2003;83:1491.
6. Falcone T, Goldberg J, Garcia-Ruiz A, et al. Full robotic assistance for laparoscopic tubal anastomosis: a case report. *J Laparoendosc Adv Surg Tech A.* 1999;9:107.
7. Anthony G, Visco MD, Arnold Advincula MD. Robotic gynecologic surgery. *Obstet Gynecol.* 2008 Dec;112(6):1369-1384.
8. Reynolds RK, Advincula AP. Robot assisted laparoscopic hysterectomy: technique and initial experience. *Am J Surg.* 2006;191:555-560.
9. Elizabeth J, Geller MD, Nazema Y, et al. Short term outcomes of robotic sacrocolpopexy compared with abdominal sacrocolpopexy. *Obstet Gynecol.* 2008 Dec;112(6):1201-1213.
10. American College of Obstetricians and Gynecologists, et al. Appropriate use of laparoscopically assisted vaginal hysterectomy. ACOG Committee Opinion No. 311. April 2005. *Obstet Gynecol.* 2005;105:929-930.
11. Wu JM, Wechter ME, Geller EJ, Nguyen TV, Visco AG. Hysterectomy rates in the United States, 2003. *Obstet Gynecol.* 2007;110:1091-1095.
12. Advincula AP, Song A. The role of robotic surgery in gynecology. *Curr Opin Obstet Gynecol.* 2007;19:331-336.
13. Manyonda I, Sinthamoney E, Belli AM. Controversies and challenges in the modern management of uterine fibroids. *BJOG.* 2004;111:95-102.
14. Goldberg JM, Falcone T. Laparoscopic microsurgical tubal anastomosis with and without robotic assistance. *Hum Reprod.* 2003;18:145.
15. Dharia Patel SP, Steinkampf MP, Whitten SJ, Malizia BA. Robotic tubal anastomosis: surgical technique and cost effectiveness. *Fertil Steril.* 2008;90:1175.
16. Veljovich DS, Paley PJ, Drescher CW, et al. Robotic surgery in gynecology oncology: program initiation and outcomes after the first year with comparison with laparotomy for endometrial cancer staging. *Am J Obstet Gynecol.* 2008;198:679.
17. Boggess JF, Gehrig PA, Cantrell L, et al. A comparative study of 3 surgical methods for hysterectomy with staging for endometrial cancer: robotic assistance, laparoscopy, laparotomy. *Am J Obstet Gynecol.* 2008;199:360.
18. Sert B, Abeler V. Robotic radical hysterectomy in early stage cervical carcinoma patients, comparing results with total laparoscopic radical hysterectomy cases. The future is now? *Int J Med Robot.* 2007;3:224.
19. Boggess JF, Gehrig PA, Cantrell L, et al. A case control study of robot-assisted type III radical hysterectomy with pelvic lymph node dissection compared with open radical hysterectomy. *Am J Obstet Gynecol.* 2008;199:357.

20. Nezhat C, Lavie O, Hsu S, Watson J, Barnett O, Lemyre M. Robotic-assisted laparoscopic myomectomy compared with standard laparoscopic myomectomy—a retrospective matched control study. *Fertil Steril.* 2009 Feb;91(2):556-559.
21. Magrina JF, Kho RM, Weaver AL, Montero RP, Magtibay PM. Robotic radical hysterectomy: comparison with laparoscopy and laparotomy. *Gynecol Oncol.* 2008;109:86-91.

Case 6

You are performing an operative laparoscopy on a 28-year-old woman with a history of pelvic pain, dyspareunia, and a left adnexal mass. She had a history of PID 2 years ago and had an exploratory laparotomy for endometriosis 10 years ago. You place the initial trocar infraumbilically using an open technique. Upon inserting the laparoscope, you find a loop of bowel adherent to the abdominal wall next to your trocar. Multiple adhesions are also present in the lower abdomen and pelvis. Additional trocars are placed under direct visualization. The procedure is tedious and challenging, but you are able to expose the pelvic organs. You free the adnexal mass from the rectosigmoid colon using sharp and blunt dissection. Hemostasis was achieved using electrosurgical devices. A left salpingo-oophorectomy was performed to remove a large endometrioma. The patient is discharged the next day. Three days later, she calls your clinic late in the afternoon complaining of lower abdominal discomfort. You see her the next morning in your clinic, and she has diffuse abdominal pain, nausea, and feels feverish. On examination, she appears ill. She has a temperature of 101°F, an HR of 120 beats/minute, and BP of 90/60 mm Hg. Her abdomen has hypoactive bowel sounds and rebound tenderness.

➤ What is the most likely diagnosis?

➤ What are the mechanisms of the condition?

➤ What factors contribute to this patient's condition?

ANSWERS TO CASE 6:
Electrocautery (Bowel Injury) with Laparoscopy

Summary: A 28-year-old white woman underwent laparoscopy for pelvic pain and a left adnexal mass. The surgery was difficult. Three days later, the patient has lower abdominal pain, nausea, fever, and rebound tenderness.

- **Most likely diagnosis:** Probable peritonitis from an unrecognized bowel injury. I would also consider an unrecognized bladder injury, a severe urinary tract infection, reactivation of PID, and a ruptured appendix.
- **Mechanism of bowel injuries in laparoscopic surgery:** Most bowel injuries occur with Veress needle insertion or initial trocar placement.[1] Other causes include electrical burns or traumatic injury during adhesiolysis or bowel manipulation.
- **What factors contributed to the risk of bowel injury:** The main risk factor for bowel injury was adhesions from previous abdominal surgery. PID and endometriosis also contributed to a difficult dissection. The use of electrosurgical devices, especially monopolar instruments, can lead to unrecognized thermal injuries.

ANALYSIS

Considerations

Initial entry into the abdomen with the laparoscope has always been a cause for concern, especially when the patient has had previous abdominal surgery. Many different techniques, such as the "open" technique, and many types of trocars have been advocated to reduce this risk, but none have been completely successful. The problem is that bowel is adherent in close proximity to the trocar and laparoscope, and injury is not completely avoidable. Currently, many authors are advocating for using the left upper quadrant as a "safe" entry point in patients at high risk for intra-abdominal adhesions.[2,3] The trocar is placed in the midclavicular line 2 cm below the costal margin. Using the left upper quadrant as an entry point is probably a better choice than the infraumbilical site. Once the trocar is safely inserted inside the abdominal cavity, the adhesions can be evaluated, and any further trocars must be inserted under direct visualization only. The use of electrosurgical instruments is commonplace with laparoscopy, but one must be cognizant of the risks and how to avoid them. Good visualization of the surgical site is critical. Certainly, the surgeon should always be able to clearly see the tips of the scissors when dissecting adhesions. Traction on the adhesions using a grasping device is helpful, but care must be taken when activating an electrode near a metal grasper, or other conductive instrument, and causing an injury due to the direct coupling effect. Such would be the concern with the segment of bowel that was adherent at the insertion site and lying close to the laparoscope. Effective smoke evacuation is necessary for good visualization. Good hemostasis is also important as small amounts of blood may obscure the operating field when viewed through the laparoscope. Once the pelvis is visualized, one must make a decision about the safest way to proceed. Dissecting an endometrioma off the rectosigmoid colon can be extremely difficult in any circumstance. The surgeon must possess the laparoscopic skills necessary to safely complete the dissection. If the surgeon does not possess those skills, a more experienced surgeon should be consulted or the case should be converted to an open laparotomy. Slow, deliberate sharp dissection using good surgical technique is important in preventing iatrogenic injury. When utilizing electrosurgical instruments, always try to keep bowel away from the active electrode and be aware of the proximity of other devices capable of conducting electrical current to the active electrode. This is especially important when dissecting adhesions away from bowel or other structures in tight spaces where additional instruments are needed to help with exposure. Electrical energy should be used judiciously, for the shortest duration, and at the lowest power settings to minimize tissue damage. At the completion of the procedure, the surgeon must carefully inspect the surgical site for any sign of injury. Serosal and partial thickness defects of the bowel wall should be repaired. Any evidence for perforation necessitates an intraoperative surgical consult. If there was a question about a possible perforation, the pelvis can be filled with fluid and air introduced into the rectum.[4] Bubbles resulting from this would indicate a perforation. Depending on the size of the defect, bowel resection, with or without a colostomy, may be indicated. The patient should be started on broad-spectrum antibiotics and the pelvis irrigated with copious amounts of irrigation fluid to reduce bacterial contamination.

Objectives

1. Discuss basic concept of an electrical current and how it applies to electrosurgery.
2. Understand the differences between cutting waveforms and coagulating waveforms.
3. Understand the differences between monopolar electrodes and bipolar electrodes.
4. Know the causes of burn injuries with electrosurgical instruments and how to avoid them.

APPROACH TO
Bowel Injuries from Laparoscopy

DEFINITIONS

ELECTROSURGERY: Term used to describe the passage of high-frequency electrical current through tissue to create a desired tissue effect

CAPACITOR COUPLING: The establishment of currents between two conductors that are separated by an insulator

DIRECT COUPLING: Intended or unintended contact between an active electrode and tissue

BIPOLAR: Electrosurgical current that is passed between two electrodes with a small volume of tissue between the two electrodes to complete the electrical circuit

MONOPOLAR: Electrosurgical current that is dispersed through the patient to a return electrode which then returns energy to the generator to complete the electrical circuit

CLINICAL APPROACH

Heat and cautery have been used for hundreds of years to control bleeding. In the early nineteenth century, a French physicist, Becquerel, used direct current electricity to heat a wire which was then used to cauterize tissue.[5] In the late 1920s, William Bovie and Harvey Cushing developed the first electrosurgical unit to be used in human surgery.[5] Nearly 100 years later, electrosurgery is still an integral part of most surgeons' practice. In laparoscopic gynecologic procedures, electrosurgery is still a mainstay for cutting tissue and obtaining hemostasis.

A basic understanding of electricity and electrical currents is necessary to understand the principles behind electrosurgery. Electrical current is generated when electrons are forced to move through a circuit. Power is the energy produced by the current.[6] Voltage is the force which drives the electrons through the circuit, and heat is generated when the electrons meet resistance within the circuit. Lastly, electricity needs a continuous circuit to flow. The electrosurgical unit provides the voltage for the flow of electrons. Modern electrosurgical generators utilize alternating current at radiofrequency levels.[5] When the electrosurgical unit is activated, current flows through the active electrode which is applied to the patient. The patient's tissue provides the resistance and heat is generated which produces the clinical effects desired by the surgeon. The current then flows either through the patient back to the electrosurgical unit through a return electrode ("grounding pad") or through another conducting instrument. The different tissue effects depend on the density of the electrical current, the time the current is applied to the tissue, the resistance of the tissue, the electrode size, and the waveform of the current.[7] Some common uses of electrosurgical energy in gynecologic laparoscopy include lysing adhesions, controlling bleeding, destroying areas of endometriosis, interrupting tubal patency for female sterilization, and treating ectopic pregnancies.

Two basic waveforms of electrical current are generated by the electrosurgical unit. They are a "cut" waveform and a "coagulation" waveform. The "cut" waveform is a continuous radiofrequency sine wave which creates higher current but lower voltage (Figure 6–1A and B).[5] This waveform produces intense local heat and is used to vaporize tissue. It is the vaporization of the tissue which creates the "cutting" effect. Cutting waveforms produce less tissue charring and less tissue damage. The "coagulation" waveform is composed of intermittent radiofrequency sine waves which have higher voltage but lower current than cutting waveforms.[5] The waveform consists of small bursts of energy followed by a "cooling-off" period. This cooling-off period allows the coagulation effect to begin. The coagulation waveform can be used to fulgurate or desiccate tissue. A "blended" waveform is a modification of the cutting waveform and allows the surgeon to both cut and coagulate tissue at the same time.[8] The ratio of voltage to current is modified by diminishing the current and increasing the voltage so that the power remains constant. This allows for more or less coagulation effects, depending on the settings.

Energy from the electrosurgical unit is delivered to the tissue by either a monopolar electrode or bipolar electrodes. With the monopolar electrode, the electrical current passes from the tip of the electrode to the tissue, then goes through the patient, and is returned to the electrosurgical generator through

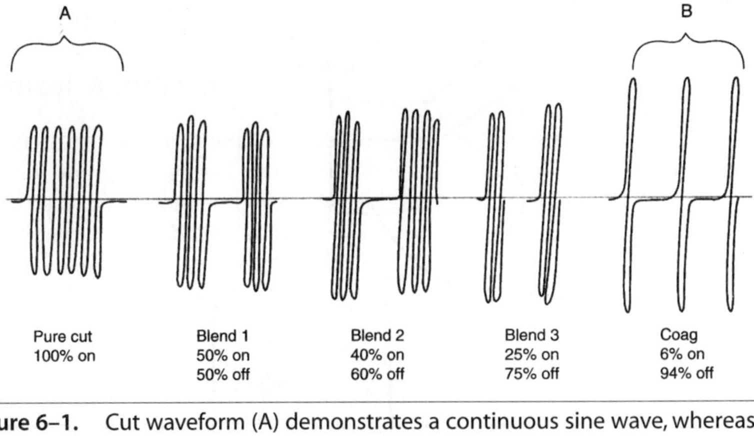

Figure 6–1. Cut waveform (A) demonstrates a continuous sine wave, whereas the coagulation waveform (B) shows an intermittent, higher peak voltage, when both are set at equal wattages. Blend currents have different proportion of "cut" and "coagulation" waveforms. (*Reproduced, with permission, from Doherty GM.* Current Diagnosis & Treatment: Surgery, *13th ed. New York: McGraw-Hill, 2010.*)

a return electrode placed on the patient's body.[5] Monopolar devices can be used for cutting tissue, fulgurating tissue, or desiccating tissue. With bipolar electrodes, the current is passed from the active electrode through the tissue to the return electrode to complete the circuit.[4] With the bipolar electrodes, the active and return electrodes are within the same instrument being used at the site of the surgery. Tissue damage is limited to the tissue between the electrodes. Bipolar electrodes are used primarily for desiccating tissue and coagulation. It requires lower power settings, but takes longer to be effective and creates more tissue charring. Both devices can utilize cutting or coagulating waveforms of current (Figure 6–2A and B).

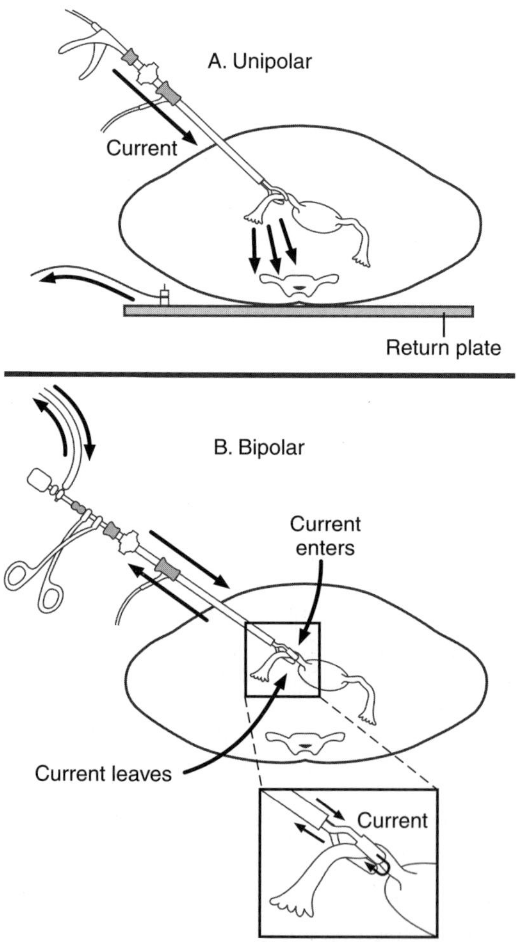

Figure 6–2. **A** demonstrates a unipolar scissors in which the current travels from the electrode through the tissue to the grounding plate. **B** shows bipolar device in which the current travels from one electrode to the other electrode.

Types of Thermal Injuries

The greatest fear with using electrosurgical instruments in laparoscopic surgery is unintended thermal injury to the patient. Electrosurgical thermal burn injuries occur primarily by misapplication of the active electrode or "stray energy" as the result of capacitor coupling, direct coupling, or insulation failure. **Misapplication** of the active electrode usually occurs when the electrode is activated away from the intended target. Poor visualization may lead to misidentification of the targeted tissue. This may be due to bleeding, smoke, or distorted anatomy due to pathologic changes or adhesive disease. Hopefully, these injuries are recognized and addressed when they occur. Injuries from "stray energy" are infrequent, usually occur out of the view of the surgeon, and may not be immediately recognizable. It is important to have some understanding of how these unrecognized transfers of electrical current occur.

Capacitor coupling involves the storage of energy between two conductors separated by an insulator.[5] An electromagnetic field is established when an insulated electrode is placed through a metal cannula/trocar and activated. Electrical current is induced into the metal cannula through a process known as *capacitance*.[9] Energy is stored in the capacitator until the generating force of the current is deactivated or a pathway to complete the electrical circuit is established. In most instances, the current stored in the metal cannula/trocar is in direct contact with the patient and dispersed through the patient back to the return electrode. If there is an insulator (ie, a plastic anchoring collar) between the metal cannula and the patient, current cannot pass through to the patient and is stored in the cannula (ie, a capacitator). When the net charge in the capacitor exceeds the insulator's capacity, current is produced and passed to other conductive material (ie, tissue). Thermal injuries can result.

Capacitative coupling is highest when voltages are high. This happens when the electrode is activated in an "open circuit" away from the targeted tissue. High voltage coagulation current creates the same problem.[9] Using all metal or all plastic cannulas/trocars avoids the problem entirely, but hybrid systems are to be avoided. Direct coupling or "probe" coupling occurs when the active electrode comes in contact with another metal instrument, thus directly passing the electrical current to the other instrument.[10] This may be intentional when a bleeding point is grasped with a metal grasper; the grasper is then touched by the active electrode to produce a cauterizing effect. Inadvertent injury occurs when the active electrode accidently touches a metal object (ie, probes, graspers, suction devices, etc) which is in contact with other nontargeted tissue.

Insulation failure occurs when there are breaks in the insulation covering the active electrode shaft, allowing current to leave the electrode and find an alternate pathway to complete its circuit back to the return electrode.[9] Thus, energy can be transferred from the shaft of the electrode to other conductive, nontargeted tissue that might be in contact with the shaft, resulting in an unrecognized injury. These injuries typically occur on the portion of the instrument that is beyond the field of view of the laparoscope but distal to the protective trocar. A recent study revealed that 20% of reusable instruments had insulation defects, and that 18% of the defects were in the portion of the electrode that is exposed but "out of sight" of the surgeon.[11] All electrodes should be examined or tested prior to use for insulation defects, although these defects may be quite small and difficult to appreciate.

Prevention of Thermal Injuries

Prevention of electrosurgical injuries is paramount. Safe laparoscopic surgery requires a common sense approach to the use of electrosurgical devices. All laparoscopic instruments should be in good working order. All OR personnel should be familiar with the electrosurgical generators, how they are to be operated, and the safety features of each particular unit. They should also know how to assemble all the electrosurgical devices and have the proper connecting cords immediately available. The surgeon should specify the type of energy source he/she would like to use and be familiar with all aspects of its use. Bipolar rather than unipolar electrosurgery should be used when possible. It minimizes damage to the surrounding tissue and avoids the problems of "stray energy." When monopolar electrodes are going to be used, the surgeon must ensure that the return electrode pad is properly placed on the patient. The surgeon should inspect the electrodes for any breaks in the insulation. The tip of the electrode should always be visible to the surgeon when it is activated, and the electrode should only be activated when the surgeon is sure of its intended target. The electrode should never be activated in an open circuit (ie, in the abdomen away from the intended target)! Care must always be taken when activating the electrode when it is in close proximity to another metal or other conductive instrument. Metal cannulas are the safest operating channels for active electrodes, and any metal/plastic hybrid cannulas should not be used.[7]

When using either monopolar or bipolar instruments, the lowest possible power settings should be used for the shortest period of time necessary to achieve the desired clinical effect. Cut waveforms should be used whenever possible because they require lower voltage settings.[5] The electrodes (or paddles with bipolar devices) should always have any coagulum removed as this increases resistance and causes the electrode to adhere more to the tissue. Finally, when the electrode is not in use, it should be placed in a protective, insulated holster rather than just left lying in the surgical field. This simple step eliminates accidental burns to the patient and reduces the risk of starting a fire in the OR.

Safety Features

The surgeon should also know which safety features are being used with their particular electrosurgical unit. The modern electrosurgical unit is an isolated solid-state generator.[5] In this system, the current can only return to the generator through the return electrode pad. This has been a major factor in reducing alternate site burns. Contact quality monitoring systems now being used also prevent the unit from being activated if the return electrode pad is not in proper contact with the patient. This eliminates patient burns at the site of an improperly placed pad.[5] An active electrode monitoring system is available which detects and shields the patient from stray energy from insulation failure or capacitor coupling.[12] Recently, tissue response technology has come into use. Vessel sealing devices using bipolar energy and tissue response technology can seal arterial vessels up to 7 mm in diameter while reducing thermal spread to surrounding tissue.[13] This technology uses computers to sense tissue resistance and then automatically adjusts the output voltage to maintain a constant effect to the targeted tissue. These devices have been associated with less blood loss, shorter operating times, and shorter hospital stays.[14]

In the end, however, nothing is more important than a well-prepared, knowledgeable surgeon who possesses good manual dexterity, excellent hand-eye coordination, and sound clinical judgment. Knowledge of electrosurgical principles and proper use of electrosurgical devices should enable the laparoscopic surgeon to operate safely and effectively.

Comprehension Questions

6.1 A 48-year-old woman is undergoing laparoscopy for assessment of a 6-cm left adnexal mass. Which of the following is the most significant risk factor for bowel injury?

A. Prior cesarean
B. Prior PID
C. Endometriosis
D. Prior cervical dysplasia with cryotherapy

6.2 A 44-year-old woman underwent a laparoscopy for chronic pelvic pain. The patient developed bowel symptoms 5 days after the surgery. Which of the following is the most likely mechanism for this complication?

A. Laceration with the Veress needle
B. Laceration with the trocar
C. Thermal injury
D. CO_2 embolism

6.3 In considering the possibility of bowel injury, which of the following can decrease the severity of these complications?

A. Bowel preparation
B. Open laparoscopy technique
C. Use of a pneumoperitoneum
D. Use of a bipolar rather than unipolar current

ANSWERS

6.1 **C.** A prior cesarean typically does not lead to significant adhesions of the bowel to the abdominal wall. Prior PID leads to adnexal adhesions and tubal scarring, but unless there was tubo-ovarian abscess, there is usually no bowel involvement. Endometriosis can lead to widespread adhesions and fibrosis.

6.2 **C.** The delay in symptoms is likely related to thermal injury, which can be manifest up to a week postoperatively. Lacerations during surgery typically cause symptoms immediately.

6.3 **A.** A bowel preparation with both cleansing the bowel (mechanical) as well as antibiotics can decrease the bacterial load of the intestinal contents. Thus, if bowel laceration or injury occurs, less contamination occurs. Neither the use of a pneumoperitoneum or Veress needle or open laparoscopy techniques has been shown to decrease the incidence of bowel injuries.

Clinical Pearls

See Table 1-2 for definition of level of evidence and strength of recommendation

- Tissue necrosis and subsequent perforation of affected bowel can occur 72-96 hours after surgery (Level B).
- The return electrode pad should be placed on a clean, dry area of skin over a large muscle mass (Level C).
- Superficial thermal injuries of the bowel should be oversewn with suture being placed in healthy tissue well beyond the area of injury (Level C).
- Insulation defects are found in 20% of reusable electrodes (Level B).
- An all metal cannula system is the safest choice for the operating cannula containing the active electrode (Level B).

REFERENCES

1. Schäfer M, Lauper M, Krähenbühl L. Trocar and Veress needle injuries during laparoscopy. *Surg Endosc*. 2001;15:275-280.
2. Parker J, Reid G, Wong F. Microlaparoscopic left upper quadrant entry in patients at high risk of periumbilical adhesions. *Aust N Z J Obstet Gynaecol*.199;39:88-92.
3. Sepilian V, Ku L, Wong H, Liu CJ, Phelps JY. Prevalence of infraumbilical adhesions in women with previous laparoscopy. *JSLS*. 11;1:41-44.
4. Shirk J, Johns A, Redwine DB. Complications of laparoscopic surgery: how to avoid them and how to repair them. *J Minim Invasive Gynecol*. 2006 Jul-Aug;13(4):352-359.

5. Wang K, Advincula AP. "Current Thoughts" in electrosurgery. *Int J Gynaecol Obstet*. 2007 Jun;97(3):245-250.
6. Jones CM, Pierre KB, Nicoud IB, Stain SC, Melvin WV. Electrosurgery. *Curr Surg*. 2006 Nov-Dec;63(6):458-463.
7. Wu MP, Ou CS, Chen SL, Yen YET, Rowbotham R. Complications and recommended practices for electrosurgery in laparoscopy. *Am J Surg*. 2000 Jan;179(1): 67-73.
8. McCauley G. Understanding electrosurgery. Bovie/Aaron Medical. Copyright 2003.
9. Nezhet C, Siegler A, Nezhat F, Nezhat C, Seidman D, Luciano A. Electrosurgery. In: *Operative Gynecologic Laparoscopy: Principles and Techniques*. 2nd ed. New York: McGraw-Hill; 2000:73-80.
10. Odell RC. Electrosurgery: principles and safety issues. *Clin Obstet Gynecol*. 1995;38:610-621.
11. Montero PN, Robinson NR, Weaver JS, Stiegmann GV. Insulation failure in laparoscopic instruments. *Surg Endosc*. 2009;24:462-465 [Epub 2009 Jul 2].
12. Safety technology for laparoscopic monopolar electro surgery; devices for managing burn risks. *Health Devices/ECRI*. 2005 Aug;34(8):259-272.
13. Hubner M, Demartines N, Muller S, Dindo D, Calvien P-A, Hahnloser D. Prospective randomized study of monopolar scissors, bipolar vessel sealer and ultrasonic shears in laparoscopic colorectal surgery. *Br J Surg*. 2008;95:1098-1104.
14. Campagnacci R, de Sanctis A, Baldarelli M, Lezoche G, Guerrieri M. Electrothermal bipolar vessel sealing device vs. ultrasonic coagulating shears in laparoscopic colectomies: a comparative study. *Surg Endosc*. 2007 Sep;21(9):1525-1531 [Epub 2007 Feb 8].

Case 7

A 37-year-old G4P3013 woman presents to your office requesting a sterilization procedure. She desires to have a sterilization and would like to have a surgical technique that would allow her to resume her daily duties in a short period of time. Her last delivery was over a year ago, and she has a negative past surgical history. She is 5 ft 4 in in height and weighs 165 lb (75 kg). She is currently using condoms for contraception.

- ➤ What is the clinical condition?
- ➤ What counseling is important for this patient?
- ➤ What is your next step?

ANSWERS TO CASE 7: Laparoscopic Tubal Occlusion

Summary: This is a 37-year-old G4P3013 woman with a negative past surgical and medical history desiring sterilization.

- **Clinical condition:** Multiparous patient desiring sterilization.
- **Counseling:** The patient should be given the options of contraception, male sterilization, and female sterilization. She should be aware of the irreversibility, failure rate, and risk of ectopic pregnancy with female sterilization.
- **Next step:** Outline the surgical options, including vasectomy, and explain the risks, benefits, and alternatives of the operation.

ANALYSIS

Objectives

1. Be able to provide proper counseling for sterilization.
2. Be familiar with different methods of surgical sterilization and methods of occlusion.
3. Be familiar with risks, complications, and failure rates.

Considerations

This is a 37-year-old G4P3013 woman who desires permanent sterilization. The first step for the physician is to provide proper counseling. It is important for the patient to understand that tubal sterilization is permanent. Despite the availability of surgical techniques that allow the reversal of tubal anatomy and in vitro fertilization, both options are complicated, costly, and not always successful. Sterilization accounts for 39% of contraceptive method used in the United States by women aged 15 to 44 years and their partners. Of those who chose sterilization, 28% had tubal sterilization and 11% had partners who had vasectomy. In comparison, in the same group, 27% use oral contraceptives, 21% use male condoms, 3% use injectable contraceptives, 2% use diaphragms, and 1% use intrauterine devices. Approximately 700,000 tubal sterilizations and 500,000 vasectomies are performed annually in the United States.[1] Laparoscopic tubal occlusion is the most common method of interval sterilization in the United States, with approximately 200,000 performed every year. *Interval sterilization* is defined as a nonpregnant state at least 4 to 6 weeks after the completion of the previous pregnancy. However, tubal sterilization can also be performed postpartum and after a spontaneous or therapeutic abortion. Postpartum sterilization is performed after 10% of hospital deliveries and approximately 3.5% after spontaneous or therapeutic abortions. Postpartum sterilization can be performed at the time of a cesarean section or after a vaginal delivery preferably through a minilaparotomy. Postpartum sterilization optimally involves counseling and informed consent during prenatal care and prior to labor and delivery. The patient should be explained that the sterilization might be postponed in cases of intra- or postpartum medical or obstetrical complications. The physician should be aware of federal and state regulations that govern the timing of consent of the procedure.

Interval sterilization can be performed at any time during the menstrual cycle, although the performance during the follicular phase and/or the use of an effective contraceptive method by the patient greatly reduces the risk of a concurrent pregnancy. In addition, the utilization of a highly sensitive pregnancy test prior to the sterilization is a wise and necessary option. The routine performance of a D&C concurrent with all interval sterilizations is not recommended.

Methods of Laparoscopic Sterilization

Bipolar Coagulation Laparoscopic sterilization has evolved in the United States from the unipolar coagulation originally described by Palmer and Steptoe, to the bipolar techniques described by Rioux and Kleppinger.[2] Unipolar sterilization has lost its initial popularity as a result of a series of mysterious bowel injuries that were reported in the 1970s. It is quite possible that these injuries were a result of capacitance coupling (as explained in Case 6) or from mechanical laceration at the time of sterilization. As a result, bipolar laparoscopic tubal occlusion became the most commonly used technique. Approximately 3 cm of the isthmic portion of the fallopian tubes are coagulated using at least 25 W of energy in a cutting waveform (see Figure 7–1). The 3 cm length of the fallopian tubes involved with the sterilization corresponds to the three applications of the bipolar forceps (Figure 7–1). It is imperative to use a current meter (ammeter) to ensure complete desiccation, and this finding of "power used until no current flowed as per ammeter" should be documented in the operative report. Visual inspection can lead to incomplete coagulation of the fallopian tube and increased failures. The tube is grasped approximately 2 to 4 cm from the uterus in order to minimize the possibility of uteroperitoneal fistula formation and ectopic pregnancy. It is probably a good practice to leave a stump of isthmus of approximately 1 to 2 cm after all techniques of sterilization. Coagulation of 3 cm of fallopian tube without division has been demonstrated to be as effective as coagulation and division. Division can lead to bleeding from underlying vessels that were not occluded during the coagulation. Also, coagulation and division may be associated with the destruction of a larger segment of the tube. Division is unnecessary as a result of the normal healing process after bipolar coagulation of the fallopian tube. Bipolar coagulation and the resulting desiccated or devitalized fallopian tissue induce the body to create a state of hypervascularization around the site with gradual absorption of dead tissue

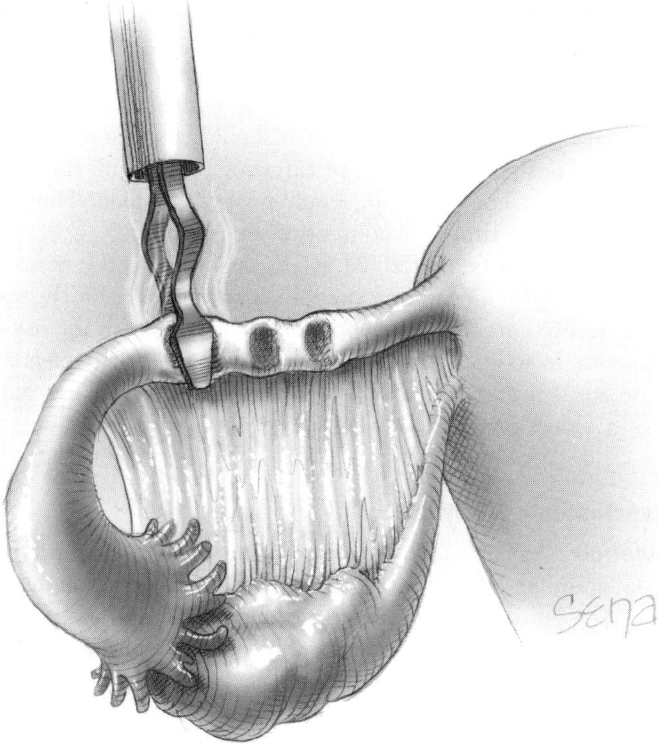

Figure 7–1. Bipolar cautery of the tube on the 3-cm segment. (*Reproduced, with permission, from Schorge JO, Schaffer JI, Halvorson LM, et al.* Williams Gynecology. *New York: McGraw-Hill, 2008:937.*)

within 3 weeks. The proximal and distal stumps of the desiccated fallopian tube are drawn together as the intervening tissue is absorbed 3 to 6 months after coagulation. Absorption of the dead tissue is usually complete by 6 months, and at that point the two stumps fall apart. Hypervascularization subsides within 1 year. Therefore, with bipolar coagulation within 1 year, there would be an absence of a small segment of the fallopian tube that would have been absorbed. Incomplete coagulation can lead to drawing the stumps together and recanalization within 3 months.

Silastic Band (Falope Ring) Nonelectrical alternatives to tubal occlusion were developed in the 1970s in response to complications mainly associated with unipolar coagulation. In 1974, Yoon and associates[3] introduced the silastic band (also called Falope or Yoon ring). It requires an applicator that contains an inner and outer cylinder and grasping hooks. The tube is grasped with the hooks of the Falope ring applicator 3 cm from the uterotubal junction and drawn into the inner lumen of the applicator. As the fallopian tube is drawn inward, the applicator is moved toward the mesosalpinx to minimize tension on the tube and avoid transaction. Thereafter, one silicone band is applied to the grasped segment of the tube by moving the outer cylinder forward. After the application, the grasping hooks are moved forward, thus releasing the occluded segment of tube (Figure 7–2A to C). Inspection is carried out and, if desired, photographic documentation could be carried out. Yoon initially recommended the instillation of indigo carmine dye through the uterine manipulator to ensure proper occlusion. I find this practice unnecessary if the surgeon has achieved a good application. One of the limitations of this surgical option lies with the size and flexibility of the tube and the high incidence of postoperative pain. The application of the ring is not possible in an enlarged or scared tube. It can be associated with transection and/or bleeding. The high incidence of postoperative pain is associated to gradual necrosis from anoxia from the knuckle of tube constricted by the silastic band. In some instances hospitalization is required for pain control and observation. As with electrocoagulation, necrotic tissue stimulates a hyperemic reaction in order to absorb the necrotic tissue adjacent to the loop. The absorption process also takes 3 to 6 months. At 6 months there is usually complete separation of the proximal and distal stumps with the

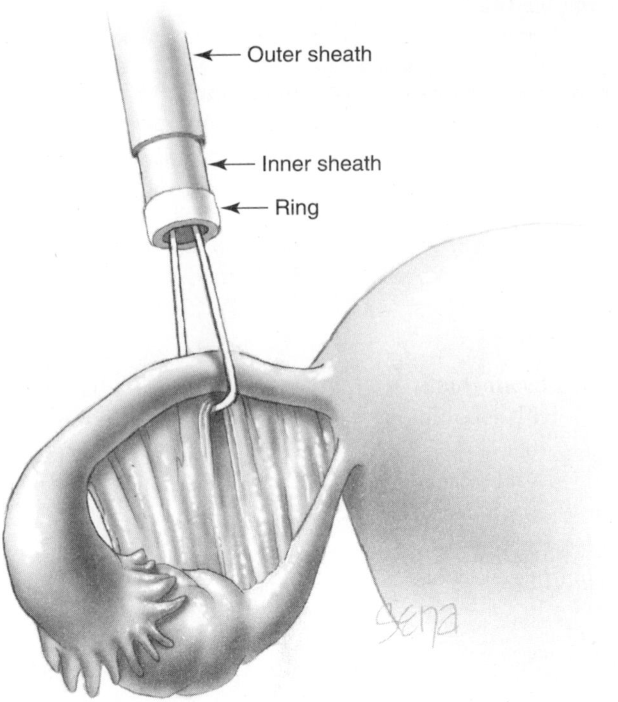

Figure 7–2A. Falope ring placed on the tube. The grasping prongs are placed in the mid-portion of the tube and carefully brought into the sheath. (*Reproduced, with permission, from Schorge JO, Schaffer JI, Halvorson LM, et al.* Williams Gynecology. *New York: McGraw-Hill, 2008:939.*)

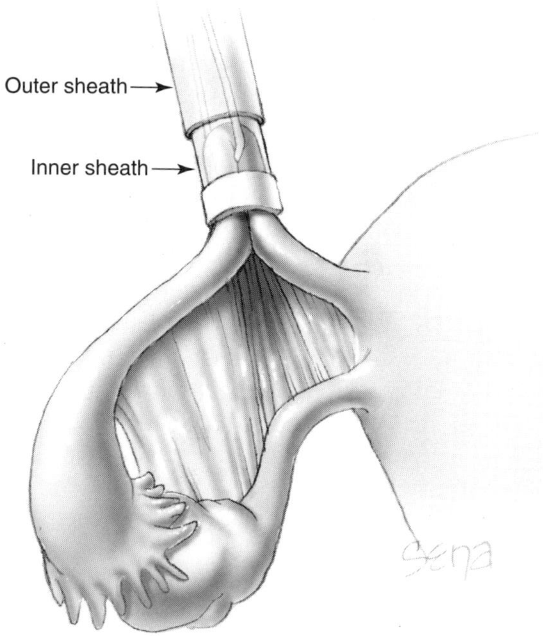

Figure 7–2B. The tube is allowed to retract from the applicator sheath, leaving an ischemic "knuckle of tube." (*Reproduced, with permission, from Schorge JO, Schaffer JI, Halvorson LM, et al.* Williams Gynecology. *New York: McGraw-Hill, 2008:939.*)

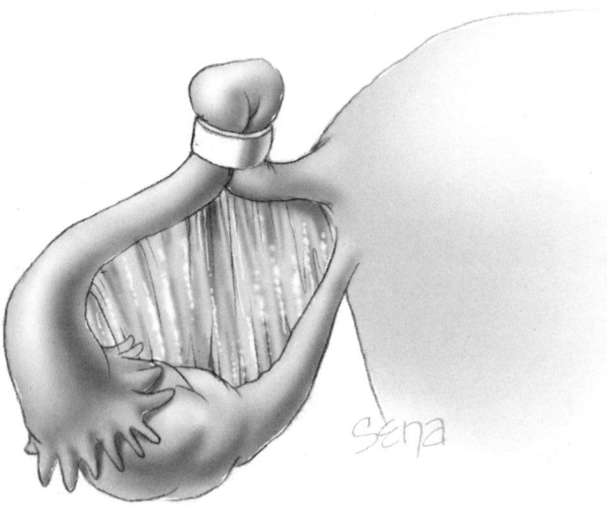

Figure 7–2C. The tube segments are separated after time, achieving the sterilization procedure. (*Reproduced, with permission, from Schorge JO, Schaffer JI, Halvorson LM, et al.* Williams Gynecology. *New York: McGraw-Hill, 2008:940.*)

band in its unstretched form covered by peritoneum. However, improper application of the band on the ampulla of the tube may not completely occlude the tube.

Spring Clip The continuous evolution of laparoscopic female sterilization has tried to improve on previous surgical techniques and associated complications of hemorrhage and bowel burns seen with the silastic band and electrocoagulation. The first application in humans took place in 1972. It was tested from 1973 to 1975 in over 1000 patients. The final version was manufactured in 1976 and is known as the Hulka-Clemens Clip (Richard Wolf Medical Instruments Corp., Knittlingen, Germany).[4-6] The application requires skill by the surgeon who needs to manipulate both the tube and the clip applicator in order to ensure a correct application across the isthmus of the tube. This task is facilitated through a double-puncture technique and the utilization of a uterine manipulator. Although the device can be applied through a double- or single-puncture technique, the clip is loaded to a clip applier which has a handle and a thumb manipulator (Figure 7–3). The clip is made of Lexan Plastic (Lexan Products Division, General Electric, Mt. Vernon, Indiana) and a gold-plated surgical

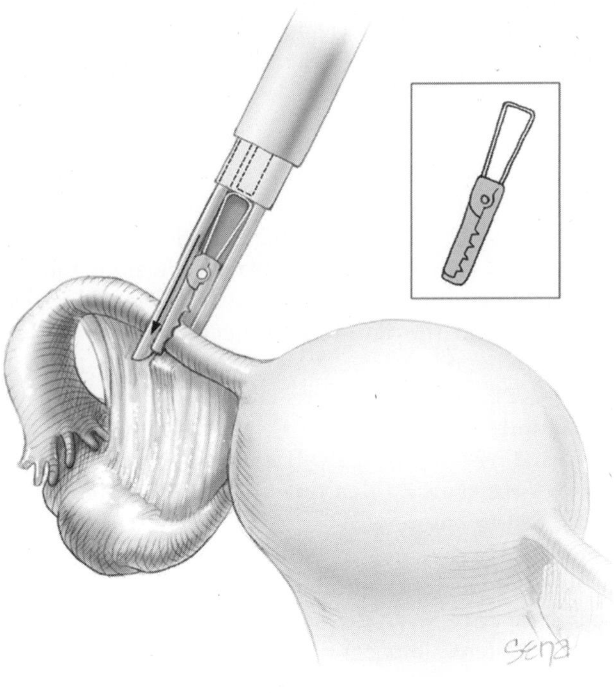

Figure 7–3. Spring-loaded clip applied to the tube using an applicator. (*Reproduced, with permission, from Schorge JO, Schaffer JI, Halvorson LM, et al.* Williams Gynecology. *New York: McGraw-Hill, 2008:938.*)

stainless steel spring. Advancing the thumb manipulator in a partial position allows for the clip to be secured firmly in the basket and preventing dislodgement during the insertion through a trocar sleeve. Upon obtaining the desired application across the isthmic portion of the tube, the lower ram is moved forward by pushing the thumb manipulator to the fully closed position, closing the C-shaped spring over the upper and lower jaws of the clip. At this point, the clip cannot be removed since it is permanently attached to the tube. Once the spring is in place over the jaws, both lower and upper jaws can be rapidly drawn back into the full open position. Correct application produces Kleppinger envelope sign. The mesosalpinx is pulled upward to the surface of the tube resembling the flat triangular shape of an envelope flap. Moving the applicator downward and away from the tube will facilitate the disengagement of the clip from the applicator. There are no reports of complications from unrecovered clips in the abdominal cavity. The spring clip allows for a gap of 1 mm between the upper and lower jaws at the time of application. The jaws contain teeth that prevent the tissue from rolling out during and after application. Over the next 24 to 48 hours the spring compresses the upper and lower jaws exerting sufficient pressure to squeeze out the fluids out of the cells, thus ensuring necrosis. The process also compresses nerves which can be associated with postoperative cramps. Healing is complete in 6 weeks. The clip is covered by peritoneum. There have been reports of patients allergic to gold that required removal of the clips due to persistent pelvic pain. It should be noted that the utilization of the clip greatly facilitates in the performance of a postpartum tubal ligation.

Additional Options In May 1996, the U.S. Food and Drug Administration (FDA) approved the sale of the Filshie clip (Avalon Medicao Corp., Williston, Vermont). The clip is a hinged titanium clip lined with silastic rubber. It is designed to be applied over the isthmic portion of the tube. Its curved upper jaw is designed to accommodate edematous tubes. It can be applied through a single- or double-puncture technique. The Falope ring, Hulka-Clemens clip, and the Filshie clip are associated with small tubal destruction, thus making tubal reversal a viable option.

In November 2002, the FDA approved the use of Essure (Conceptus Incorporated, Mountain View, California), a new transcervical sterilization device that is placed hysteroscopically. Backup contraception is required for 3 months after the procedure. At that time a confirmatory test (hysterosalpingogram) is performed to ensure occlusion of the fallopian tubes. The procedure can be performed in the office or the hospital. Short-term efficacy studies suggest a rate equal or greater than other methods. The limiting steps seems to be the need of expertise in hysteroscopy surgery and the need for backup contraception and hysterosalpingogram 3 months after the procedure.[7]

In the Essure procedure, a microinsert is placed into the interstitial portion of the fallopian tube under hysteroscopic guidance. The insert consists of an inner coil of stainless steel and polyethylene terephthalate (PET) fibers, and an outer coil of nickel-titanium (nitinol). Therefore, insertion of the device is contraindicated in patients with known nickel sensitivity by skin testing.

The PET fibers elicit a benign tissue response that promotes the invasion of macrophages, fibroblasts, foreign body giant cells, and plasma cells. The tissue reaction and the resulting fibrotic ingrowth around the device produce complete tubal occlusion. Bilateral tubal placement rate is 94.6%, although rates as high as 99% have been reported. Essure is highly efficacious with no pregnancies reported in combined data from the phase II and pivotal trials.

In 2009, the FDA approved the second method of transcervical sterilization, Adiana® Permanent Contraception System (Hologic, Inc., Bedford, MA). The Adiana sterilization method consists of a combination of controlled thermal damage to the lining of a small segment of the fallopian tube followed by insertion of a non-absorbable biocompatible silicone elastomer matrix within the tubal lumen. Under hysteroscopic guidance, the delivery catheter is introduced into the tubal ostium. The distal tip of the catheter delivers radiofrequency (RF) energy for 1 minute, creating a 5-mm lesion in the lining of the fallopian tube. Following the thermal injury, the 3.5-mm silicone matrix is deployed within the lesion. Proper deployment of the matrix is identified by the black marker at the tubal ostia and through the position array (PDA). The PDA is a series of 4 sensors that are designed to monitor uniform tissue contact throughout the ablation portion. When the catheter is withdrawn, there are no material visible protruding from the ostia. Occlusion of the tube is achieved by fibroblast ingrowth into the matrix. The system requires the utilization of electrolyte free distending solution such as Glycine or Sorbitol. This raises the risk of excessive absorption and the requirement for a fluid management system and/or careful fluid deficit monitoring. Proper occlusion of the tubes is assessed by performing a HSG 3 months after the procedure. Back up contraception is required. The matrix is visible by ultrasound examination but is not visible through x-ray or HSG. The Adiana system is effective in over 98% cases. However, the 2-year cumulative failure rate is 1.8%, which is higher than all forms of sterilization reported by the CREST study, except for the spring clip application (2.38%), for the same time interval.

Failure of sterilization persists for years after the procedure and varies by method, age, and ethnicity. The younger the patient undergoing the procedure, the higher the failure rate. The U.S. Collaborative Review of Sterilization (CREST) data reported that the 10-year cumulative probability for sterilization failure varied by method and ranged from 7.5 per 1000 to 36 per 1000 procedures. The 5- and 10-year cumulative pregnancy rates per method are as follows:[8]

Postpartum partial salpingectomy: 6.3 per 1000 and 7.5 per 1000 procedures
Bipolar coagulation: 16.5 per 1000 and 24.8 per 1000 procedures
Silicone band: 10 per 1000 and 17.7 per 1000 procedures
Spring clip: 31.7 per 1000 and 36.5 per 1000 pregnancies

A secondary analysis of the 5-year failure rates with bipolar coagulation has shown a higher rate of 19.5 per 1000 procedures from 1978 to 1982, as compared to a rate of 6.3 per 1000 procedures from 1985 to 1987. This could be explained on the basis of utilization of an ammeter during bipolar coagulation of the fallopian tubes.

The risk of an ectopic pregnancy is higher after bipolar coagulation than postpartum salpingectomy. It could be a reflection of the technique. The overall risk of an ectopic pregnancy by any method is 7.3 per 1000 procedures. The probability of an ectopic pregnancy is greater for women sterilized before the age of 30 years. If a patient has a positive pregnancy test after tubal sterilization, the presence of an ectopic pregnancy should be ruled out.[8]

There has been a perception that there is higher rate of menstrual irregularities after sterilization. However, prospective studies have found little or no difference at 1 to 2 years of follow-up. The incidence of regret and subsequent desire for reversal seems to be related to age (< 25 years), lack of preoperative information regarding the procedure, lack of information on contraceptive options, pressure from a spouse, and due to medical indications. In terms of sexual interest or pleasure after sterilization, most prospective studies have shown either no consistent change or no improvement.[9,10]

Comprehension Questions

7.1 A 32-year-old G4P4 woman has had a bilateral tubal occlusion via laparoscopy 2 years previously. She understands that she is at risk for ectopic pregnancy. As compared to women who do not have sterilization, which of the following is most accurate?

A. Female sterilization is associated with a greater risk of ectopic pregnancy.
B. Female sterilization is associated with the same risk of ectopic pregnancy.
C. Female sterilization is associated with a lower risk of ectopic pregnancy.

7.2 Which of the following method of female sterilization is associated with the highest failure rate?

A. Unipolar cautery at laparoscopy
B. Bipolar cautery at laparoscopy
C. Tubal ligation at the time of cesarean
D. Falope ring via laparoscopy
E. Spring clips

7.3 A 37-year-old woman strongly desires female sterilization. She has had numerous abdominal surgeries in the past and has had a ruptured appendicitis previously. Which of the following is the best surgical approach in this patient?

A. Laparoscopic Falope ring
B. Laparoscopic electrocautery
C. Hysteroscopic approach
D. Minilaparotomy with tubal occlusion

ANSWERS

7.1 **C.** Women who have female sterilization have a lower rate of ectopic pregnancy since there are far less pregnancies than in the nonsterilized cohort. However, if a woman who has had a tubal occlusion does become pregnant, the risk of ectopic pregnancy is fairly high.

7.2 **E.** Spring clips are associated with the highest failure rate, in other words, the highest pregnancy rate.

7.3 **C.** Hysteroscopic use of coils in the tubal ostia (Essure) is a good option for patients to avoid the abdominal cavity, given her abdominal adhesions and multiple prior abdominal surgeries. A hysterosalpingogram is recommended following the procedure to ensure that the tubes are occluded.

Clinical Pearls

See Table 1-2 for definition of level of evidence and strength of recommendation

- Sterilization by tubal occlusion is chosen by women at a rate of approximately three times that of vasectomy (Level B).
- Laparoscopic tubal occlusion is the most common type of female sterilization (Level A).
- Bipolar sterilization is best performed using a 3-cm segment of tube (three applications of the bipolar device) and an ammeter to determine that the tissue is adequately desiccated (Level B).
- Division of the tube after bipolar cautery is unnecessary and may lead to bleeding (Level B).
- The spring clip device is associated with the highest risk of sterilization failure (Level B).
- The hysteroscopic placement of coils in the tubal ostia (Essure system), and the insertion of a non-absorbable biocompatible silicone elastomer matrix (Adiana) seems to be effective and can be performed in the office. A hysterosalpingogram needs to be performed to ensure tubal occlusion (Level B).
- The incidence of regret after sterilization seems to be associated with age, especially younger than the age of 25 years (Level B).

REFERENCES

1. Piccinino LJ, Mosher WD. Trends in contraceptive use in the United States: 1982-1995. *Fam Plann Perspect.* 1998;30:10,46.
2. Pollack AE, Soderstrom RM. Female tubal sterilization. In: Corson SL, Derman RJ, Tyler LB, eds, *Fertility Control.* 2nd ed. London, ON: Goldin Publishers; 1994:293-317.

3. Yoon IB, King TM, Parmley TH. A two-year experience with the Falope ring sterilization procedure. *Am J Obstet Gynecol.* 1977;127:109-112.
4. Hulka JF, Mercer JP, Fishburne JI, et al. Spring clip sterilization: one year follow-up of 1,079 cases. *Am J Obstet Gynecol.* 1976;125:1039-1043.
5. Sokal D, Gates D, Amatya R, Dominik R. Two randomized controlled trials comparing the tubal ring and Filshie clip for tubal sterilization. *Fertil Steril.* 2000;74:525-533.
6. Dominik R, Gates D, Sokal D, et al. Two randomized controlled trials comparing the Hulka and Filshie Clips for tubal sterilization. *Contraception.* 2000;62:169-175.
7. Bradley L. Long-term follow-up of hysteroscopic sterilization with the Essure Microinsert. Supplement to the *Journal of Minimally Invasive Gynecology. Fertil Steril.* 2008;15(6):S14-S15.
8. Peterson HB, Jeng G, Folger SG, Hillis SA, Marchbanks PA, Wilcox LS. The risk of ectopic pregnancy after tubal sterilization. U.S. Collaborative Review of Sterilization Working Group. *N Engl J Med.* 1997;336:762-767.
9. Peterson HB, Ory HW, Greenspan JR, Tyler CW Jr. Deaths associated with laparoscopic sterilization by unipolar electrocoagulating devices, 1978 and 1979. *Am J Obstet Gynecol.* 1981;139:141-143.
10. Peterson HB, DeStefano F, Rubin GL, Greenspan JR, Lee NC, Ory HW. Deaths attributable to tubal sterilization in the United States, 1977-81. *Am J Obstet Gynecol.* 1983;146:131-136.
11. Magnani RJ, Haws JM, Morgan GT, Gargioullo PM, Pollack AE, Koonin LM. Vasectomy in the United States, 1991 and 1995. *Am J Public Health.* 1999;89:92-94.
12. Kleppinger RK. Female outpatient sterilization using bipolar coagulation. *Bull Postgrad Comm Med Univ Syd.* 1977 Nov;33(8):144-154.
13. Soderstrom RM, Levy BS, Engel T. Reducing bipolar sterilization failures. *Obstet Gynecol.* 1989;74:60-63.
14. Fishburne JI Jr, Hulka JF. Tubal healing following laparoscopic electrocoagulation. *J Reprod Med.* 1976;16:129-134.
15. Rulin MC, Davidson AR, Philliber SG, et al. Changes in menstrual symptoms among sterilized and comparison women: a prospective study. *Obstet Gynecol.* 1989;74:149-154.
16. Shain RN, Miller WB, Mitchell GW, et al. Menstrual pattern change 1 year after sterilization: results of a controlled prospective study. *Fertil Steril.* 1989;52:192-203.
17. Wilcox LS, Chu SY, Eaker ED, et al. Risk factors for regret after tubal sterilization: 5 years of follow-up in a prospective study. *Fertil Steril.* 1991;55:27-33.
18. Jamieson DJ, Hillis SD, Duerr A, Marchbanks PA, Costello C, Peterson HB. Complications of interval laparoscopic tubal sterilization: findings from the United States Collaborative Review of Sterilization. *Obstet Gynecol.* 2000;96(6): 997-1002.
19. Moore CL, Vasquez NF, Lin H, Kaplan LJ. Major vascular injury after laparoscopic tubal ligation. *J Emerg Med.* 2005;29(1):67-71.
20. Vancaille TG, Anderson TL, Johns DA. A 12-month prospective evaluation of transcervical sterilization using implantable polymer matrices. *Obstet Gynecol.* 2008;112:1270-1277.
21. Levy B, Levie MD, Childers ME. A summary of reported pregnancies after hysteroscopic sterilization. *J Minim Invsive Gynecol.* 2007;14:271-274.
22. Connor VF. Essure: a review six years later. *J Minm Invasive Gynecol.* 2009; 16:282-290.

Case 8

A 35-year-old G2P2002 Hispanic woman presents to your office complaining of abdominal pain, nausea, and vomiting. Her abdominal pain has become progressively worse, and for the past 6 hours, she has had vomiting. She is postoperative day 3 from a right salpingo-oophorectomy for an 8-cm complex mass that was diagnosed as a mature teratoma on pathology. Some moderately dense adhesions of the omentum and small bowel were noted to be adherent to the mass and were dissected down. No complications were noted during the surgery, and the patient was discharged home the same day. Her past medical history is significant for pelvic inflammatory disease (PID) and two previous cesarean deliveries. Her vitals are temperature 101.4°F, pulse 110 beats/min, respiratory rate (RR) 22 breaths/min, and BP 120/70 mm Hg. On abdominal examination, the trocar sites are without erythema or induration and are well reapproximated. She has marked tenderness throughout the abdomen with rebound and guarding.

- ➤ What is the most likely diagnosis?
- ➤ What imaging modality is most helpful to confirm the diagnosis?
- ➤ What is the best treatment for this patient?

ANSWERS TO CASE 8: Laparoscopic Complications

Summary: A 35-year-old G2P2002 Hispanic woman presents with fever and abdominal pain with rebound tenderness. She is postoperative day 3 from a right salpingo-oophorectomy for an 8-cm complex mass. Some moderately dense adhesions of the omentum and small bowel were noted adherent to the mass and were dissected down.

- **Most likely diagnosis:** Peritonitis from bowel injury.
- **Most helpful imaging modality:** Abdominal and pelvic computed tomography (CT) with water-soluble contrast.
- **Best treatment for this patient:** The patient should receive broad-spectrum antibiotics that cover anaerobic and aerobic organisms. She should then undergo a laparotomy. Meticulous inspection of the bowel should be carried out. Further treatment should take into consideration the location of the injury (small bowel or the large bowel), the cause of the injury (thermal, laceration, puncture), the size of the injury, and presence of fecal contamination. She may need a simple closure of the bowel wall defect or a colostomy.

ANALYSIS

Objectives

1. List the different types of laparoscopic injuries.
2. Know techniques to prevent laparoscopic injuries.
3. Know the intra- and postoperative presentation of laparoscopic injuries.
4. Know techniques for the management of various injuries.

Considerations

This is a patient who underwent a difficult laparoscopy. The patient had multiple risk factors for complications from surgery such as prior PID and prior cesareans. The surgical findings noted omentum and small bowel adherent to the ovarian mass. The patient's surgery occurred 3 days previously, and now she presents with peritonitis. The most important goals in the approach to this patient are broad-spectrum antibiotics and expeditious exploratory laparotomy. Affected patients can become septic and hypotensive; intravenous fluid hydration and blood pressure support are important.

APPROACH TO
Laparoscopic Complications

DEFINITIONS

ENTEROTOMY: Full-thickness opening in the bowel wall where the lumen is entered.

URETEROURETEROSTOMY: Anastomosis of the two transected ends of the ureter.

URETERONEOCYSTOSTOMY WITH PSOAS HITCH: When the ureter is transected within 6 cm of the ureterovesical junction, this is the treatment of choice. The distal ureter segment is ligated. The bladder is mobilized and elongated toward the proximal injured ureter. The proximal ureter is anastomosed to the bladder. The bladder is attached to the psoas muscle to keep tension off the proximal ureter.

ILEAL INTERPOSITION: When a ureter injury takes place in the upper or middle third of the ureter and length for reanastomosis is lacking, the proximal ureter is anastomosed to a segment of ileum which in turn is anastomosed to the distal ureter.

URETEROILEONEOCYSTOSTOMY: When a ureter injury takes place in the upper or middle third of the ureter and the length for a tension-free reanastomosis is lacking, the proximal ureter is anastomosed to a segment of ileum which in turn is anastomosed to the bladder.

BOARI BLADDER FLAP: A flap of bladder wall shaped into a tube to replace a missing ureter segment.

TAMPON TEST: Helps to differentiate between a ureteral and bladder fistula. The patient wears the largest size tampon that is comfortable. She then takes oral Phenazopyridine HCl (Pyridium) and liquids for 30 minutes. Orange-stained urine on the tampon indicates a ureteral or a cephalad bladder fistula. A fresh tampon is then placed in the vagina, and 300 cc of methylene blue–stained sterile water is placed into the bladder via transurethral catheter. If there is no blue stain on the tampon, the fistula is from the ureter. An exception is a very small vesicular fistula.

CLINICAL APPROACH

Complications of laparoscopic surgery include injury to the gastrointestinal tract, vessels, urinary tract; related to the pneumoperitoneum; and incisional hernia. It is essential to recognize the injuries intraoperatively. The injury can occur during insertion of Veress needle or trocars, or at the time of the operative laparoscopy.[1] The management of the injury may include laparoscopic repair or laparotomy, depending on the level of surgeon comfort and expertise. Consultations with specialists in general surgery, urology, or vascular surgery may be invaluable.

Pneumoperitoneum

If the Veress needle fails to enter the peritoneal cavity and causes extraperitoneal insufflation, it may result in mediastinal emphysema and pneumothorax. If the gas from the extraperitoneal insufflation extends to the mediastinum, mediastinal emphysema will be seen. The anesthesiologist will have difficulty ventilating the patient. As much gas as possible should be released, and the patient should be carefully monitored. The patient may require assisted ventilation in severe cases. A pneumothorax can occur if the Veress needle is placed in the pleural cavity, and may be more likely if an upper abdomen site is chosen for insufflation. A penetrating injury into a blood vessel can cause a gas embolism. The anesthesiologist may note a "mill-wheel" murmur over the precordium. In this case, a central venous catheter can be placed in the right atrium or the superior vena cava and the CO_2 gas can be aspirated.[1]

Vascular Injuries

The insertion of the Veress needle or the trocar can cause trauma to the omental or mesenteric blood vessels and major abdominal or pelvic vessels. Small vessels in the omentum can be coagulated. Injury to the mesenteric vessels may compromise blood supply to the bowel, which may lead to bowel resection. Large vessels require immediate laparotomy, blood transfusion, and vascular repair.

The most common complication of laparoscopic surgery is the injury of the superficial or inferior epigastric vessels.[2] Laceration of these vessels is minimized by transillumination of the abdominal wall, directly visualizing the inferior epigastric vessels and inserting the trocar 6 to 7 cm lateral to the midline.[1] However, transillumination identifies the superficial epigastric artery only 64% of the time, and it is less helpful in patients with dark skin and body mass index (exceeding 25 kg/m^2).[2] The inferior epigastric is seen 80% of the time with transillumination.[4] Injury to these vessels can present with bleeding from the trocar site. Techniques that can help control the bleeding from these vessels include direct pressure, tamponade from the trocar, bipolar coagulation of the vessel, placing sutures cephalad and caudad to the sleeve, and compression with an inflated 12-Fr Foley catheter that is clamped to the skin.[2] If a hematoma forms, it should be evacuated, the incision explored, and the bleeding vessel ligated.[1]

Dixon and Carrillo studied a small series of pelvic vessel injuries that occurred from Veress needle and trocar placement. They reported that right-sided iliac vessel injuries were more common, and the right iliac vein was the most common site of injury.[5] This injury can be prevented by aiming the Veress needle and trocar toward the hollow of the sacrum with the patient's bed in the horizontal position. Large vessel injury may present with rapid pooling of blood in the operative field, welling of blood from the Veress needle or trocar, or with a hemodynamically unstable patient. If large vessel injury is suspected, the needle or trocar should be kept in place to help identify the site of the injury and immediate laparotomy should be performed. The injured area should be identified and compressed. The repair is based on the location of the injured vessel, whether it is arterial or venous, and the degree of the hemorrhage.

Bonjer and colleagues performed a retrospective comparison of open and closed laparoscopy. They reported rates of 0.075% of vascular injury with closed laparoscopy and 0% with open laparoscopy. Visceral injury rates were 0.083% and 0.048%, respectively.[6] Although this study found statistical significance between open and closed laparoscopy for rates of vascular and bowel injuries, a meta-analysis found that open laparoscopy was not superior or inferior to any other entry technique.[7]

Gastric Injuries

Injury to the gastrointestinal tract can involve the stomach, small bowel, or large bowel. The injury can be sharp or thermal. A gastric injury may occur during gynecologic surgery from distention of the stomach during a difficult intubation. This can be minimized by gastric decompression prior to entry. If gastric juices are aspirated after the placement of the Veress needle or if a gastric injury is suspected, the Veress needle should be removed. The stomach should be decompressed with a nasogastric tube, and the Veress needle should be replaced. Gastric injuries may be recognized after the placement of the periumbilical trocar. The surgeon may visualize gastric contents or the rugal folds of the stomach.[8] If the puncture is less than 5 mm in diameter and is hemostatic, the injury will usually resolve spontaneously. If the injury is larger, it may require a more extensive closure.[1]

Intestinal Injuries

A recent meta-analysis found that the incidence of bowel injuries to be 0.33% with major operative laparoscopy.[9] Women with previous abdominal surgeries and pelvic adhesions are at greatest risk.

Bowel perforation with the Veress needle is often undiagnosed because the perforation seals off spontaneously. If perforation is suspected, the needle is removed and replaced at another site. Once the laparoscope is in place, the bowel should be inspected carefully. Most needle injuries to the small bowel do not require a laparotomy, but should be monitored closely. A hemostatic serosal injury does not need to be repaired.[1]

Trocar injuries are usually larger and require repair. A bowel injury is suspected if the trocar obturator has fecal matter upon removal from the sleeve or if the bowel lumen is visualized via the laparoscope. If the trocar or the laparoscope creates an enterotomy, it should be left in place to decrease contamination and for identification of the injured site; a laparotomy should then be performed. A small enterotomy that occurs during the surgical procedure can be repaired laparoscopically. Colon injuries can be repaired laparoscopically if the patient has undergone a bowel preparation or if fecal spill is minimal. Copious irrigation and broad-spectrum antibiotics are essential in prevention of peritonitis. Depending on the site and nature of the injury, a colostomy may be necessary.[1]

A thermal bowel injury can result from direct contact of electrical, thermal, or laser energy. The area of tissue destruction is larger than the initial area of contact due to thermal spread. Unrecognized thermal injury can result in tissue necrosis and subsequent perforation up to 72 to 96 hours after the surgery. One should suspect thermal bowel injury in a patient who presents several days after operative laparoscopic surgery with fever and abdominal pain. Significant thermal bowel injury should be treated with wide resection and reanastomosis.[1]

Approximately 15% of bowel injuries are not recognized at the time of laparoscopy. Brosens and associates reported that one in five cases of delayed diagnosis of bowel injury resulted in death.[9]

Bladder Injuries

Bladder injury can take place with trocar insertion. Women with previous pelvic surgery are at highest risk. To avoid this complication, the bladder should be drained prior to initiating the surgical procedure. If the surgery is anticipated to take longer than 30 minutes, a catheter should be placed for continuous drainage. The size of the injury will determine the treatment. A Veress needle puncture can be managed expectantly. Lacerations less than 5 mm will resolve spontaneously with continuous bladder drainage for 4 to 5 days postoperatively. Larger injuries should be closed in two layers. The mucosa should be reapproximated with 2-0 chromic suture, and the detrusor muscle should be reapproximated with 2-0 polyglycolic acid suture. Care should be taken to avoid involvement of the ureteral orifices in the repair. The repair should be tension free with a good seal. A catheter should be placed in the bladder for continuous drainage for 5 to 7 days.[1]

Ureteral Injuries

Ureteral injuries occur less frequently than those involving the bladder. The best way to prevent ureteral injury is to identify the course of the ureter prior to clamping the pedicle.

Leonard and associates performed a review of ureteral injuries during total laparoscopic hysterectomies and found an incidence of 0.3% with all injuries occurring at the level of the uterine artery and the uterosacral ligament.[10] Laparoscopic ureteral injuries are more likely to result from thermal injuries. Furthermore, these injuries have a significant delay of diagnosis.[1] If patients present with flank pain, fever, retroperitoneal fluid collection, or ileus in the postoperative period, an injury to the ureter should be suspected. A creatinine elevation of 0.8 mg/dL may be related to a unilateral ureteral ligation. A CT scan will be most helpful at this time. It will provide information about the integrity and function of the renal collecting system while identifying urinomas and surrounding postoperative anatomy. If intrinsic renal damage is present and there is concern for the use of contrast medium, a renal and proximal ureter ultrasound can be performed. However, it has a 25% false-negative rate.[1] A retrograde stent, anterograde stent, or a percutaneous nephrostomy tube should be performed if an obstruction is noted and cannot be immediately relieved. If the obstruction is not relieved, permanent renal damage may result. If there is no ureteral obstruction but leakage of urine is noted, a ureteral stent should be placed. The best chance of healing after repair is when reoperation occurs within the first 48 hours. With increasing delay, more edema, necrosis, and tissue damage decrease the likelihood of a successful primary repair.

An intraoperative ureteral transection or ligation injury may be suspected if the ureter seems to enter a clamped or cut pedicle, a tubular structure is noted in a cut pedicle, there is lack of peristalsis from the ureter, and no urine output if both ureters are transected. If a ureteral injury is suspected intraoperatively, indigo carmine can be injected intravenously. A cystoscopy will show dye from the ureteral orifices after 5 minutes. If the ureteral injury is suspected immediately postoperatively, an intravenous pyelogram should be obtained. Up to 50% of cases of unilateral ureteral injury are asymptomatic postoperatively.[11] Patients may also present with urine leakage from the vagina, indicating that an undetected ureteral or bladder injury has caused a fistula. A fistula can be diagnosed with a tampon test.

If a ureteral injury does occur, the management is based on the location, mechanism of the injury,[4] and time of diagnosis. Repair of ureters is most often done via laparotomy. If the ureter is kinked by a ligature, simple dissection of the ureter away from the ligature is needed. In cases where the ureter is partially or completely ligated, the suture is removed and a stent is placed. If there is a question of ureteral viability, especially in cases of devascularization or thermal injury, the portion of concern must be resected. If a partial ureteral transection has taken place, a stent is introduced via the ureterotomy and the ureter is reapproximated over the stent with 5-0 polyglycolic acid suture. A closed suction drain should be placed at the base of the repair. If a complete transection has occurred in the upper or middle third of the ureter, a ureteroureterostomy over a stent is recommended. Care must be taken to ensure the repair is tension free and the ends are spatulated to increase the lumen size. If a transection of the ureter has occurred in the upper or middle third and the repair cannot be performed in a tension-free manner, a ureteroileal interposition or a ureteroileoneocystostomy is carried out. If a ureteral injury takes place within 6 cm of the ureterovesical junction, there is concern for vascular compromise of the distal portion of the ureter. The repair of choice in this situation is a ureteroneocystostomy with psoas hitch over a stent.

Trocar Hernia

Incisional hernia after laparoscopy is rare. With the use of bladed trocars, the incidence of hernia was found to be 0.23% at the 10-mm site and 3.1% at the 12-mm site.[12] The recommendation is to close the fascia at trocar sites 10 mm or larger. With the use of bladeless trocars, the incidence of hernia is 0% to 0.2% at the 10- and 12-mm sites, respectively. The lower rate of hernia is thought to result from a smaller residual defect after the bladeless trocars are removed.[13]

Comprehension Questions

8.1 A 34-year-old woman is undergoing a tubal sterilization procedure. Bipolar cautery is planned to be used to cauterize the isthmic portion of the tubes. Which of the following statements regarding this patient is most accurate?

A. In general unipolar cautery is safer than bipolar cautery in avoiding thermal injury.
B. A thermal injury to the bowel is usually not apparent immediately and takes several days to a week to manifest.
C. The most likely cause of death to this patient related to the surgery is hemorrhage.
D. The ampulla of the tube is a more appropriate location rather than the isthmic portion.

8.2 A 29-year-old woman has chronic pelvic pain that has been worsening over the past 6 months despite medical therapy. The patient has had a thorough work-up, and is being scheduled for a diagnostic laparoscopy. In consenting the patient for complications, the gynecologist explains that vascular injury can occur. Which of the following is the most common vessel to be injured in this procedure?

A. Deep (inferior) epigastric artery
B. Aorta
C. Vena cava
D. Common iliac artery
E. Internal iliac artery

8.3 A 29-year-old woman undergoes extensive lysis of adhesions and ablation of endometriosis via laparoscopy. Postoperatively, she has abdominal distention and some leakage of yellowish fluid from her incision site. The fluid is sent for analysis. Which of the following statements is most accurate regarding this patient's condition?

A. If the fluid has a sodium level of 140 mEq/L, it is likely to be urine.
B. If the fluid has a creatinine level of 0.8 mg/L, it is unlikely to be urinary in origin.
C. If the fluid has a pH of 7.40, it is likely to be urine.
D. If the fluid has a cloudy appearance, it is likely to be peritoneal fluid (ascites).

ANSWERS

8.1 **B.** Thermal injury often does not manifest itself until several days to a week after the initial surgery, due to the ischemia and necrosis that takes place. Bipolar is in general safer since the current passes from one paddle to another, whereas unipolar current can arc from the device to adjacent tissue. The most common cause of death due to female sterilization is anesthetic in nature. The isthmus of the tube is the most appropriate location for tubal ligation/occlusion.

8.2 **A.** In general, the deep epigastric artery is the most commonly injured vessel in laparoscopy that is associated with significant hemorrhage. This vessel is located between the rectus muscle and the parietal peritoneum of the anterior abdominal wall.

8.3 **B.** If the creatinine level is 0.8 mg/dL, it is unlikely to be urinary in origin, since the creatinine concentration is typically in the range of 40 to 50 mg/dL in the ureteral/bladder due to the concentrating ability of the kidneys. The sodium concentration is usually between 20 to 50 mEq/L. The pH varies and is not a good differentiating criterion.

Clinical Pearls

See Table 1-2 for definition of level of evidence and strength of recommendation

- Early detection of laparoscopic complication is the key to preventing patient morbidity and mortality (Level A).
- Fascia should be closed at trocar sites 5 mm or larger to prevent hernias (Level B).
- Repair of the ureter or bladder must be tension free for optimal healing (Level B).
- Thermal injuries may not be noted intraoperatively. Urinary and gastrointestinal tract injuries can present days later. An unrecognized bowel injury can present 72 to 96 hours from surgery (Level A).
- Although not consistent, some studies have noted decreased visceral and vascular complications with open laparoscopy compared to closed laparoscopy (Level B).

REFERENCES

1. Namnoum AB, Murphy AA. *Diagnostic and Operative Laparoscopy in TeLinde's Operative Gynecology*. 9th ed. Philadelphia, PA: Lippincott Williams & Wilkins; 2003.
2. Donnez J, Nisolle M. *An Atlas of Operative Laparoscopy and Hysteroscopy*. 2nd ed. New York, NY: The Parthenon Publishing Group Inc.; 2001.
3. Hurd WW, Amesse LS, Gruber JS, et al. Visualization of the epigastric vessels and bladder before laparoscopic trocar placement. *Fertil Steril*. 2003;80:209-212.
4. Stany MP, Farley JH. Complications of gynecologic surgery. *Surg Clin North Am*. 2008;88:343-359.
5. Dixon M, Carrillo EH. Iliac vascular injuries during elective laparoscopic surgery. *Surg Endosc*. 1999;13:1230-1233.
6. Bonjer HJ, Hazebroek, EJ, Kazemier G, et al. Open versus closed establishment of pneumoperitoneum in laparoscopic surgery. *Br J Surg*. 1997;84:599-602.
7. Vilos Ga, Ternamian A, Dempster J, et al. Laparoscopic entry: a review of techniques, technologies, and complications. *J Obstet Gynaecol Can*. 2007;29:434-465.
8. Mateus J, Pezzi C, Somkuti SG. Recognition and prevention of gastric injury during gynecologic laparoscopy. *Obstet Gyencol*. 2006;108:804-806.
9. Brosens I, Gordon A, Campo R, et al. Bowel injury in gynecologic laparoscopy. *J Am Assoc Gyencol Laparosc*. 2003;10:9-13.
10. Leonard F, Fotso A, Borghese B, et al. Ureteral complications from laparoscopic hysterectomy indicated for benign uterine pathologies: a 13-year experience in a continuous series of 1300 patients. *Hum Reprod*. 2007;22:2006-2011.
11. Nezhat FNC, Nezhat CR. Averting complications of laparoscopy: pearls from 5 patients. *OBG Management*. 2007;19:69.
12. Kadar N, Reich H, Liu CY, et al. Incisional hernias after major laparoscopic gynecologic procedures. *Am J Obstet Gynecol*. 1993;168:1493-1495.
13. Liu CD, McFadden DW. Laparoscopic port sites do not require fascial closure when nonbladed trocars are used. *Am Surg*. 2000;66:853-854.

Case 9

A 37-year-old G4P3013 woman presents to your office with menorrhagia and pelvic pain. The patient also has some feeling of incomplete emptying of her bladder. The patient has been seen by another gynecologist and placed on medical therapy, including nonsteroidal anti-inflammatory drugs (NSAIDs) and oral contraceptives without alleviation. She desires a permanent solution as future fertility is not an issue and would like to have a surgical technique that would allow her to resume her daily duties in a short period of time. She has a negative past surgical history. She is 5 ft 4 in in height and weighs 165 lb (75 kg). The abdominal examination reveals an irregular midline pelvic mass. She also has left uterosacral ligament tenderness without nodularity. Grade 1 uterine prolapse is noted.

➤ What is the clinical condition?

➤ What is your next step?

ANSWERS TO CASE 9: Total Laparoscopic Hysterectomy

Summary: This is a 37-year-old G4P3013 woman with menorrhagia and pelvic pain, which has failed medical therapy. Examination reveals a fibroid uterus of 16-week size just below the umbilicus and left uterosacral ligament tenderness without nodularity. Grade 1 prolapse is noted, and upon further questioning some urinary retention is mentioned.

- **Clinical condition:** Multiparous patient with symptomatic fibroids causing menorrhagia, and possible endometriosis and minimal prolapse.
- **Next step:** Office ultrasound of the pelvis. Then, outline the surgical options and explain the risks, benefits, and alternatives of the operation. Unfortunately, the symptoms of urinary retention are seldom volunteered by the patient seeking hysterectomy and should be ascertained by the physician during the history. The simple question is "Do you feel like you are completely emptying your bladder or do you feel that you still have to go after urinating?"

ANALYSIS

Objectives

1. Be familiar with what total laparoscopic hysterectomy (TLH) means.
2. Be familiar with a TLH technique.
3. Be familiar with complications of this operation.

Considerations

This is a 37-year-old G4P3013 woman who desires relief from menorrhagia and pelvic pain. Additionally, she would be grateful if she did not feel that she has to urinate immediately after doing so. The first step for the physician is to be able to provide proper counseling. It is important for the patient to understand that a laparoscopic approach is almost always possible. After surgical therapy is chosen, the route of surgery should be discussed. Vaginal hysterectomy (VH) is superior to the abdominal approach due to shorter hospital stay, quicker recovery, and less pain. When the VH is difficult due to lack of descensus, a laparoscopic approach is useful. Evidence-based medicine suggests that VH is the best method and should be performed when possible. Yet, VH is done in less than 20% of cases.

Most problems with VH can be solved by TLH, especially if we do the original version of TLH which includes vaginal cuff suspension by laparoscopic suturing!

Recent studies suggest that the incidence of pelvic organ prolapse (POP) surgery is high after all modes and routes of hysterectomy for benign indications. In a large study from Sweden, overall risk of subsequent prolapse surgery increased by 50% after TAH, doubled after subtotal hysterectomy, and quadrupled after vaginal hysterectomy.

Indications for TLH include whenever abdominal hysterectomy is considered and VH not possible or available, including limited vaginal access, large fibroid uterus, endometriosis, extensive adhesions, most endometrial cancer hysterectomies, and pelvic support procedures. Of course, LAVH is the wrong operation for cul-de-sac endometriosis. TLH should include vaginal cuff suspension from above usually by high McCall cuff suspension.

APPROACH TO Total Laparoscopic Hysterectomy

DEFINITIONS

Many physicians use the phrase "laparoscopic hysterectomy" as an umbrella term encompassing all types of laparoscopically associated surgical procedures in which the uterus is removed.

In reality, laparoscopic hysterectomy (LH) is a distinct procedure. Its sine qua non is laparoscopic ligation of the uterine arteries by means of electrosurgical desiccation or suture ligature. All the following maneuvers or methods of laparoscopic-associated hysterectomy (LAH) can be accomplished either vaginally or laparoscopically.

TOTAL LAPAROSCOPIC HYSTERECTOMY (TLH): TLH means laparoscopic dissection and ligation of all vascular pedicles continuing until the uterus lies free of all attachments in the peritoneal cavity. The uterus is removed through the vagina, often with laparoscopic and/or vaginal morcellation. The vagina is closed with laparoscopically placed suspension sutures. No vaginal surgery except for morcellation is done.

The surgical technique for TLH with a classification system for LAH was published in 1993 by Reich and colleagues, describing all LAHs performed from April 1983 to July 1992. The conclusion of that paper was that LH is a substitute for abdominal hysterectomy and not for vaginal hysterectomy. Laparoscopic vaginal cuff closure with incorporation of the uterosacral ligaments was an integral part of the TLH operation since its inception and still remains so.

LAPAROSCOPIC HYSTERECTOMY (LH): LH is the laparoscopic ligation of the blood supply to the uterus, including both uterine arteries either by electrosurgery desiccation, suture ligature, or staples. All surgical steps after the uterine vessels have been ligated can be done either vaginally or laparoscopically, including anterior and posterior vaginal entry, cardinal and uterosacral ligament division, uterine removal (intact or by morcellation), and vaginal closure (vertically or transversely). Laparoscopic ligation of the uterine vessels is the sine qua non for laparoscopic hysterectomy. Ureteral identification often by isolation, and more recently by cystoscopy, has always been advised.

LAPAROSCOPIC-ASSISTED VAGINAL HYSTERECTOMY (LAVH): LAVH is a vaginal hysterectomy after laparoscopic adhesiolysis, endometriosis excision, or oophorectomy.

This term is also used when the upper uterine ligaments (eg, round, infundibulopelvic or utero-ovarian ligaments) of a relatively normal uterus are ligated with staples or bipolar desiccation before vaginal hysterectomy. Most of these cases can be done without the laparoscope as completely vaginal hysterectomies.

CLINICAL APPROACH

While it is important that these different procedures are clearly delineated, some overlap is present, especially between LAVH and LH (LAVH is more vaginal hysterectomy) and between LH and TLH with cuff suspension. We need to make clear what we mean.

What is a TLH? Today, much unwarranted confusion exists. After 20 years there is finally a CPT code for billing this procedure. This coding further confuses the issue making one wonder where it came from, certainly not from the experts doing this operation.

58570 Laparoscopy, surgical, with total hysterectomy, for uterus 250 g or less

58571 Laparoscopy, surgical, with total hysterectomy, for uterus 250 g or less; with removal of tube(s) and/or ovary(ies)

58572 Laparoscopy, surgical, with total hysterectomy, for uterus greater than 250 g

58573 Laparoscopy, surgical, with total hysterectomy, for uterus greater than 250 g; with removal of tube(s) and/or ovary(ies)

Although it is not noted in the literature, there seems to be significant difference between closing the vagina vaginally, closing the vagina laparoscopically, and closing the vagina and its supportive ligaments laparoscopically. Seemingly, small differences in technique may lead to substantial differences in outcome, and are not usually included in the nomenclature.

For instance, during a vaginal hysterectomy, we know that tagging the uterosacral-cardinal complex vaginally helps in its identification for vaginal cuff repair, and affixing the uterosacral ligaments to the vaginal cuff helps to ensure its secure suspension. However, if the ligaments are divided laparoscopically and the vagina closed vaginally, it is much more difficult to identify these ligaments and incorporate them into the repair. Likewise, suturing just the vagina closed laparoscopically, often with expensive disposable devices, does little for support. These nuances may certainly lead to an increased risk of vaginal vault prolapsed.

Since the first LH in January 1988, the vast majority of surgeons have been slow to embrace this alternative to the costlier abdominal hysterectomy and LAVH, often citing concerns about patient selection as the primary reason. There are few absolute contraindications specific to LH. The procedure shouldn't be performed when vaginal hysterectomy can be accomplished with little vaginal repair necessary. Also, the LH should not be performed when the patient has a potentially cancerous pelvic mass too large to fit intact into an impermeable sack. Stage III ovarian cancer, which requires a large abdominal incision, is another contraindication, as is a surgeon's inexperience. But uterine weight and size, degree of endometriosis, and similar factors should not preclude a skilled surgeon from choosing LH.

Perhaps the greatest advantage TLH offers is the surgeon's ability to obtain better support for the vagina and to suture stretched ligaments to the top of the vagina at a point far higher than would be possible with other types of hysterectomy.

Total Laparoscopic Hysterectomy Technique

There are various techniques to this procedure, and the following is one such rendition. These steps are designed to prevent complications.

Since hysterectomy is usually an elective procedure, the patient should be counseled extensively regarding the range of currently available options appropriate to her individual clinical situation. In 2010, it is clearly not acceptable to advocate hysterectomy without detailing the risks and benefits of other intermediary procedures, such as myomectomy and/or excision of endometriosis with uterine preservation.

Whereas conversion to laparotomy when the surgeon becomes uncomfortable with the laparoscopic approach has never been considered a complication, conversion rates should be monitored to ensure that the patient has reasonable expectations. For instance, when half of attempted laparoscopic hysterectomies are converted to abdominal procedures, neither the patient nor the surgeon is well served.

Preoperative Preparation The patient's coexisting medical problems should be best optimized. Patients are encouraged to hydrate on clear liquids the day before surgery. Fleet Phospho-soda 3 oz divided into two doses are given at 3:30 pm and 7:30 pm to evacuate the lower bowel. If the patient is prone to nausea, promethazine (Phenergan) 25 mg orally is taken 25 minutes before the bowel preparation. Lower abdominal, pubic, and perineal hair is not shaved.

All laparoscopic procedures are performed using general endotracheal anesthesia with orogastric tube suction to minimize bowel distension. The patient's arms are placed at her side and shoulder braces at the acromioclavicular joint are positioned. Trendelenburg position up to 40 degrees is available. I use one dose of prophylactic antibiotics optimally 30 to 60 minutes prior to incision.

Incisions Three laparoscopic puncture sites including the umbilicus are used. Pneumoperitoneum 25 to 30 mm Hg is obtained before primary umbilical trocar insertion and reduced to 15 mm afterward. The lower quadrant trocar sleeves are placed under direct laparoscopic vision lateral to the rectus abdominis muscles and just beside the anterior superior iliac spines in patients with large fibroids. The left lower quadrant puncture is my major portal for operative manipulation as I stand on the patient's left.

Sometimes, however, special entry techniques are necessary. When a patient has had numerous prior abdominal surgical procedures, may have adhesions around the umbilicus, or is extremely overweight, I insert the Veress needle in the left ninth intercostal space and the trocar at the left subcostal margin. I do this because in such a patient the peritoneum often is stuck to the undersurface of the ribs and can't tent away from the Veress needle. The stomach must be decompressed with this entry location.

Reduction in wound morbidity and scar integrity as well as cosmesis is enhanced using 5-mm sites. The use of 12-mm incisions when a 5-mm one will suffice is not an advance in minimally invasive surgery.

Vaginal Preparation Every year, new innovations for uterine and vaginal manipulation appear. The Valtchev uterine manipulator (Conkin Surgical Instruments, Toronto, Canada) has been around for more than 20 years and allows anterior, posterior, and lateral manipulation of the uterus so that the surgeon can visualize the posterior cervix and vagina. Although newer devices are currently available that have been developed by Pelosi, Wattiez, Hourcabie, Koninckx, Koh, McCartney, Donnez, and Reich, I still use the Valtchev and the Wolf tube.

Exploration The upper abdomen is inspected, and the appendix is identified. Clear vision is maintained throughout the operation using the I.C. Medical smoke evacuator (Phoenix, Arizona). Endometriosis is excised before starting TLH. Bleeding is controlled with microbipolar forceps.

Retroperitoneal Dissection The peritoneum is opened early with scissors in front of the round ligament to allow CO_2 from the pneumoperitoneum to distend the retroperitoneum. The tip of the laparoscope is then used to perform "optical dissection" of the retroperitoneal space by pushing it into the loosely distended areolar tissue parallel to the uterus to identify the uterine vessels, ureter, or both. The uterine artery is often ligated at this time, especially in large uterus patients.

Ureteral Dissection (Optional) The ureter is identified medially, superiorly, or laterally (pararectal space). Stents are not generally used as they may cause hematuria and ureteric spasm. The laparoscopic surgeon should dissect (skeletonize) either the ureter or the uterine vessels during the performance of a laparoscopic hysterectomy.

Bladder Mobilization The round ligaments are divided at their midportion, and scissors or a spoon electrode is used to divide the vesicouterine peritoneal fold starting at the left side and continuing across the midline to the right round ligament. The upper junction of the vesicouterine fold is identified as a white line firmly attached to the uterus, with 2 to 3 cm between it and the bladder dome. The initial incision is made below the white line while lifting the bladder. The bladder is mobilized off the uterus and upper vagina using scissors or blunt dissection until the anterior vagina is identified. The tendinous attachments of the bladder in this area may be desiccated or dissected (Figures 9–1 to 9–4).

Upper Uterine Blood Supply When oophorectomy is indicated or desired, the peritoneum is opened on each side of the infundibulopelvic ligament with scissors and a 2-0-Polyglycolic acid (Vicryl) free ligature is passed through the window and created and tied extracorporeally using the Clarke-Reich (Cook Medical Group, Bloomington, IN) knot pusher. This maneuver is repeated until two proximal and one distal ties are placed and the ligament divided. This maneuver helps develop suturing skills. The broad ligament is divided to the round ligament just lateral to the utero-ovarian artery anastomosis using scissors or cutting current through a spoon electrode. I rarely desiccate the infundibulopelvic ligament as it results in too much smoke early in the operation.

When ovarian preservation is desired, the utero-ovarian ligament and fallopian tube are compressed and coagulated until desiccated with bipolar forceps, at 25 to 35 W cutting current, and then divided. Alternatively, the

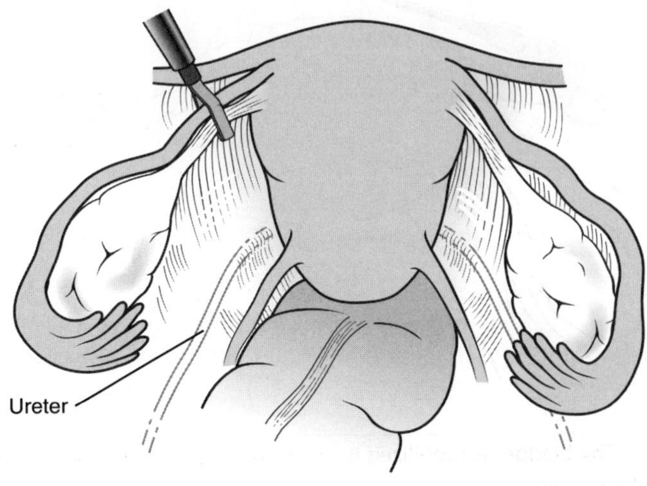

Figure 9–1. Atraumatic graspers are used to elevate the left tube and ovary to help identify the left ureter.

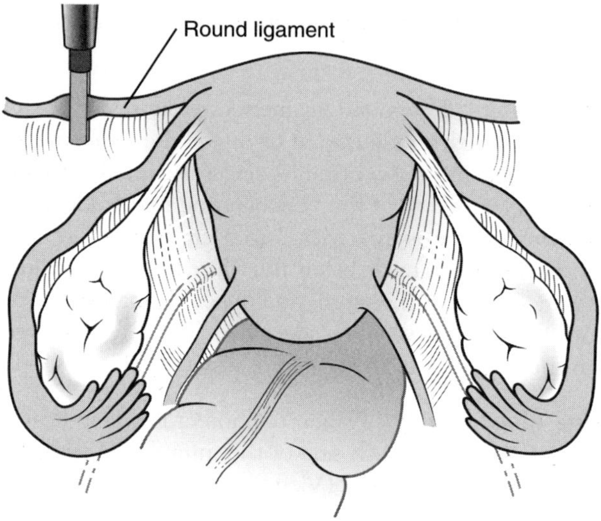

Figure 9–2. The left round ligament is cauterized using bipolar electrocautery, after which it will be divided."

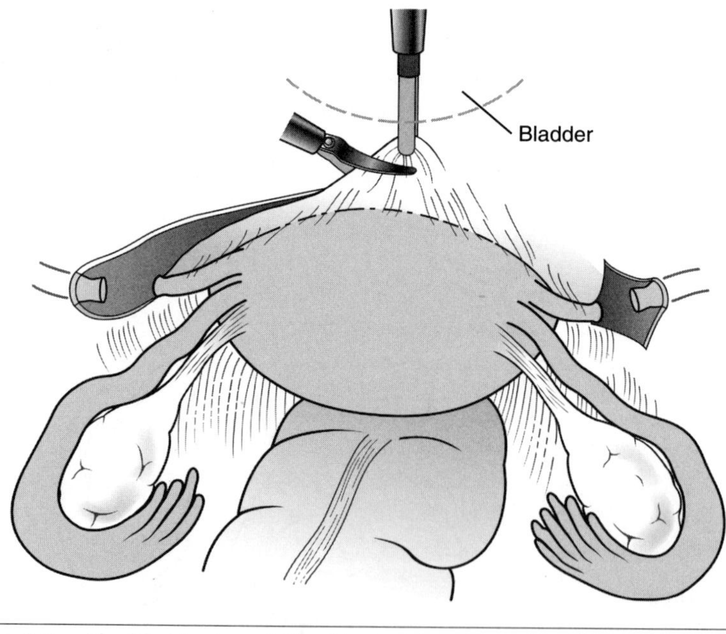

Figure 9–3. The bladder is mobilized by incising the vesicouterine peritoneal fold using unipolar scissors.

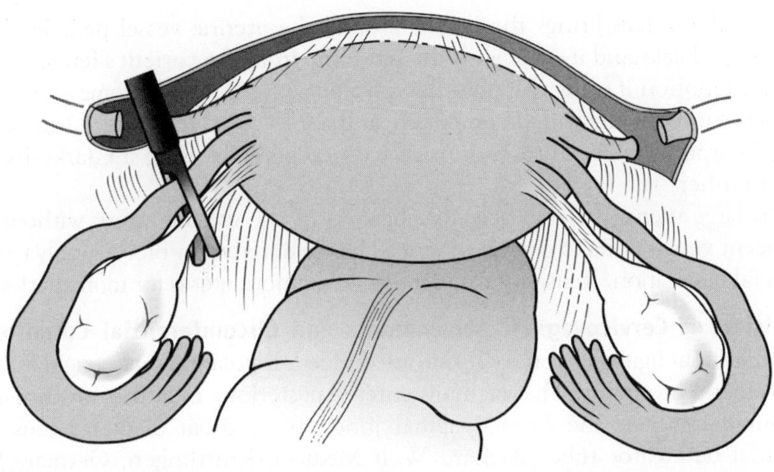

Figure 9–4. The utero-ovarian ligament is ligated and divided. This can be accomplished in a number of different ways such as with bipolar cautery, endoscopic stapler, or harmonic scalpel.

utero-ovarian ligament and fallopian tube pedicles are suture-ligated adjacent to the uterus with 2/0-Vicryl, using a free ligature that is passed through a window that is created, enabling the ligature to be positioned around the ligament. Stapling devices are rarely used.

If the ovary is to be preserved and the uterus is large, the utero-ovarian ligament/round ligament/fallopian tube junction may be divided with a 30- or 45-mm gastrointestinal anastomosis (GIA)-type stapler. This may be time saving for this portion of the procedure, thus justifying its increased cost.

The use of staplers may decrease operative time, but can increase the risk for postoperative hemorrhage and injury to the ureter. Ligation or coagulation of the vascular pedicles generally is safer.

Uterine Vessel Ligation The uterine vessels may be ligated at their origin, at the site where they cross the ureter, where they join the uterus, or on the side of the uterus (see Figure 9–1). Most surgeons use bipolar desiccation to ligate these vessels, but in our center, we prefer suture because it can be removed if ureteral compromise is suggested at cystoscopy.

In most cases, the uterine vessels are suture-ligated as they ascend the sides of the uterus. The broad ligament is skeletonized to the uterine vessels. Each uterine vessel pedicle is suture-ligated with 0-Vicryl on a CTB-1 blunt needle (Ethicon JB260, Ethicon Inc, Somerville, NJ) (27 in), as a blunt needle reduces surrounding venous bleeding. The needles are introduced into the peritoneal cavity by pulling them through a 5-mm incision. A short, rotary movement of the needle holder brings the needle around the uterine vessel pedicle. This motion is backhand if done with the left hand from the patient's left side and forward motion if using the right hand from the right side. In some cases, the vessels can be skeletonized completely and a 2-0-Vicryl free suture ligature is passed around them. Sutures are tied extracorporeally using a Clarke-Reich knot pusher.

In large uterus patients, selective ligation of the uterine artery without its adjacent vein is done to give the uterus a chance to return its blood supply to the general circulation. It also results in a less voluminous uterus for morcellation.

Division of Cervicovaginal Attachments and Circumferential Culdotomy The cardinal ligaments on each side are divided. Bipolar forceps coagulate the uterosacral ligaments. The vagina is entered posteriorly over the uterovaginal manipulator near the cervicovaginal junction. A 4-cm diameter reusable vaginal delineator tube (Richard Wolf Medical, Knittlingen, Germany) is placed in the vagina to prevent loss of pneumoperitoneum and to outline the cervicovaginal junction circumferentially as it is incised using the CO_2 laser to complete the circumferential culdotomy with the delineator as a backstop. The uterus is morcellated, if necessary, and pulled out of the vagina.

Morcellation (Laparoscopic and Vaginal) Morcellation can be done laparoscopically or vaginally. Vaginal morcellation is done with a no. 10 blade on a long knife handle to make a circumferential incision into the uterus while pulling outward on the cervix and using the cervix as a fulcrum. The myometrium is incised circumferentially parallel to the axis of the uterine cavity with the scalpel's tip always inside the myomatous tissue and pointed centrally, away from the surrounding vagina.

Morcellation through anterior abdominal wall sites is done when vaginal access is limited or supracervical hysterectomy requested. Reusable electromechanical morcellators are motorized circular saws. Using claw forceps or a tenaculum to grasp the fibroid and pull it into contact with the fibroid, large pieces of myomatous tissue are removed piecemeal until the myoma can be pulled out through the trocar incision. With practice, this instrument can often be inserted through a stretched 5-mm incision without an accompanying trocar. The new Sawalhe II Supercut Morcellator (Karl Storz, Tuttlingen, Germany) comes with 12-, 15-, and 20-mm diameter circular saws.

Laparoscopic Vaginal Vault Closure and Suspension With McCall Culdoplasty The vaginal delineator tube is placed back into the vagina for closure of the vaginal cuff, occluding it to maintain pneumoperitoneum. The uterosacral ligaments are identified by bipolar desiccation markings or with the aid of a rectal probe. The first suture is complicated as it brings the uterosacral and cardinal ligaments as well as the rectovaginal fascia together. This single suture is tied extracorporeally, bringing the uterosacral ligaments, cardinal ligaments, and posterior vaginal fascia together across the midline. It provides excellent support to the vaginal cuff apex, elevating it and its endopelvic fascia superiorly and posteriorly toward the hollow of the sacrum. The rest of the vagina and overlying pubocervicovesicular fascia are closed vertically with one or two 0-Vicryl interrupted sutures.

If a high cystocele is present causing urinary retention, two or more additional sutures can be placed as follows: The second suture is placed through the uterosacral ligaments closer to the sacrum and then through the endopelvic fascia just above the uterine vessel pedicle. The third suture is placed through the uterosacral ligaments even closer to the sacrum and through the endopelvic fascia well above the cardinal ligament, resulting in a vertical vaginal closure. The last suture is usually placed into the anterior vagina/pubocervicovesicular fascia above the cuff at 12 o'clock to bring the anterior vagina much higher than the posterior wall. All sutures after the first are nonabsorbable synthetic polyester suture (0-Ethibond). The last suture also is placed at the highest level toward the sacral area. As with any suspension, special care must be taken to ensure the integrity of the rectum and ureters. The sutures must not constrict the rectum, which is identified throughout the procedure with a rectal probe inside it. This suspension achieves a physiologic position of the vagina. In addition, it provides the vagina with good depth since the vagina can go high toward the sacral region where the uterosacrals ligaments originate. The closure of the vagina in a vertical fashion avoids the ureters as the sutures stay in the midline.

Cystoscopy Cystoscopy is done after vaginal closure to check for ureteral patency in most cases, after intravenous administration of indigo carmine dye. This is necessary when the ureter is identified but not dissected and especially necessary when the ureter has not been identified. Blue dye should be visualized through both ureteral orifices. The bladder wall should also be inspected for suture and thermal defects.

Underwater Examination At the close of each operation, an underwater examination is used to detect bleeding from vessels and viscera tamponaded during the procedure by the increased intraperitoneal pressure of the CO_2 pneumoperitoneum. The CO_2 pneumoperitoneum is displaced with 2 to 4 L of Ringer lactate solution, and the peritoneal cavity is vigorously irrigated and suctioned until the effluent is clear of blood products. Any further bleeding is controlled underwater using microbipolar forceps to coagulate through the electrolyte solution, and 2 L of lactated Ringer solution are left in the peritoneal cavity.

Skin Closure The vertical intraumbilical incision is closed with a single 4-0 Vicryl suture opposing deep fascia and skin dermis, with the knot buried beneath the fascia. This will prevent the suture from acting like a wick, transmitting bacteria into the soft tissue or peritoneal cavity. The lower quadrant 5-mm incisions are loosely approximated with a Javid vascular clamp (V. Mueller, McGaw Park, Illinois) and covered with Collodion (AMEND, Irvington, New Jersey) to allow drainage of excess Ringer lactate solution.

Endometriosis Hysterectomy with excision of all visible endometriosis usually results in relief of the patient's pain. Oophorectomy may not be necessary at hysterectomy for advanced endometriosis if the endometriosis is removed carefully.

Endometriosis nodules in the muscularis of the anterior rectum can usually be excised laparoscopically without entering the rectum. Full-thickness penetration of the rectum can occur during hysterectomy surgery, especially when excising rectal endometriosis nodules. Following identification of the nodule or rent in the rectum, a closed circular stapler (Proximate ILS Curved Intraluminal Stapler [Ethicon, Stealth] Ethicon Inc, Somerville, NJ) is inserted into the lumen just past the lesion or hole, opened 1 to 2 cm, and held high to avoid the posterior rectal wall. The proximal anvil is positioned just beyond the lesion or hole, which is invaginated into the opening, and the device closed. The instrument is fired and removed.

Complications

Complications of laparoscopic hysterectomy are those of hysterectomy and laparoscopy combined: anesthetic accidents; respiratory compromise; thromboembolic phenomenon; urinary retention; injury to vessels, ureters, bladder, and bowel; as well as infections, especially of the vaginal cuff. Ureteral injury is more common when staplers or bipolar desiccation are used without ureteral identification. Complications unique to laparoscopy include large vessel injury, epigastric vessel laceration, subcutaneous emphysema, and trocar site incisional hernias.

Infection Experience with serious wound infection after laparoscopic hysterectomy is rare. Morcellation during laparoscopic or vaginal hysterectomy results in a slightly increased risk of fever, especially if prophylactic antibiotics are not used.

Hemorrhage Intraoperative hemorrhage occurs when a previously nonanemic patient loses greater than 1000 mL of blood or requires a blood transfusion. By doing careful laparoscopic dissection, most profuse hemorrhage situations are avoided or controlled as they occur.

Ureter Complications I remain committed to prevention of ureteral injury intraoperatively by ureteral identification often with dissection and by cystoscopy at the conclusion of hysterectomies.

The ureters are commonly injured at the level of the infundibulopelvic ligament, uterosacral ligament, or pelvic sidewall due to adhesions resulting from endometriosis, pelvic inflammatory disease, or previous abdominal surgery. During laparoscopic hysterectomy, ureteral injury may occur while cutting dense adhesions and fibrotic scar tissue, trying to stop bleeding close to the ureter with bipolar cautery, or in the process of ligating the uterine vessels with bipolar electrosurgery, staples, or suture.

Most ureteral injuries are not identified or even suspected without cystoscopy. The bottom line is that an aggressive approach to ureteral protection can reduce but not eliminate ureteral injury. However, prompt recognition and management can prevent multiple surgical procedures and significant patient morbidity, including organ loss.

Urinary retention is a common undetected complication. More studies are necessary to determine how common and whether long-term compromise can occur.

Bladder Injury Bladder injury can occur during dissection of the bladder off the uterus and cervix or from an inflamed adnexa. In these cases the bladder is repaired using 3-0 Vicryl usually in two layers, with prolonged bladder drainage.

Bowel Injury Small bowel injury during laparoscopic hysterectomy is uncommon and is usually associated with extensive intraperitoneal adhesions. Small bowel injuries can be suture-repaired. Small bowel enterotomy may require mobilization from above, delivery through the umbilicus by extending the incision 1 cm, and repair or resection. If the hole is confined to the antimesenteric portion, the bowel can be closed with interrupted 3-0 silk or Vicryl. All enterotomies are suture-repaired transversely to reduce the risk of stricture. If the hole involves greater than 50% of the bowel circumference, resection is done. An extracorporeal segmental enterectomy with side-to-side stapled anastomosis is preferred.

Rectal injury may occur during rectal endometriosis excision or during vaginal morcellation of a large fibroid uterus. Repair is with a circular stapler.

Long-Term Complications

Bowel obstruction from adhesions: Among benign gynecologic operations, TAH was the most common cause of small bowel obstruction. The median interval between TAH and obstruction was 4 years. The adhesions were adherent to the previous laparotomy incision in 75% and to the vaginal vault in 25%. Obstruction did not occur after laparoscopic supracervical hysterectomy. TAH incisions may result in adhesions and bowel obstruction many years later.

Pelvic pain: Adhesions, adnexal remnants, and endometriosis may cause chronic pelvic pain after hysterectomy.

ADDITIONAL COMMENTS

It took 5 years for laparoscopic cholecystectomy to be universally adopted! Laparoscopic hysterectomy has been available for the last 20 years with sporadic acceptance. The low level of reimbursement has curbed the enthusiasm for training in minimally invasive surgery in our specialty in the United States. Practitioners faced with shrinking reimbursement and rising costs must spend more time in the office and less in surgery.

Abdominal hysterectomy is the preferred method of treatment based on training and economics, and this poses an ethical dilemma. Are we offering the best choices to our patients? We as specialists need to answer this question. Why would physicians take time to learn a new technique if they are going to be poorly reimbursed?

Because the reimbursement of hysterectomy is so low, there is a natural disincentive to putting forth the effort in learning new techniques. These are important issues that must be addressed.

Laparoscopic hysterectomy is clearly beneficial for patients in whom vaginal surgery is contraindicated or can't be done. When indications for the vaginal approach are equivocal, laparoscopy can be used to determine if vaginal hysterectomy is possible. With this philosophy, patients avoid an abdominal incision with resultant decrease in length of hospital stay and recuperation time. The laparoscopic surgeon should be aware of the risks and how to minimize them and, when they occur, how to repair them laparoscopically.

A randomized trial comparing TLH to TAH may not be possible, unless the patients have no real concern about the cosmetics of incision size. If the patient has a preference, it may take a long time to explain why the trial is needed and why randomization is ethical. Recruitment to trials is very difficult when minimally invasive therapy is an available option.

I do not pretend to understand studies comparing TLH and VH as they have different indications. TLH is a substitute for TAH, not for VH. And, as discussed, there are many different variations of TLH that may give the wrong conclusions. Presently, the studies show that if the surgeon can do a VH, it is the best possible operation. That is, unless future studies prove this wrong.

I don't think vaginal hysterectomy is better than laparoscopic hysterectomy. Vaginal and abdominal surgery will never be as precise as laparoscopic surgery. In the latter, the surgeon is right on top of the tissue with a scope and can focus it for magnification. You can see better with a laparoscope in the peritoneal cavity than with an operating room light directed toward the proximal vagina. I think we should work on removing the technical barriers to successfully accomplishing laparoscopic hysterectomy in a majority of patients. Because TLH mimics abdominal hysterectomy in almost all respects, it should be easier to assimilate its practice for the majority of patients.

LAVH practitioners add the potential complications of laparoscopic surgery to those of vaginal surgery; that is why it seems as though there are more complications with laparoscopy. In actuality, ureteral and bladder injuries occur more often during the vaginal part of the LAVH. Peripheral nerve injuries occur secondary to stirrup changes going from above to below.

If they are recognized, most complications of laparoscopic hysterectomy can be corrected by laparoscopic surgery. Check the bladder and ureters by including cystoscopy in the procedure. Check the rectum and rectosigmoid by filling them with blue dye underwater. Check for bleeding by looking underwater at low pressure while irrigating.

Remember that laparoscopic hysterectomy used to be a substitute for abdominal hysterectomy but not for vaginal hysterectomy. In the future, the possibilities of better pelvic support from above may make TLH the best choice.

Comprehension Questions

9.1 A 43-year-old woman is counseled by her gynecologist regarding the need for hysterectomy due to significant menorrhagia that has not responded to medical therapy. A TLH is recommended. Which of the following is the best situation for a TLH?

A. 4-week-size uterus with second-degree descensus
B. 6-week-size uterus with first-degree prolapse
C. 16-week-size uterus that is irregular
D. 12-cm adnexal mass

9.2 A 28-year-old woman undergoes an LAVH. The surgeon is concerned about whether the right ureter was possibly ligated, although on laparoscopy it appears to be close but not included in the staple ligature. Which of the following is the best next step?

A. Surgical dissection of the ureter
B. Deligation of the stapling
C. Intravenous pyelogram
D. Cystoscopy

9.3 A 37-year-old woman is undergoing laparoscopic hysterectomy. The surgeon is attempting to dissect the bladder away from the uterus. Which of the following is the appropriate surgical technique on where to make the incision of the vesicouterine peritoneum?

A. Above the white line
B. At the white line
C. Below the white line

ANSWERS

9.1 **C.** Since TLH is most appropriate for patients who would undergo abdominal hysterectomy, the patient with a 16-week-size uterus is most appropriate for this procedure.

9.2 **D.** Cystoscopy is the best modality to ensure normal function of the ureter. Typically, the use of indigo carmine intravenously allows visualization of the ureteric orifices of the bladder.

9.3 **C.** The correct location is to incise below the white line where the vesicouterine peritoneum is adherent to the uterus.

Clinical Pearls

See Table 1-2 for definition of level of evidence and strength of recommendation

- TLH should be considered to be a substitute for abdominal hysterectomy, not vaginal hysterectomy (Level C).
- Uterine vessels may be ligated by bipolar cautery, but suture ligation has the advantage that it can be removed if ureteral kinking is suspected (Level B).
- An aggressive approach to ureteral protection can reduce but not eliminate ureteral injury; however, prompt recognition and management can prevent multiple surgical procedures and significant patient morbidity, including organ loss (Level B).
- For patients who may have adhesions around the umbilicus due to prior abdominal surgery, an entry in the left midclavicular line in the subcostal region may be advantageous. The stomach must be decompressed (Level C).

REFERENCES

1. Altman D, Falconer C, Cnattingius S, et al. Pelvic organ prolapse (POP) surgery following hysterectomy on benign indications. Karolinska. *Am J Obstet Gynecol.* 2008;198:572.e1.
2. Al-Sunaidi M, Tulandi T. Adhesion-related bowel obstruction after hysterectomy for benign conditions. *Obstet Gynecol.* 2006;108(5):1162-1166.
3. Clayton RD. Hysterectomy: best practice and research. *Clin Obstet Gynecol.* 2006;20:1-15.
4. Johnson N, Barlow D, Lethaby A, et al. Surgical approach to hysterectomy for benign gynaecological disease. *Cochrane Database Syst Rev.* 2005;(1):CD003677.
5. Johnson N, Barlow D, Lethaby A. Methods of hysterectomy: systematic review and meta-analysis of randomized controlled trials. *BMJ.* 2005;330:1478-1481.

6. Reich H, DeCaprio J, McGlynn F. Laparoscopic hysterectomy. *J Gynecol Surg.* 1989;5:213-216.
7. Reich H, McGlynn F, Sekel, L. Total laparoscopic hysterectomy. *Gynaecol Endosc.* 1993;2:59-63.
8. Reich H. Laparoscopic hysterectomy. *Surgical Laparoscopy & Endoscopy*. New York, NY: Raven Press; 1992;2:85-88.
9. Reich H, Roberts L. Laparoscopic hysterectomy in current gynecological practice. *Rev Gynaecol Pract.* 2003;3:32-40 .
10. Reich H, Clarke HC, Sekel L. A simple method for ligating in operative laparoscopy with straight and curved needles. *Obstet Gynecol.* 1992;79:143-147.
11. Ribeiro S, Reich H, Rosenberg J. The value of intra-operative cystoscopy at the time of laparoscopic hysterectomy. *Hum Reprod.* 1999;14:1727-1729.
12. Reich H. Letters to the editor. Ureteral injuries after laparoscopic hysterectomy. *Human Reprod.* 2000;15:733-734.

Case 10

A 45-year-old G3P3003 woman presents to your office complaining of right lower quadrant pain occurring over the last 6 months which seemed to have increased in intensity during the last 30 days. She is afebrile and her vital signs are stable. She is not in acute distress but presents with tenderness to deep palpation over the right lower abdomen. On pelvic examination, her uterus is non-tender, but has a painful mass of approximately 5 × 6 cm in the right adnexa. Vaginal ultrasound reveals an enlarged right ovary measuring 7 × 7 × 8 cm containing a 5.0 × 5.4 × 1-cm cyst which has diffuse internal echoes with possible calcifications. Cervical cytology is benign and cultures are negative. Cancer antigen (CA) 125 was 41 U/mL. Her past surgical history is significant for three vaginal deliveries and tubal sterilization. She is interested in laparoscopic surgery if possible.

- What is the clinical condition?
- What is your next step?

ANSWERS TO CASE 10: Laparoscopic Surgery of an Adnexal Mass

Summary: This is a 45-year-old G3P3003 woman with a painful right adnexal mass desiring laparoscopic surgery if intervention is indicated.

- **Clinical condition:** Multiparous patient with a painful complex adnexal mass.
- **Next step:** Outline the surgical options and explain the risks, benefits, and alternatives of the operation.

ANALYSIS

Objectives

1. Be familiar with the workup of an adnexal mass.
2. Be familiar with different methods of surgical management of adnexal mass, including risks and benefits.
3. Be familiar with the proper patient selection for laparoscopic management of an adnexal mass.

Considerations

This 45-year-old patient has a tender 5-cm complex adnexal mass. The CA-125 tumor marker is somewhat elevated. The differential diagnosis of the adnexal mass in this patient is an endometrioma, or a serous or mucinous cystadenoma, or less likely cystadenocarcinoma. A germ cell tumor is also a possibility, but less likely due to the patient's age. A functional cyst such as a corpus luteal cyst is possible, but less likely due to the 6-month nature of her symptoms. Due to the patient's symptoms, as well as importance of assessing whether this adnexal mass is a neoplastic process, surgery should be recommended to the patient. The patient should be informed about the various surgical approaches, and the benefits of laparoscopy—outpatient setting, easier recovery time, and cosmetic ramifactions.

APPROACH TO Laparoscopic Surgery of an Adnexal Mass

DEFINITIONS

RISK OF MALIGNANCY INDEX (RMI): Use of menopausal status, CA-125, and ultrasound characteristics to determine the likelihood of an adnexal mass being malignant.

GERM CELL TUMOR MARKERS: The serum lactate dehydrogenase (LDH), α-fetoprotein (AFP), and human chorionic gonadotropin (hCG) levels are elevated with germ cell tumors.

EPITHELIAL TUMOR MARKERS: The serum CA-125, serum carcinoembryonic antigen (CEA), and CA-19-9 are the tumor markers which can be elevated with epithelial neoplasms.

CLINICAL APPROACH

The management of an adnexal mass provides unique challenges to the treating physician; the decision making is based on the characteristics of the mass, age, and expectations of the patient. The almost universal availability of the Internet provides vast medical information to our patients, including articles about the etiology and also treatment of a particular condition. Laparoscopic treatment is an appealing option due to its shorter hospitalization, less discomfort, faster return to normal activity, and superior cosmetic results.[1-4] In addition, laparoscopic management of adnexal mass is a cost-effective surgical option associated with decreased indirect and also direct costs. However, all these benefits should not compromise the clinical outcome in women with ovarian malignancy. Proper patient selection and planning is very important in considering a laparoscopic approach. It is argued that the puncture or spillage of the contents of a malignant mass can compromise the survival of the patient. It definitely worsens the staging and has the potential of diffuse intra-abdominal dissemination with the CO_2 gas. However, a multivariate analysis, and a retrospective study, on stage I ovarian epithelial cancers did not show an impact on survival when intraoperative spillage occurred in properly staged patients. It seems that patients with preoperative rupture or positive washings have a worst prognosis than the patients who suffer intraoperative spillage with negative washings. It seems that the delay in definitive surgery carries the worst outcome. It should also be noted that cyst aspiration done percutaneously or during laparoscopy carries a poor correlation between cytology and histology. Thus, a biopsy should accompany a cyst aspiration. In certain types of pathology, such as ovarian endometriomas, the recurrence rate is very high. It should also be noted that as many as 56% of aspirates do not contain diagnostic cells. A patient with a highly suspicious lesion should be treated by laparotomy if the mass cannot be removed intact. Consultation with a gynecologic oncologist should be considered when the patient is suspected of having a strong likelihood of a malignancy, since early and thorough surgical debulking is paramount in the treatment of this condition. In inconclusive cases, the laparoscope can aid the surgeon in identifying the type of pelvic mass, thus allowing for the proper abdominal incision and treatment. The laparoscopic visualization of a mass coupled with frozen section readings carries a sensitivity and specificity of over 92%.[5]

Although the majority of adnexal masses are benign, the workup should exclude or at least minimize the possibility of a malignant neoplasm. Adnexal masses are a common clinical problem. It is estimated that a woman in the United States has a 5% to 10% lifetime risk of undergoing surgery for a suspected ovarian neoplasm, and within that group 13% to 21% will be diagnosed with a malignant lesion. A woman has a lifetime risk of 1 in 70 of developing ovarian cancer in her lifetime. Unfortunately, of the 22,430 new cases of ovarian cancer diagnosed in the United States, 65% to 70% are diagnosed in an advanced stage, with a survival rate of 30% to 55%. Obviously, early diagnosis of ovarian carcinoma is paramount. It will require more specific ancillary tests, physician suspicion, and patient education. The minimally invasive nature of laparoscopy can also play an important role in early diagnosis of ovarian malignancy.[1-2]

In the evaluation and subsequent management of an adnexal mass, age of the patient plays an important role. In the reproductive age, the majority of the ovarian lesions are benign, and conservative management with ovarian preservation is very important. In contrast, in the postmenopausal patients, malignant lesions are more frequent and adnexal removal is indicated. The differential diagnosis should include gynecologic and nongynecologic lesions both of the benign and malignant variety. In the gynecologic and benign subtypes, the following entities should be considered: simple ovarian cysts, endometriomas, mature teratomas, leiomyomas, tubo-ovarian abscesses, hydrosalpinx, paratubal cyst, ectopic pregnancy, serous and mucinous cystadenomas, just to mention a few. In the gynecologic malignant subtype, ovarian carcinoma should be considered. In the nongynecological benign subtype, the following entities should be considered: diverticular abscess, appendiceal abscess or mucocele, urological lesions such as pelvic kidney, ureteral diverticulum, and bladder diverticulum. In the nongynecologic malign subtype, the following entities should be considered: gastrointestinal carcinomas, retroperitoneal sarcomas, and metastatic lesions. Metastatic cancers from breast, colon, or stomach may first appear as adnexal masses.

Pelvic examination should be part of the clinical evaluation although it carries a very low sensitivity and specificity in the preoperative diagnosis of an adnexal mass. Pelvic examination coupled with transvaginal ultrasound greatly aids in the correct diagnosis of an adnexal mass. No alternative imaging modality has demonstrated a superior diagnostic sensitivity and specificity to transvaginal ultrasound. Although the only limitation of transvaginal ultrasound lies with its lack of specificity and low positive predictive value for cancer in the premenopausal group of patients; however, a mass that is less than 10 cm in diameter, unilateral, with smooth borders, no excrescences or solid parts, and no free fluid almost excludes the possibility of an ovarian malignancy.[6]

The measurement of CA-125 aids in the diagnosis of nonmucinous epithelial ovarian cancers, but it is of no value in the diagnosis of other type of ovarian malignancies.[7] Measurement of β-hCG, L-lactate dehydrogenase (LDH), and AFP can be useful in the diagnosis of certain malignant germ cell tumors, while inhibin A and B can be markers for granulose cell tumors. CEA can be useful with endodermal sinus tumors and immature teratomas. CA-125 has a sensitivity of 61% to 90%, with a specificity of 71% to 93%, a positive predictive value of 35% to 91%, and a negative predictive value of 67% to 90%. Sensitive and specific methods for preoperative diagnosis of ovarian cancer would provide a rational basis for referral and timely treatment. Jacobs et al. proposed a risk of malignancy index (RMI) incorporating levels of CA-125, ultrasound findings, and menopausal status.[4] An RMI of 200 or more has a sensitivity of 85% and a specificity of 97%.

The RMI = ultrasound (U) × menopausal status (M) × levels of serum CA-125.

Ultrasound determines the following five characteristics:

- Multiloculated cysts
- Evidence of solid areas
- Evidence of metastasis
- Presence of ascites
- Bilateral lesions

Ultrasound: points for U

0 points = no characteristics
1 point = 1 characteristic
3 points = 2 or more characteristics
M = 1 point for menopausal, 3 points for postmenopausal

Despite our best intentions and workup, an adnexal mass can be ultimately found to be malignant. We should be prepared to offer the patient an adequate and timely surgical staging and treatment. It is also appropriate to consider referring the patient with high probability of ovarian malignancy to a physician with advanced training in gynecologic cancer. The Society of Gynecologic Oncologists and American College of Obstetricians and Gynecologists have developed the following referral guidelines for a newly diagnosed pelvic mass.[8]

Premenopausal (age < 50 years)

- CA-125 levels greater than 200 U/mL
- Ascites
- Evidence of abdominal or distant metastasis (by results of examination or imaging study)
- Family history of breast or ovarian cancer (in a first-degree relative)

Postmenopausal (age > 50 years)
- Elevated CA-125 levels
- Ascites
- Nodular or fixed pelvic mass
- Evidence of abdominal or distant metastasis (by results of examination or imaging study)
- Family history of breast or ovarian cancer (in a first-degree relative)

Adnexal masses in pregnancy have an incidence of around 4%. This is a recent increase which might be attributable to the more liberal utilization of ultrasonography, and maybe ovulation induction. However, the great majority of adnexal masses in pregnancy will resolve spontaneously by 16 weeks' of gestation. In approximately 1 in 1300 live births, an adnexal mass will require surgical management during pregnancy. It is estimated that 3% to 13% of persistent adnexal masses in pregnancy are found to be malignant. Indication for surgical management for a persistent adnexal mass in pregnancy includes the presence of a mass 6 cm or greater at 16 to 18 weeks' of gestation or symptoms due to a mass during any time during pregnancy.[9-13]

The most frequent pathology is mature cystic teratomas (dermoids), and serous cystadenomas, followed by corpus luteum cysts, mucinous cystadenomas, paraovarian cysts, endometriomas, and malignancies. In the past, surgical management of an adnexal mass in pregnancy consisted solely of a laparotomy. Laparoscopy was considered a contraindication due to the unknown effects of pneumoperitoneum on the fetus and the gravid uterus. However, several studies comparing laparoscopy to laparotomy in pregnancy have shown no difference in fetal outcomes between the two surgical procedures. In animal studies, it seems that an intra-abdominal pressure of 20 mm Hg has no effect on fetal placental perfusion and pH. Human studies are not available. Because of the concern of pneumoperitoneum on the fetus and the gravid uterus, gasless laparoscopy might be a safer alternative. If fetal monitoring is requested, transvaginal fetal monitoring with ultrasound is an option. If fetal distress is detected, the intra-abdominal pressure is decreased and the patient is hyperventilated.[9]

Surgical Technique

Laparoscopic management of an adnexal mass requires the same intraoperative concerns as any other procedure, including proper positioning with appropriate stirrups, arms positioned to the side, insertion of a Foley catheter, and sturdy uterine manipulator if the patient is not pregnant. After the insertion of an umbilical port, inspection of the upper abdomen is carried out in order to exclude the possibility of metastatic lesions or any other pathology. The patient is then placed in a steep Trendelenburg position, and two 5-mm trocars are introduced at the level of the anterior and superior iliac spine and lateral to the inferior epigastric vessels. An irrigator is introduced through the ports in the lower abdomen and pelvic washings are obtained. Inspection of the pelvis is carried out.[1]

In cases of adnexal pathology, such as an ovarian tumor, ectopic pregnancy, and hydrosalpinx, which may be associated with complete or partial adnexal removal, evaluation of the opposite side is recommended. In this case the patient presents with a whitish mass involving the entire right ovary. The mass is highly suggestive of a mature cystic teratoma (dermoid). No signs of malignancy were observed. Because of the location of uterus, involvement of the ovary, age of the patient, and the history of previous sterilization, it was decided to proceed with a right salpingo-oophorectomy. The course of the right ureter was visualized. The right fallopian tube was retracted with an atraumatic grasper and pulled toward the left side, placing the infundibular pelvic (IP) ligament under tension and away from the ureter. The IP ligament is desiccated with the bipolar forceps in three adjacent areas and transected in the middle. Through a blunt and sharp dissection and proper hemostatic technique, dissection is carried toward the proximal portion of the tube and the utero-ovarian ligament which is transected freeing the right adnexa (Figures 10–1 and 10–2).

The specimen is deposited in the cul-de-sac. There are several options for specimen removal including posterior colpotomy placement in an endoscopic bag with removal from the umbilicus or lower abdominal port and via a mini-laparotomy. For the removal of the specimen through the lower ports, it is

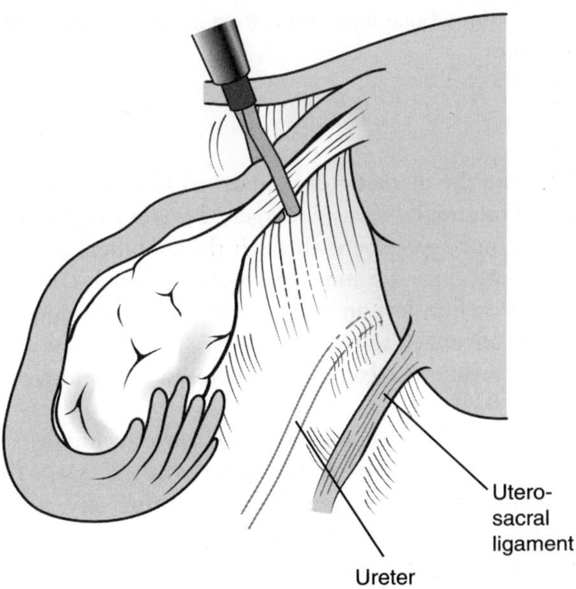

Figure 10–1. The tube and ovary are removed by using bipolar cautery and then incising on the utero-ovarian ligament.

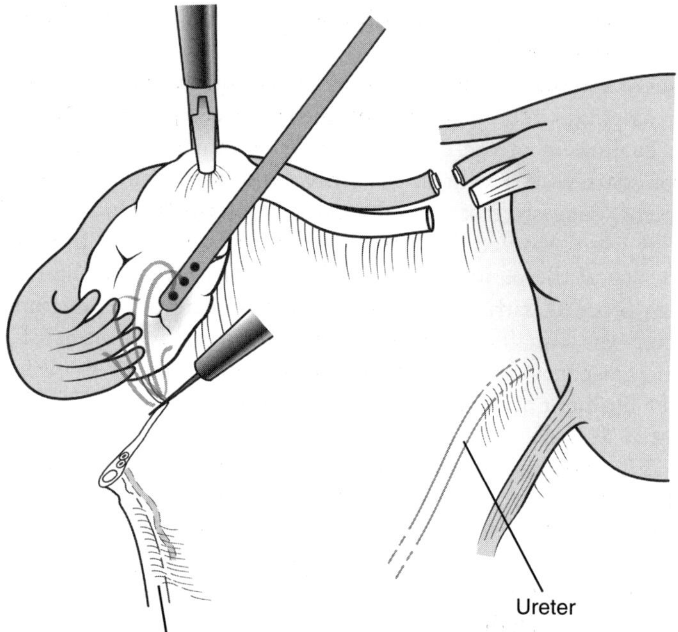

Figure 10–2. The infundibular ligament is then cauterized and divided, with care to identify the ureter.

necessary to increase the diameter of the port to 12 mm or greater. To adhere to the principle of minimally invasive surgery, I prefer to remove specimens or perform morcellation of specimens through the umbilical port which can be easily widened. I introduce a 5-mm laparoscope through the left lower port, and under direct visualization an endoscopic bag is introduced through the umbilical port and advanced toward the pelvis. The assistant grasps the specimen and places it inside the bag which is closed and removed through the umbilicus.

The specimen can be decompressed by introducing a Veress needle attached to a syringe and aspirating the contents of the cyst, while the specimen sits inside the endoscopic bag thus preventing any spillage into the abdominal cavity.[14-16] Alternatively, the endoscopic bag can be introduced through the posterior colpotomy incision placing the specimen in the bag and removing it through the vagina. A large mass might require decompression prior to removal in order to avoid gross contamination even in benign cases such as endometriomas or dermoid cysts. This can be accomplished by placing the specimen inside the bag and decompressing it with the suction irrigator probe, or by using endoscopic cyst aspirators. Any suspicious masses are sent for frozen section. Frozen section is a highly sensitive and specific test, except with very large masses.[17-19]

Comprehension Questions

10.1 An adnexal mass is diagnosed in a multiparous patient. Laparoscopic management is contemplated. Which of the following is more likely to indicate benign rather than a malignant process?

A. Septations
B. Size of 10 cm
C. Cystic mass
D. Papillations

10.2 A 28-year-old woman is noted to have a 12-cm adnexal mass. Which of the following tumor markers is most useful in this patient?

A. α-Fetoprotein
B. CEA
C. CA-125
D. CA-19-9

ANSWERS

10.1 **C.** A cystic mass is more likely associated with a benign process. Septations, complexities, solid component, larger size, ascites, and papillations are more indicative of a malignant process.

10.2 **A.** In a patient who is premenopausal, particularly less than age 30, germ cell tumors are likely. These tumor markers include AFP, hCG, and LDH.

Clinical Pearls

See Table 1-2 for definition of level of evidence and strength of recommendation

- The patient's age together with the CA-125 and ultrasound characteristics of the adnexal mass can help to determine the likelihood of malignancy (Level B).
- Pregnancy is not a contraindication to laparoscopic ovarian surgery (Level B).
- A variety of techniques may be used to remove an adnexal mass laparoscopically such as through a colpotomy incision, with a specimen bag through the umbilical incision, or a lateral port incision (Level C).

REFERENCES

1. Papasakelariou C, Saunders D, De La Rosa A. Comparative study of laparoscopic oophorectomy. *J Am Assoc Gynecol Laparosc.* 1995;2(4):407-410.
2. Dembo AJ, Davy M, Stenwig AE, et al. Prognostic factors with stage I epithelial cancer. *Obstet Gynecol.* 1990;75:263-273.
3. Sevelda P, Dittrich C, Salzar H. Prognostic value of the rupture of the capsule in stage I epithelial ovarian carcinoma. *Gynecol Oncol.* 1989;35:321-322.
4. Jacobs I, Oram D, Fairbanks J, et al. A risk of malignancy index incorporating Ca 125, ultrasound and menopausal status for the accurate preoperative diagnosis of ovarian cancer. *Br J Obstet Gynaecol.* 1990;97:922-929.
5. National Institutes of Health Consensus Development Conference Statement. Ovarian cancer: screening, treatment, and follow up. *Gynecol Oncol.* 1994;55: S4-S14.
6. Schutter EM, Kenemans P, Sohn C, et al. Diagnostic value of pelvic examination, ultrasound, and serum CA 125 in postmenopausal women with pelvic mass. An international multicenter study. *Cancer.* 1994;74:1398-1406.
7. Maggino T, Gadducci A, D'Addario V, et al. Prospective multicenter study on CA 125 in postmenopausal pelvic masses. *Gynecol Oncol.* 1994;54:117-123.
8. Manjunath AP, Pratapkumar, Sujatha K, et al. Comparison of three risks of malignancy indices in evaluation of pelvic masses. *Gynecol Oncol.* 2001;81:225-229.
9. Yuen PM, Chang AMZ. Laparoscopic management of adnexal mass during pregnancy. *Acta Obstet Gynecol Scand.* 1997;76:173-176.
10. Whitecar MC, Turner S, Higby K. Adnexal masses in pregnancy: a review of 130 cases undergoing surgical management. *Am J Obstet Gynecol.* 1999;181:19-24.
11. Platek DN, Henderson CE, Goldberg GL. The management of a persistent adnexal mass in pregnancy. *Am J Obstet Gynecol.* 1995;173:1236-1240.
12. Buttery BW, Beisner NA, Fortune DW, et al. Ovarian tumors in pregnancy. *Med J Aust.* 1973;1:345-349.
13. Curet MJ, Voght DA, Schob O, et al. Effects of CO_2 pneumoperitoneum in pregnant ewes. *J Surg Res.* 1996;63:339-344.
14. Higgens RV, Matkins JF, Marroum MC. Comparison of fine needle aspiration cytologic findings of ovarian cysts with ovarian histologic findings. *Am J Obstet Gynecol.* 1999;180:550-553.

15. Mulvany NJ. Aspiration cytology of ovarian cysts and cystic neoplasms. A study of 235 aspirates. *Acta Cytol.* 1996;40:911-920.
16. Vercellini P, Oldani S, Felicette I, et al. The value of cyst puncture in the differential diagnosis of benign ovarian tumors. *Hum Reprod.* 1995;10:1465-1469.
17. Smorgick N, Barel O, Halperin R, Schneider D, Pansky M. Laparoscopic removal of adnexal cysts: is it possible to decrease inadvertent intraoperative rupture rate? *Am J Obstet Gynecol.* 2009 Mar;200(3):237.e1-3.
18. Whiteside JL, Keup HL. Laparoscopic management of the ovarian mass: a practical approach. *Clin Obstet Gynecol.* 2009 Sep;52(3):327-334.
19. Tinelli R, Malzoni M, Cosentino F, et al. Feasibility, safety, and efficacy of conservative laparoscopic treatment of borderline ovarian tumors. *Fertil Steril.* 2009 Aug;92(2):736-741 [Epub 2008].

Case 11

A 37-year-old African American nulliparous woman complains of fatigue, loss of productivity, and regular heavy prolonged menses during the last 9 months, which worsens with time. She mentions that an asymptomatic myoma less than 4 cm was incidentally detected by transvaginal ultrasound examination during her annual visit to her gynecologist 1 year ago. She has always had normal Pap smear tests and she denies sexually transmitted diseases or abnormal mucopurulent vaginal discharge. Her pregnancy test is negative despite her wish to conceive during the last 12 months. Heart and lung examinations are normal. On examination, her blood pressure is 105/70 mm Hg, heart rate 98 beats/min, and temperature 97°F. On palpation, her abdomen presents a firm, round, nontender palpable midline mass 2 cm above the pubic symphysis. On bimanual examination, an anteverted, enlarged 15-week-size uterus is revealed with a hard painless protruding fundal mass with irregular contour, approximately 7 cm in diameter that moves together with uterus during pushing the cervix upward or laterally. No adnexal masses are palpable. On speculum examination, no abnormalities are detected in the vagina and cervix. Transvaginal ultrasound examination demonstrates a solitary fundal intramural myoma protruding into the uterine cavity. Her hemoglobulin level is 8.1 g/dL, leukocyte count 10,500/mm^3, and platelet count 160,000/mm^3.

➤ What is the most likely diagnosis?

➤ What is your next step?

ANSWERS TO CASE 11: Uterine Leiomyoma

Summary: An African American 37-year-old nulliparous woman, with a history of a known asymptomatic intramural leiomyoma less than 4 cm the last year, complains of menometrorrhagia. She has also been trying to become pregnant unsuccessfully for the last 12 months. Her pregnancy test is negative. On examination, a midline hard mass seems to be contiguous to an enlarged anteverted uterus with irregular contour. Also, she has anemia and mild tachycardia.

- ➤ **Most likely diagnosis:** Symptomatic uterine leiomyoma and infertility
- ➤ **Next step:** Ultrasound examination to confirm the clinical diagnosis, and then discussion with the patient about various options, including surgery including laparoscopic myomectomy

ANALYSIS

Objectives

1. Know that most myomas are asymptomatic and require intervention when they cause clinical symptoms.
2. Understand that the location and size of a myoma are the most crucial determinants of its potential to become symptomatic.
3. Know that the most common symptoms associated with uterine leiomyomas in reproductive age women are abnormal uterine bleeding manifested as menorrhagia or hypermenorrhea.
4. Describe the treatment options for uterine leiomyomata, including conservative, minimally invasive surgical procedures, medical therapies, and hysterectomy.

Considerations

This 37-year-old woman complains of fatigue, loss of productivity, and irregular menstrual pattern due to hypermenorrhea and menorrhagia. Clinical examination and history are consistent with a fundal myoma, because of the presence of a midline hard mass contiguous with the uterus that also explains its irregular contour. The prevalence of myomas in African American women is two to three times higher in comparison to white Caucasian women. Moreover, this uterine abnormal mass may be a possible cause of her infertility. The movement of this mass together with the uterus during lateral or upward displacement of cervix is another argument that this mass is of uterine origin. Furthermore, the absence of pelvic tenderness and fever with normal leukocyte count excludes pelvic inflammatory disease as a cause of abnormal uterine bleeding. The normal clinical findings on speculum examination and, also, the negative Pap smear tests make the diagnosis of vaginal or cervical pathology such as cervical or vaginal endometriosis, ectropion, cervical polyps, endometrial pedunculated myomas or polyps protruding through the external cervical os, cervical intraepithelial neoplasia, or malignancy remote. Dysfunctional uterine bleeding is excluded from the differential diagnosis, as it is frequent in adolescent and perimenopausal women and is a manifestation of anovulatory cycles in the absence of any uterine pathology or medical illness. Furthermore, in this case the patient seems to have ovulatory cycles because she has regular menses. Ectopic pregnancy as a cause of abnormal uterine bleeding is impossible due to her negative pregnancy test. Benign or malignant ovarian tumors are absent on bimanual examination. The clinical differential diagnosis between leiomyoma and adenomyoma as causes of menorrhagia is difficult without the use of transvaginal ultrasound or preferably magnetic resonance imaging (MRI) (ill-defined borders of the adenomyoma within myometrium in contrast to the pseudocapsule of myomas with clear contour). However, the main dominant symptom of adenomyoma or endometriosis is chronic pelvic pain and not menorrhagia that is the main complaint of women with symptomatic myomas. Adenomyosis is presented in the fourth or fifth decade of life and affects 1% of usually multiparous women. In general, endometrial sampling is performed with abnormal vaginal bleeding in women older than age 35 years. Finally, a Pipelle office endometrial biopsy is mandatory when the ultrasound findings raise the suspicion of endometrial hyperplasia or carcinoma, though they appear in peri- or postmenopausal women with metrorrhagia and not with menorrhagia. They are rarely found as a cause of abnormal uterine bleeding in women of reproductive age and especially younger than 40 years without the coexistence of risk factors such as excessive BMI, diabetes, or hypertension, which are not present in our case. Finally, the workup of menorrhagia except from platelet count should include further investigation of the thyroid function and clotting factors in order to exclude hyperthyroidism or coagulation disorders such as von Willebrand disease.

APPROACH TO Uterine Leiomyoma

DEFINITIONS

HYPERMENORRHEA: It is defined as heavy, profuse periods that exceed 80 mL blood loss.

MENORRHAGIA: It is defined as heavy and prolonged periods that exceed 7 days.

METRORRHAGIA: It is defined as abnormal uterine bleeding at irregular intervals, particularly between the expected menstrual periods.

LEIOMYOMA: Benign smooth muscle tumor, which arises from the myometrium, also called myoma or fibroma. It is classified by its location in relation to the uterine wall: serosal (which may be broad-based or pedunculated), intramural, and submucosal. The latter is further distinguished as type 0 (pedunculated, totally protruding in the uterine cavity), type I (> 50% protrudes in the uterine cavity), and type II (< 50% protrudes in the uterine cavity or has an intramural portion of > 50%).

ADENOMYOSIS: It is the presence of heterotopic endometrial glands and stroma in the myometrium at least 2.5 mm below the endometrial-myometrial interface with adjacent smooth muscle hyperplasia. It can be either diffuse or focal, leading to the formation of the so-called "adenomyoma."

ADENOMYOMA: It is a circumscribed nodule of hypertrophic and distorted endometrium and myometrium, which is usually embedded within the myometrium.

CLINICAL APPROACH

Uterine leiomyomas are among the most frequent pathologic entities encountered in gynecologic clinical practice. Myomas are the most common benign gynecologic neoplasms and the primary indication for hysterectomy, accounting for over 200,000 hysterectomies per year in the United States. Although in the pathology reports of hysterectomy specimens leiomyomas can be identified in up to 77%, they are clinically apparent in approximately 20% to 35% of women of reproductive age. Despite the high prevalence of these tumors, there is paucity of data available regarding the natural clinical history of myomas. They are monoclonal-independent lesions, such that multiple tumors from the uterus arise independently and may have distinct chromosomal abnormalities, while their growth is estrogen and progesterone dependent. Increased prevalence of leiomyomas is observed two- to threefold higher in African American women, who have earlier age at first diagnosis with multiple and larger myomas in comparison to that in white women. The prevalence of myomas increases with age until 50 years and then declines sharply. In pregnant women, the prevalence of myomas has been reported to be approximately 1.4%. Oral contraceptives, parity, and smoking decrease the risk of myoma development due to low oestrogen levels. On the other hand, obesity with higher oestrogen levels, diastolic hypertension with cytokine release, or injury of uterine smooth muscle as well as pelvic inflammatory disease with intrauterine irritation are associated with increased risk of fibroids. Malignant transformation of leiomyomas is extremely rare, and according to cytogenetic studies it has been documented that leiomyosarcomas arise de novo and rarely from a specific subset of myomas. However, the incidence of uterine sarcoma in symptomatic premenopausal women undergoing surgical removal is less than 0.3%. Current studies do not support any association between rapid growth of a leiomyoma and increased risk of malignancy. So, the rapid growth of an asymptomatic myoma that gains 6 weeks or more in gestational size within an interval of 1 year or less is an outdated indication for surgical intervention.

Most uterine myomas cause no symptoms. Approximately 62% of women with symptomatic myomas present with multiple symptoms, which correlate with their location, number, size, or concomitant degenerative changes. Excessive menstrual bleeding that leads to iron deficiency and subsequent anemia is the most common and often the sole symptom associated with myomas, particularly when there is protrusion in the endometrial cavity or distortion of it. Metrorrhagia, that is, alteration of the menstrual regularity, is not characteristic of myomas, and it should be worked up to exclude other pathologies. Pelvic pressure due to increased uterine size is responsible for the mass effect symptoms to the adjacent organs such as urinary frequency, urinary incontinence, hydronephrosis, constipation, tenesmus, infertility, and pregnancy complications (painful red degeneration, spontaneous miscarriage, and obstetric complications). Pelvic pain is attributed to degeneration changes or torsion of pedunculated myomas. Leiomyomas are considered to impair fertility by interference with sperm or embryo transport, causing anatomic distortion of the uterine cavity or cervix, by obstruction of tubal ostia, or by altering the uterine contractility and endometrial environment, but their precise role has not been clearly demonstrated.[1]

The gold standard for assessing the number, location, and size of uterine myomas is the transvaginal ultrasound. The combination of transvaginal and abdominal ultrasound is necessary for mapping myomas of an enlarged uterus with size greater than 10 weeks' of gestation and especially for subserosal ones. Of course, its diagnostic accuracy for the detection of submucosal myomas and in the mapping of multiple ones is operator dependent and is enhanced by the addition of sonohysterography. Although MRI has the same accuracy in the detection of uterine myomas with ultrasound, it is much more expensive and it certainly consists of a reasonable disadvantage. However, MRI is a superior imaging technique in the mapping of multiple leiomyomas and in diagnostic differentiation from leiomyosarcomas or adenomyomas due to the precise depiction of well-defined pseudocapsule margins of benign myomas.[2]

The symptomatology of leiomyomas dictates the need and the urgency for medical or surgical intervention. But, regarding the impact of myomas on reproductive outcome, there are no definitive answers. However, submucosal and intramural leiomyomas distorting the uterine cavity and/or measuring larger than 5 to 7 cm seem to reduce pregnancy rates and pregnancy outcome and therefore they should be removed, especially if they are associated with multiple failed in vitro fertilization (IVF) cycles.

The target of medical treatment is to relieve the symptoms and regress the uterine or myoma volume by manipulating ovarian steroids due to its hormonal responsiveness. Gonadotropin-releasing hormone agonists (GnRH-a) are the most well-established agents for medical treatment of myomas, achieving temporary amenorrhoea and reduction in uterine or myoma size by

30% to 65% within 3 months of treatment. Add-back therapy, especially with raloxifene or tibolone, is necessary due to the significant side effects of hypoestrogenism caused by GnRH-a. However, prolonged use (6 months) should be avoided in premenopausal women, except in perimenopausal ones or in the preoperative period for the control of anemia. In addition, GnRH-a facilitate the ability to perform a hysterectomy laparoscopically or vaginally instead of abdominally, as well as permit a smaller or Pfannenstiel skin incision in a woman having an abdominal approach by reducing the size and vascularity of myomas. Exclusion criteria involve women with multiple small myomas that might subsequently be missed during myomectomy. Nonsteroidal anti-inflammatory agents and oral contraceptives with progestins only help to control the symptoms, without reducing the size of myomas or uterus. GnRH-antagonists, mifepristone, aromatase inhibitors, steroid receptor modulators, and levonorgestrel intrauterine device need further investigation before reaching definite conclusions about their effects on myomas.[1,2]

Although hysterectomy is considered the definitive treatment of uterine myomas, there is increasing demand for more conservative surgical approaches of myomas, which allow to preserve the uterus in situ. Abdominal myomectomy remains the treatment of choice for solitary myomas larger than 10 cm. When more than four multiple fibroids measuring greater than 7 cm are present, these must be removed if concomitant pathology that involves major surgery is encountered. Laparoscopic myomectomy compared with abdominal myomectomy has clear advantages in terms of postoperative pain relief, recovery time, hospital stay and demand for fewer transfusions, less postoperative fever, and de novo adhesion formation, but with no significant difference in terms of pregnancy and miscarriage rates in the few prospective, well-designed published studies. Of course, its application depends on gynecologist's skills and mastering in endoscopic suturing, and also availability of the necessary instrumentation. Under these prerequisites, the need for conversion to laparotomy is reported only in 1.4% of cases.[3,4,5]

Adhesion formation can be eliminated by performing the incision (transverse incision is preferable to vertical in order to avoid incoming arcuate vessels, except from the corneal areas) on the anterior uterine wall or fundus in order to remove myomas, even if they are located posterior, by reducing the use of electrocautery and by using absorbable adhesion barriers. The risk of uterine rupture following myomectomy is ranged from 0.002% to 5% and usually occurs between 29 and 36 weeks' of gestation. This is related to the following factors: (1) single instead of multilayer suturing, which minimizes the hematoma formation and maximizes the strength of uterine wall, (2) the excessive use of bipolar electrocoagulation for hemostasis that might impair the healing process, and (3) the poor suturing skills of the gynecologist to achieve uniform closure of the uterine defect by symmetric hickness of the scar in relation to the adjacent myometrium. Finally, hysteroscopic myomectomy is established as the gold standard for the treatment of submucosal myomas types 0 and I due to the advantage of no incision or suturing on the

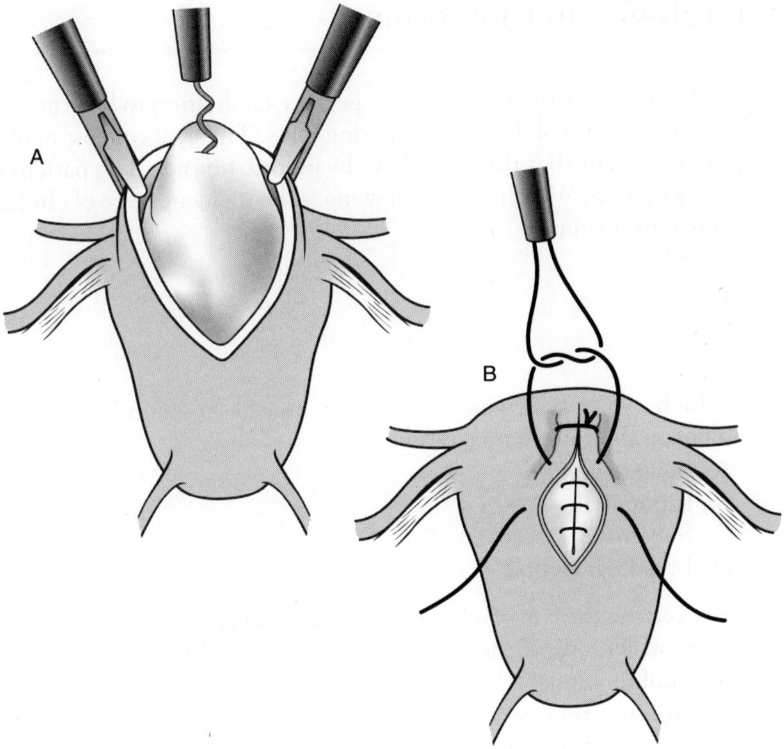

Figure 11–1. A myomectomy is performed laparoscopically. The myoma is grasped with a corkscrew and dissected from the myometrium (A), and then the uterine defect is sutured closed (B).

normal myometrium (Figure 11–1). However, this approach can be rarely complicated by perforation, bleeding, infection, and intracavitary adhesion formation. Other techniques such as electromyolysis, uterine and ovarian artery ligation, or embolization have been proposed as conservative minimally invasive approaches with short-term results in women who desire to preserve their uterus, but with unknown effect on their fertility potential and risk of recurrence.

The recurrence of fibroids is diagnosed by ultrasound demonstrating myomas at least 2 cm in diameter. The 5-year risk of recurrence is 62% with a 9% risk of additional major surgery, a crucial issue when counselling patients for myomectomy. The majority of recurrences (75%) occur between 10 and 30 months after surgery. This risk is greater in patients with multiple myomas and large size of uterus. Moreover, the decreased tactile ability of laparoscopy may account for the increased rate of recurrence at laparoscopy.

Comprehension Questions

11.1 A 42-year-old woman is noted on pelvic examination to have an irregularly shaped mobile midline uterine mass. The gynecologist explains to the patient that this is likely to be uterine fibroids. The patient has no symptoms. Which of the following is the incidence rate of clinically apparent myomas?

A. 5%
B. 30%
C. 70%
D. 90%

11.2 Which type of myoma should be removed in infertile women to increase their pregnancy rates?

A. Submucosal
B. Intramural
C. Subserosal
D. Broad ligamental

11.3 To decrease the risk of adhesion formation with laparoscopic myomectomy, which one of the following incisions should be avoided?

A. Midline fundal
B. Anterior transverse
C. Anterior horizontal
D. Posterior

11.4 A gynecology case manager is reviewing charts for appropriate surgery. This month the focus is on myomectomy. Which of the following cases would most likely be flagged as an inappropriate indication for surgery?

A. Patient complains of pain
B. Patient complains of vaginal bleeding
C. Patient has pressure symptoms
D. Patient is informed that surgery would help protect against malignant transformation

ANSWERS

11.1 **B.** It is estimated that myomas are clinically apparent in approximately one out of every three or four women of the reproductive age. However, the prevalence of uterine myomas is higher in pathology reports of hysterectomy specimens.

11.2 **A.** Neither intramural nor subserosal myomas seem to affect fertility rates and removal has not been shown to increase fertility. Broad ligament myomas are outside the uterus.

11.3 **D.** Posterior uterine incision should be avoided, if possible, to decrease the risk of adhesion formation. The midline fundal incision has been popularized to decrease the risk of extending the uterine incision into the cornua. A horizontal incision has been advocated to avoid sectioning the blood vessels that run transversely to minimize blood loss.

11.4 **D.** Malignant transformation of uterine myomas is not acceptable indication for myomectomy in otherwise asymptomatic women. The risk of malignant transformation in an otherwise asymptomatic patient is less than 1:1000. However, if the uterus is noted to be growing in a postmenopausal woman, or uterine fibroids are noted in a patient with prior pelvic irradiation, surgery should be strongly considered.

Clinical Pearls

See Table 1-2 for definition of level of evidence and strength of recommendation

- Most myomas are asymptomatic common benign tumors of the myometrium with the highest incidence in women of reproductive age, affecting African American population three times as often as Caucasian women (Level A).
- The clinical suspicion of myomas can be confirmed by ultrasonography. MRI and sonohysterography are complementary diagnostic tools in complicated cases (Level A).
- Large intramural myomas (> 5 cm) and/or those distorting the endometrial cavity may adversely affect fertility (Level B).
- Medical treatment of myomas with GnRH-agonists is indicated for symptom relief during the preoperative period or in perimenopausal women (Level A).
- Laparoscopic myomectomy is a conservative surgical treatment in women who desire to preserve their uterus. However, hysterectomy is the definitive treatment of myomas (Level B).

REFERENCES

1. Arici A, Rayburn W. Myomas. In: *Obstetrics and Gynecology Clinics of North America*. Philadelphia, PA: Elsevier Saunders; 2006;33(1):1-225.
2. Nowak R. Fibroids: pathophysiology and current medical treatment. *Baillieres Best Pract Res Clin Obstet Gynaecol.* 1999;13(2):223-238.
3. Parker W. Laparoscopic myomectomy and abdominal myomectomy. *Clin Obstet Gynecol.* 2006;49(4):787-797.
4. Carter JE, McCarus SD. Laparoscopic myomectomy. Time and cost analysis of power vs. manual morcellation. *J Reprod Med.* 1997 Jul;42(7):383-388.

5. Alessandri F, Lijoi D, Mistrangelo E, et al. Randomized study of laparoscopic versus minilaparotomic myomectomy for uterine myomas. *J Minim Invasive Gynecol.* 2006 Mar-Apr;13:92-97.
6. Walker C, Stewart E. Uterine fibroids: the elephant in the room. *Science.* 2005;308: 1589-1592.
7. Hurst BS, Matthews ML, Marshburn PB. Laparoscopic myomectomy for symptomatic uterine myomas. *Fertil Steril.* 2005 Jan;83(1):1-23.
8. Palomba S, Zupi E, Falbo, A, et al. A multicenter randomized, controlled study comparing laparoscopic versus minilaparotomic myomectomy: reproductive outcomes. *Fertil Steri.* 2007 Oct;88:933-941.
9. Sinha R, Hegde A, Warty N, Patil N. Laparoscopic excision of very large myomas. *J Am Assoc Gynecol Laparosc.* Nov 2003;10(4):461-468.
10. Parker W. Uterine myomas: management. *Fertil Steril.* 2007 Aug;88:255-271.

Case 12

A 28-year-old thin and nulliparous woman with a history of progressive dysmenorrhea not responding to medical therapy is taken to surgery for laparoscopy and possible excision of endometriosis. The Veress needle is introduced through an infraumbilical incision and the abdomen filled with 2 L of CO_2 gas. A 10/11-mm trocar is introduced into the abdominal cavity without much effort. Upon inserting the laparoscope, large amount of blood is visualized. The anesthesiologist alerts you that the patient is currently hypotensive.

➤ What is the most likely diagnosis?

➤ What is your next step?

ANSWERS TO CASE 12: Laparoscopic Vascular Complications

Summary: This is a 28-year-old woman who, during a laparoscopy, developed hypotension and intra-abdominal bleeding.

- **Most likely diagnosis:** Major vascular injury.
- **Next step:** Proceed with a laparotomy and obtain the assistance of a vascular surgeon.

ANALYSIS

Objectives

1. Be familiar with the definition and consequences of major vascular injury.
2. Learn the differences between closed versus open technique in laparoscopy.
3. Learn strategies to minimize the incidence of major vascular injury.
4. Be familiar with the management of major vascular injury.

Considerations

This is a 28-year-old thin woman who suffered a major vascular injury during laparoscopic surgery. Sometimes surprising to the surgeon, it is the thin patient who is at greatest risk for vascular injuries, because of the decreased distance from the skin to the retroperitoneal space. This patient had a hypotensive episode immediately upon injury to her major vessels. It is unclear at this point whether it is the aorta or vena cava that is injured. The surgeon should immediately perform a laparotomy via vertical incision to put pressure on the vascular injury. Large bore IVs should be placed, and crystalloid resuscitation should be initiated. Blood should be immediately ordered, and likely, the patient will need uncross-matched O negative blood. A vascular surgeon should be immediately summoned. Time is of the essence, and may mean survival or death for this patient. Major vascular injury is defined as one that threatens the patient's life almost immediately upon its occurrence.

APPROACH TO Laparoscopic Vascular Injury

Vascular injury associated with laparoscopy has an incidence of less than 1 per 1000 cases (0.1%). Despite its low incidence, it remains one of the most feared complications in laparoscopic procedures. It is a complication that can occur even to the most experienced laparoscopic surgeon. However, timely diagnosis and proper management are paramount for a good outcome. Laparoscopy is particularly associated with vascular injury due to the blind introduction of either the Veress needle to produce the pneumoperitoneum or the trocar to introduce the initial laparoscope.[1]

Perhaps counterintuitive, it is the thin patient rather than the obese patient who is at greater risk for these injuries, especially in those patients with well-developed abdominal walls. In the thin athletic patients, the distance from the abdominal wall to the retroperitoneal structures is less than that in obese patients. Certain anatomical considerations and surgical techniques can minimize vascular injuries. An intraumbilical incision at the deepest point represents the shorter distance to the abdominal cavity. In a retrospective review by Hurd and associates,[2] the vertical distance from the base of the umbilicus to the peritoneum remained very constant despite an increase in the BMI of the subjects. It was a distance of 6 cm or less in nearly all subjects. In contrast, the distance at 45 degrees from the lower margin and base of the umbilicus to the peritoneum increased to a much larger degree with an increase in the BMI. The introduction of the initial umbilical trocar remains a blind entry. Despite the utilization of an open technique, major vascular complications can occur.[3-5] Thus, even with open trocar introduction, the surgeon should be vigilant and should exercise careful technique.

Clinical trials comparing closed versus open entry technique have not demonstrated a superiority of one over the other. A study by the American Association of Gynecologic Laparoscopists showed more visceral lesions with open laparoscopy entry but not significantly fewer vascular lesions.[3] It is important to note that visceral lesions are potentially more life threatening since they are commonly missed during laparoscopy and only recognized when the patient is admitted with peritonitis and sepsis. I prefer the closed technique. In the establishment of pneumoperitoneum, filling the abdomen to a specific pressure rather than a set volume allows for different intra-abdominal distensibility and volume capacity. In our setting, I typically insufflate the abdomen to a pressure of 20 mm Hg. This offers a tight abdomen which allows for an easier insertion of the trocar. The patient should be kept in a completely horizontal position. Premature Trendelenburg position such as by the anesthesiologist or even the surgeon direction can alter the anatomy, bringing the major vessels into closer proximity to the site of the trocar insertion. In this case the insufflation of the abdominal cavity with 2 L was inadequate and may have been the contributing factor to the major vascular injury. The utilization of sharp/disposable trocars allows for an easier and controlled insertion.

Avoidance of Injury

The abdominal and pelvic examinations should be performed preoperatively not only to assess for disease but also to assess the distance between the abdominal wall and the retroperitoneal vessels. A very easily palpable abdominal aortic pulse, a sharply inclined sacral promontory, or pronounced lumbar lordosis can all be hints of bony variations that push the aorta or vena cava toward the abdominal wall, putting the patient at risk for vascular injury. Additionally, patients who have had abdominal surgery or pelvic adhesive disease may also be at risk due to a "solid interface" between the anterior abdominal wall and the retroperitoneum. This lack of space does not allow the trocar sheath guard to engage, and, thus, the surgeon may make multiple attempts to push the trocar deeper and deeper trying to get the trocar sleeve to activate. Furthermore, if the surgeon deviates off the midline even slightly upon introducing the trocar, the iliac vessels can be injured. Thus, the laparoscopic surgeon must be much disciplined to place the trocar in the midline. During the surgical aspect of laparoscopy, injury to vascular structures can occur due to dissection near the retroperitoneal vessels. Ablation of endometriosis for instance can lead to vascular injury due to the distorted anatomy from the endometriotic implants.[6] The surgeon should ensure that the patient is horizontal and not in Tredelenburg position (Figure 12-1 A and B) since the change in position can lead to inadvertent directing of the trocar into the retroperitoneal vessels.

Recognition of Vascular Injury

At times, the vascular injury is obvious with bright red blood filling the abdominal cavity. Sometimes, though, the findings are more subtle. For instance, vena cava laceration may be associated with a "hematoma" in the retroperitoneal space that can deceptively "appear stable." As a rule of thumb, any hematoma in the retroperitoneal area should be fully investigated and should be considered a major vascular injury until proven otherwise. A common scenario is that a venous injury may appear stable in the operating room, only to lead to further hemorrhage postoperatively, and even exsanguination. Abdominal wall vessels can also be injured such as the inferior epigastric artery. Visualization with the laparoscope of these vessels as they course between the rectus muscle and the parietal peritoneum can direct lateral ports away from these vessels (Figure 12–1A and B).

Treatment

As soon as a major vascular injury is recognized, the surgeon should proceed with an immediate laparotomy through a midline incision, while anesthesia secures additional IV lines, experienced cardiovascular surgeon is summoned, and arrangements are being made in making blood available for transfusion. Once laparotomy has begun, the first priority is to compress the aorta to prevent exsanguination. This is accomplished by placing hand compression over the aorta or a vascular clamp. If the compression lasts for over 15 minutes, systemic anticoagulation with heparin should be considered once the repair is complete and the patient is stable. Injury to the vena cava is generally more difficult to repair due to the thin wall and friable tissue. Gentle constant pressure to help decrease blood loss, while awaiting a vacular surgeon, is the most prudent action. Because the vena cava can tear more easily, the pressure

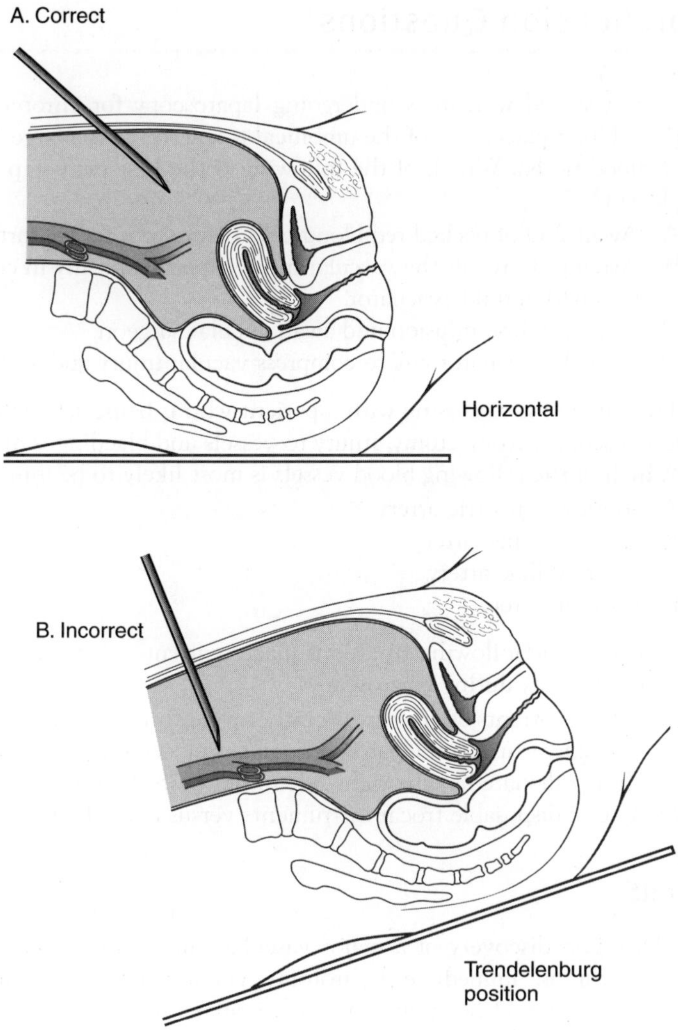

Figure 12–1. Placement of laparoscope with care to stay in the midline directed into the hollow of the sacrum (A), whereas incorrect positioning deviating from the midline can cause inadvertent injury to the retroperitoneal vessels (B).

should be directed downward without excessive movement that may cause further vessel laceration. A number of techniques are used to address injury to the inferior epigastric artery, including bipolar cautery via laparoscopy, the use of a Foley bulb placed into the trocar site into the abdominal cavity with traction and held in place such as with a small clamp on Foley catheter against the anterior abdominal wall. Various needles have been designed to allow for deep surgical ligatures, and finally enlarging the surgical incision to isolate and ligate the vessel may be employed.[7-10]

Comprehension Questions

12.1 A 43-year-old woman is undergoing laparoscopy for chronic pelvic pain. Upon placement of the umbilical trocar, there is a large amount of blood noted. Which of the following is the best next step for this patient?

A. Await 2 U of packed red blood cells before proceeding further.
B. Attempt to repair the vascular injury laparoscopically in conjunction with a fluid evacuator.
C. Normal saline infusion and await vacular surgeon.
D. Immediate laparotomy to compress vacular injury and aorta.

12.2 The surgeon is discussing with a patient who is being scheduled for a laparoscopic myomectomy. Injury to vessels and bleeding is discussed. Which of the following blood vessels is most likely to be injured?

A. Inferior epigastric artery
B. Common iliac artery
C. Internal iliac artery
D. Ovarian artery

12.3 Which of the following situations places patients at increased risk of vascular injury during laparoscopy?

A. Obese patients at greater risk rather than thin patients
B. Closed versus open laparoscopic trocar placement
C. Trocar deviated to the right side rather than the midline
D. Use of disposable trocar instruments versus reusable instruments

ANSWERS

12.1 **D.** Upon discovery of a major vascular injury, the surgeon should perform an immediate laparotomy via a vertical skin incision. Pressure should be applied at the vascular injury site, and also the aorta should be compressed. The anesthesiologist should place two large bore IVs and normal saline should be infused, while blood be cross-matched.

12.2 **A.** The inferior epigastric artery is the most commonly injured vessel causing major hemorrhage. The inferior epigastric artery is located between the rectus muscle and the peritoneum, and at the medial aspect of the rectus muscle. Injury can be avoided by transilluminating through the intra-abdominal region, to try to locate the vessels prior to placement of the lateral ports.

12.3 **C.** Vascular injuries are more common with thin patients rather than obese ones. The best technique is to aim at the hollow of the sacrum in the midline to avoid injury of the common iliac vessels. Because thin patients have less distance from the skin to the retroperitoneal space, the retroperitoneal vessels are more often injured.

Clinical Pearls

(See Table 1-2 for definition of level of evidence and strength of recommendation)

- The most common vessel injured during laparoscopy is the inferior epigastric artery (Level B).
- The most commonly injured retroperitoneal vessel is the common iliac artery or vein (Level B).
- In a hypotensive patient when a major artery is lacerated, pressure at the vessel injury site and compression of the aorta are paramount (Level B).
- A closed versus open technique for laparoscopic trocar entry has not been shown to affect the incidence of vascular injury (Level A).

REFERENCES

1. Loffer F, Pent D. Indications, contraindications and complications of laparoscopy. *Obstet Gynecol Surv.* 1975;30:407-427.
2. Hurd WW, Bude RO, Delancey JOH, Gauvin JM, Aisen AM. Abdominal wall characteristics by MRI and CT imaging: the effect of obesity on laparoscopic approach. *J Reprod Med.* 1992;36:473-476.
3. Phillips JM, Hulka JF, Peterson HB. American Association of Gynecologic Laparoscopists' 1982 membership survey. *J Reprod Med.* 1984;29:592-594.
4. Frenkel Y, Oelsner G, Ben-Baruch G, Menczer J. Major surgical complications of laparoscopy. *Eur J Obstet Gynecol Reprod Biol.* 1981;12:107-111.
5. Chamberlain G, Brown JC, eds. Gynecological laparoscopy: the report of the confidential inquiry into gynaecological laparoscopy. London: Royal College of Obstetricians and Gynaecologists. 1978:114.
6. Mintz M. Risks and prophylaxis in laparoscopy: a survey of 100,000 cases. *J Reprod Med.* 1977;18:269.
7. Jansen FW, Kolkman W, Bakkum E, de Kroon C, Trimbos-Kemper TC, Trimbos JB. Complications of laparoscopy: an inquiry about closed-versus open-entry technique. *Am J Obstet Gynecol.* 2004;190:634-638.
8. Reich H. New techniques in advanced laparoscopic surgery. *Baillieres Clin Obstet Gynaecol.* 1989;3:655-681.
9. Pring CM. Aortic injury using the Hasson trocar: a case report and review of the literature. *Ann R Coll Surg Engl.* 2007 Mar;89(2):W3-W5. Review.
10. Nezhat C, Childers J, Nezhat F, Nezhat CH, Seidman DS. Major retroperitoneal vascular injury during laparoscopic surgery. *Hum Reprod.* 1997 Mar;12(3):480-483.

Case 13

A 32-year-old G0P0 woman complains of painful menses during the last year as well as pelvic nonmenstrual pain and dyspareunia of recent onset. Although she stated that her menarche was at age 13 and her menses were painless and regular, have recently become somewhat irregular. She denies vaginal discharge or prior sexually transmitted disease. Also, she has stopped using any contraceptive method since being married. Her blood pressure is 110/70 mm Hg, heart rate 85 beats/min, and temperature 95°F. Heart and lung examinations are normal. On palpation, she had slight abdominal tenderness at the right iliac fossa, but without guarding. On pelvic examination, a retroverted and displaced uterus seems to move together with a palpable cystic mass of her right adnexa. Her pregnancy test is negative. Her hemoglobulin level is 11 g/dL, leukocyte count 8500/mm^3, and platelet count 230,000/mm^3. Ultrasound examination reveals a smooth 9-cm homogenic hypoechoic cystic mass of the right ovary attached to the posterior surface of a retroverted uterus with a small quantity of free hypodense fluid in the pouch of Douglas.

- ➤ What is the most likely diagnosis?
- ➤ What is your next step?

ANSWERS TO CASE 13: Endometriosis with Ovarian Endometrioma Formation

Summary: This is a 32-year-old nulliparous woman with a history of recent onset of dysmenorrhoea, dyspareunia, nonmenstrual pelvic pain, and perhaps infertility, because she has never become pregnant despite her unprotected sexual intercourse. Her past gynecological and medical history were unremarkable. Complete blood count is within the normal range. Pregnancy test is negative. The right adnexa have a cystic mass on palpation and is attached to the retroverted uterus.

➤ **Most likely diagnosis:** Endometriosis with ovarian endometrioma formation

➤ **Next step:** Laparoscopy

ANALYSIS

Objectives

1. Know the symptoms of endometriosis.
2. Understand the mechanism of the symptoms.
3. Differential diagnosis of endometriomas from other adnexal cystic masses in reproductive aged women.

Considerations

The history of this 32-year-old woman is highly suggestive of endometriosis with concurrent endometrioma formation because dysmenorrhea begins after years of pain-free menses and is gradually accompanied by nonmenstrual pain, dyspareunia, and possible infertility. Proposed mechanisms that explain the pain in patients with endometriosis are the alteration of peritoneal environment due to inflammatory reaction of pelvic peritoneum associated with increased concentration of macrophages, prostaglandins, angiogenesis-promoting substances, and cytokines in the peritoneal fluid. This inflammatory response results in adhesion formation as a sort of healing process, fibrotic thickening of the invaded organs, and collection of shed menstrual blood in endometriotic implants with subsequent painful traction with the physiological movements of tissues. So, in this case the retroverted displacement and attachment of the uterus to the right adnexal mass in conjunction with the absence of previous laparotomies, as well as the negative history of previous pelvic inflammatory disease or vaginal discharge are additional arguments in favor of endometriosis with endometrioma formation. In addition, adhesion formation due to endometriosis appears in the advanced stage of disease and chronic pelvic pain appears later as it progresses. However, either the hostile peritoneal environment and/or the anatomical changes of pelvic structures are often associated with ovarian dysfunction and/or tubal obstruction due to adhesions. These factors, in relation to the use of no contraceptive method, could possibly justify the nulliparity of this woman. Furthermore, ruptured corpus luteum cyst is excluded because this condition is clinically characterized by sudden onset of severe abdominal pain with various degrees of hemoperitoneum. Moreover, the diagnosis of borderline or invasive adnexal mass is quite remote in this case due to the reproductive age of this woman, the protective role of oral contraceptives use in the past, and the ultrasound findings, which are not pathognomonic but strongly indicative of the endometriotic feature of this cyst. Of course, a negative pregnancy test is mandatory in every woman of reproductive age with pelvic pain, adnexal mass, and free fluid in Douglas pouch to exclude ectopic pregnancy. In contrast to postmenopausal women, CA-125 tumor marker cannot provide additional information to ultrasonographic findings as a diagnostic tool for endometriomas. But CA-125 measurements could be useful to detect the recurrence of endometriosis during the posttreatment follow-up period. Finally, laparoscopy has been established as the "gold standard" for definitive visual diagnosis and staging of endometriosis with simultaneously histological confirmation of uncertain lesions and exclusion of rare instances of malignancy.

APPROACH TO Endometriosis With Ovarian Endometrioma Formation

DEFINITIONS

ENDOMETRIOSIS: The presence of functional endometrial glands and stroma outside the uterine cavity that responds to cyclical changes of ovarian steroid hormones. According to epidemiological, surgical, and pathological data, it manifests as peritoneal, ovarian, and deep endometriosis.

PERITONEAL OR SUPERFICIAL ENDOMETRIOSIS: It appears as typical red, black, and white superficial endometrial implants on serosal surface of organs or peritoneum according to the degree of cellular activity and fibrosis. According to its location, it is distinguished in pelvic and extrapelvic endometriosis.

OVARIAN ENDOMETRIOSIS OR ENDOMETRIOMA: It is defined as a pseudocyst formation, with ectopic endometriotic lining within the ovary after invagination of the ovarian cortex. Implantation theory and metaplasia of coelomic epithelium covering the ovary or secondary involvement of functional ovarian cysts (induction theory) have been proposed as possible pathogenetic mechanisms.

DEEP RECTOVAGINAL ENDOMETRIOSIS: It is defined as endometriotic nodular or polypoid mass invading the retroperitoneal space, more than 5 mm underneath the peritoneum. This lesion consists essentially of dense fibrotic tissue, hyperplasia of smooth muscle with active endometrial glands, and scanty stroma. Metaplasia of müllerian remnants into endometriotic glands often involves the rectovaginal septum or secondary infiltration of the pouch of Douglas by peritoneal endometriotic implants.

ADENOMYOSIS: It is defined as the presence of endometrial glands and stroma deep within the myometrium. It is considered as a separate pathological entity as it affects a different population of women and has a different etiology.

CLINICAL APPROACH

Although endometriosis is the second most common gynecological condition, its exact cause and pathogenesis are still controversial. It is estimated that the prevalence of endometriosis in the general population is 7% to 10% with a peak incidence between 35 and 40 years and is associated with pelvic pain and infertility. In women with infertility or pelvic pain, various incidences have been reported, ranging between 20% and 90%. This discrepancy is justified because a significant proportion of affected women are asymptomatic.[1]

Nulliparity, heavy and long menstrual flow, or short cycle length are considered risk factors for retrograde menstruation. A relative risk of 7.2 is found among first-degree relatives as it is inherited in polygenic-multifactorial manner.[1,2]

Extrapelvic endometriosis should be suspected when symptoms of pain or a palpable mass outside the pelvis present a cyclical pattern. Pelvic pain and infertility raise the suspicion for underlying endometriosis, but those symptoms alone do not establish the diagnosis, because there are other gynecological, urological, and gastroenterological conditions that can cause the same symptoms. As a result, there is often a delay in diagnosis of 8 to 12 years. There is no relation between the severity of symptoms and the location or stage of disease. Rectovaginal examination during menstruation is sometimes informative of uterosacral or rectovaginal painful nodules, and lesions of posterior vaginal fornix are visible during speculum inspection.[3]

Transvaginal and transrectal ultrasounds are useful noninvasive diagnostic tools for the diagnosis of ovarian endometriomas and deep infiltrating retroperitoneal nodules but not conclusive. Round-shaped homogenous cyst with low-level echoes, thick capsule with pericystic flow at the level of the ovarian hilus, and scattered vascularity are considered typical sonographic features of endometriomas that differentiated them from corpus luteum or other cysts. Elevated CA-125 may be indicative of advanced stage or recurrence but has no value as a diagnostic tool. MRI and barium enema studies are useful for mapping the extent of deep endometriosis when there is strong clinical suspicion.[2,3]

Laparoscopy is the "gold standard" for the diagnosis and treatment of endometriosis. It facilitates direct visual inspection of endometriotic lesions under magnification and determines the stage of disease, the type, the site, and extent of all lesions and adhesions according to the American Society of Reproductive Medicine classification system (r-AFS). Superficial peritoneal lesions typically have blue-black powder burn appearance and represent advanced, active lesions. Subtle lesions include red early active implants (petechial, vesicular, polypoid, hemorrhagic, red flame-like) and serous or clear vesicles. Moreover, white plaques or scarring, yellow-brown discoloration of the peritoneum, and subovarian adhesions occur in healed and inactive lesions. Neoangiogenesis is observed in active lesions. Laparoscopic features of ovarian endometrioma include (1) ovarian cyst not greater than 12 cm in diameter, (2) adhesions to the pelvic side wall and/or the posterior broad ligament, (3) burns and minute red or blue spots adjacent puckering on the surface, and (4) tarry, thick, chocolate-colored fluid content. Biopsies are recommended only from suspicious areas in peritoneal disease, and should be obtained in all cases of ovarian endometriomas and in deep infiltrating nodules to exclude malignancy. Negative histology is possible in 24% of cases due to the limited experience of the surgeon or pathologist to recognize subtle or atypical endometriotic lesions.[4-8]

The rationale for treatment of endometriosis is to treat symptoms, to remove the lesions, and to prevent recurrences. Considering that endometriosis is a chronic inflammatory disease, NSAIDs are effective in reducing endometriosis-associated pain. In addition, as an oestrogen-dependent disease, suppression of ovarian function or a pseudopregnancy status is induced by oral contraceptives, danazol, gonadotropin-releasing hormone agonists (GnRH-a), progestins, and medroxyprogesterone acetate. All of them are equally effective in pain reduction but with different side effects.[5]

Laparoscopic treatment of endometriosis can be either conservative as in most cases preservation of reproductive function is desirable or radical procedures such as oophorectomy or total abdominal hysterectomy with bilateral salpingo-oophorectomy in refractory severe cases, in which postoperative hormone replacement therapy (HRT) regimen with progestin is necessary.

Laparoscopic excision, electrocoagulation, or laser vaporization are comparable alternatives in the treatment of superficial-peritoneal or serosal endometriosis and should be treated at the same time during diagnostic laparoscopy. However, laparoscopic cystectomy of endometriomas (Figure 13–1), in terms of symptoms recurrence and pregnancy rate, seems to be the method of choice in comparison to laparoscopic electrocoagulation or laser vaporization of the inner cyst lining after one-step procedure or after drainage followed by administration of 12 weeks of GnRH-a in the three-step procedure. However, there is great concern about the impact of excisional methods on ovarian reserve and function due to inadvertent damage to healthy ovarian tissue. Interdisciplinary approach by laparotomy or laparoscopy is applied for excision of rectovaginal

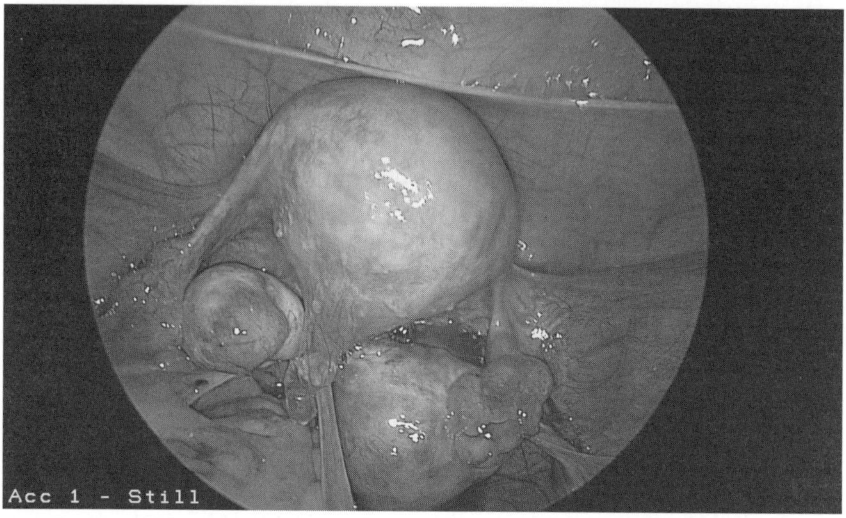

Figure 13–1. Right ovarian endometrioma is seen. Note the adhesions also of the uterus to the cul-de-sac. (*Courtesy of Dr. Cristo Papasakelariou.*)

or rectosigmoidal nodules, but it can be associated with bowel, ureteral perforations, and peritonitis in 2% to 3% of cases though treated by experts. Preoperative hormonal treatment does not improve the success or ease of surgery. Postoperative medical treatment only with GnRH-a for 3 to 6 months achieved greater pain relief scores and fewer recurrences, but it is not recommended in patients with infertility because it prevents pregnancy. Concerning endometriosis-associated fertility, laparoscopic treatment especially in advanced stages improves pregnancy rates, and the highest spontaneous pregnancy rates occur during the first 6 to 12 months after conservative surgery.[7-9]

Comprehension Questions

13.1 A 34-year-old woman is noted to have chronic pelvic pain. The gynecologist has evaluated the patient and on the basis of history does not believe that this patient's symptoms are due to endometriosis. Which of the following is present in this patient that would be *inconsistent* with endometriosis?

A. Parity
B. Short cycles length
C. Early menarche
D. Heavy menstruation

13.2 In a nulliparous woman, unilateral endometrioma should not be treated by

A. Oophorectomy
B. One-step procedure: drainage and electrocoagulation/laser vaporization at the same time
C. Three-step procedure: drainage, GnRH-agonist for 3 months, and then laser vaporization
D. Cystectomy

13.3 Which of the following statements regarding endometriosis is most accurate?

A. Deep endometriosis is typically a straightforward diagnosis by laparoscopy.
B. Endometriosis-related ovarian cancer usually affects older, multiparous women.
C. There is no clear justification to treat minimal endometriosis in women with infertility.
D. Endometriosis once treated surgically has a low risk of recurrence provided all the lesions were excised.

ANSWERS

13.1 **A.** Parity is inversely related to the risk of endometriosis, whereas the other findings are found with endometriosis.

13.2 **D.** Oophorectomy is contraindicated in women of reproductive age if there is no malignancy. However, the best conservative laparoscopic approach in nulliparous women is a controversial issue.

13.3 **C.** There is no proven benefit to treating minimal endometriosis in women with infertility. Deep endometriosis is often not a peritoneal disease and may be difficult to diagnose. Endometriosis associated ovarian cancer typically affects younger, nulliparous women and is usually well differentiated with a good prognosis. Endometriosis has a high recurrence risk approaching 40% in 5 years post therapy.

Clinical Pearls

See Table 1-2 for definition of level of evidence and strength of recommendation

- Peritoneal, ovarian, and deep endometriotic lesions constitute different manifestations of a single disease (Level B).
- Nulliparity, heavy menstruation, short cycle length, and early menarche are considered risk factors for endometriosis (Level B).
- The best means to diagnose peritoneal endometriosis is by direct laparoscopic visualization with histological confirmation where uncertainty persists (Level A).
- Transvaginal ultrasound is the preferred noninvasive diagnostic tool for confirming endometriomas, and MRI can be useful for diagnosing the presence and extent of deep endometriosis (Level B).
- The medical treatment based on induction amenorrhoea to prevent cyclical changes and menstruation and the choice of drug are determined by side effects and cost (Level B).
- Laparoscopy is indicated in all cases with ovarian endometriomas and rectovaginal adenomyotic nodules (Level C).

REFERENCES

1. D'Hooghe T, Hill J. Endometriosis. In: Berek J, ed. *Berek and Novak's Gynaecology*. 14th ed. Philadelphia, PA: Lippincott Williams &Wilkins; 2007:1137-1182.
2. Kennedy S, Bergqvist A, Chapron C, et al. on behalf of the ESHRE Specialist Interest Group for Endometriosis and Endometrium Guideline Development Group. ESHRE guideline for the diagnosis and treatment of endometriosis. *Hum Reprod.* 2005;20(10):2698-2704.
3. Shaw R. Endometriosis. In: Shaw R, Soutter P, Stanton S, eds. *Gynaecology*. 3rd ed. Philadelphia, PA: Churchill Livingstone; 2003:493-510.
4. Arulkumaran S, Brosens I. Endometriosis. *Best Pract Res Clin Obstet Gynaecol.* 2004;18(2):177-371.
5. Pados G, Tsolakidis D, Bontis J. Laparoscopic management of the adnexal mass. *Ann N Y Acad Sci.* 2006;1092:211-228.
6. Catenacci M, Sastry S, Falcone T. Laparoscopic surgery for endometriosis. *Clin Obstet Gynecol.* 2009 Sep;52(3):351-361.
7. Yeung PP Jr, Shwayder J, Pasic RP. Laparoscopic management of endometriosis: comprehensive review of best evidence. *J Minim Invasive Gynecol.* 2009 May-Jun;16(3):269-281.
8. Wykes CB, Clark TJ, Khan KS. Accuracy of laparoscopy in the diagnosis of endometriosis: a systematic quantitative review. *BJOG.* 2004 Nov;111(11):1204-1212.
9. Garry R. The effectiveness of laparoscopic excision of endometriosis. *Curr Opin Obstet Gynecol.* 2004 Aug;16(4):299-303.

Case 14

A 25-year-old G1P1001 woman presents to the emergency room complaining of worsening right lower quadrant pain for approximately 12 hours. The pain started around the umbilicus, then moved to the right lower quadrant region. She reports nausea and vomiting that started approximately 6 hours previously. She denies any vaginal discharge. Her past medical and surgical history is negative. She reports one vaginal delivery without complications. She has been with the same partner for 7 years. The vital signs include temperature 100.6°F, pulse rate 90 beats/min, RR 20 breaths/min, and BP 110/60 mm Hg. On examination, she appears to be in moderate distress. Her abdomen is tender to palpation in the right lower quadrant with guarding and possible rebound tenderness. The pelvic examination is within normal limits. Laboratory evaluation shows a white blood (cell) count (WBC) 15,000/mm^3, urinalysis is negative, and the serum β human chorionic gonadotropin (β-hCG) is negative.

➤ What is the most likely diagnosis?

➤ What radiological imaging should be considered to help confirm the diagnosis?

➤ What is the best treatment for this patient?

ANSWERS TO CASE 14: Laparoscopic Appendectomy

Summary: This is a 25-year-old woman with new-onset, worsening, right lower quadrant pain associated with nausea and vomiting. She has a low-grade fever and the abdomen is tender to palpation on examination. The serum leukocyte count is elevated and the pregnancy test is negative.

➤ **Most likely diagnosis:** Appendicitis.

➤ **Imaging test to help confirm the diagnosis:** Helical CT.

➤ **Best treatment:** The patient should be started on broad-spectrum antibiotics to cover gram-positive and -negative as well as anaerobic bacteria. She should then undergo a laparoscopic appendectomy.

ANALYSIS

Objectives

1. Know the pathophysiology of appendicitis.
2. Know the most common presentation of appendicitis.
3. Know the best diagnostic test for appendicitis.
4. Know the advantages and disadvantages of incidental laparoscopic appendectomy.

Considerations

This is a 25-year-old woman in the reproductive years with the acute onset of right lower quadrant abdominal pain. The pregnancy test is negative. The pelvic examination is unremarkable, which is helpful. The possibility of acute appendicitis, gastroenteritis, ruptured ovarian cyst, atypical pelvic inflammatory disease, or urinary tract infection should be considered. A CT scan of the abdomen and pelvis may be helpful in the diagnosis. General surgery consultation should be considered. If the patient is taken to the OR, the gynecologist should be available to view the pelvis should the patient have a tubal or ovarian pathology.

APPROACH TO Laparoscopic Appendectomy

DEFINITIONS

PSOAS SIGN: Increase in pain in the right lower quadrant of the abdomen as the right leg is extended at the hip when the patient is in the left lateral decubitus position is a positive psoas sign. This is a result of the inflamed appendix irritating the psoas muscle.

ROVSING SIGN: Pain in the right lower quadrant of the abdomen when palpating the left lower quadrant.

OBTURATOR SIGN: Increased pain in the right lower quadrant of the abdomen with passive flexion of the right leg at the hip and knee with internal rotation of the leg is a positive obturator sign. This is a result of the inflamed appendix causing irritation of the obturator muscle.

MCBURNEY POINT: One-third of the distance from the right anterior superior iliac spine to the umbilicus. The inflamed appendiceal serosa causes irritation of the parietal peritoneum at this location, resulting in pain from appendicitis.

ELECTIVE COINCIDENTAL APPENDECTOMY (INCIDENTAL APPENDECTOMY): The removal of a normal appendix at the time of another surgical procedure. This is distinguished from the removal of a normal appendix in a patient who undergoes surgery for right lower quadrant pain.

LAPAROSCOPIC APPENDECTOMY

Background

Appendectomy for acute appendicitis is the most common emergency surgery performed in the United States. Women have a lifetime risk of 7% for having appendicitis, and their overall lifetime risk of undergoing appendectomy is 25%. Women are twice as likely to undergo a negative appendectomy during which a normal appendix is removed for suspected appendicitis as compared to men.[1]

Pathophysiology

Acute appendicitis results from occlusion of the appendiceal lumen in 85% of the cases and from unknown causes in 15% of the cases. Any process that obstructs the drainage of the appendiceal secretions can cause appendicitis.[2] Hyperplasia of lymphoid follicles, fecaliths, intestinal parasites, torsion of the appendiceal artery can all cause obstruction of the appendix.[2,3] The appendix continues to secrete mucus causing increased intraluminal pressure distal to the obstruction. The increased pressure obstructs lymphatic and venous drainage, which causes the appendix to become edematous. Mucosal ulceration allows bacteria to penetrate the wall of the appendix and cause inflammation of the serosa. With continued increase in pressure, blood flow through the appendiceal artery is obstructed; and since there is no collateral circulation, ischemic necrosis and gangrene cause perforation of the appendix. Bacterial contamination from the perforated appendix causes peritonitis. As long as the rupture of the appendix has not occurred at the base, further fecal contamination of the peritoneal cavity is prevented by the primary obstruction. In young healthy patients, the infection can be walled off and contained in an abscess; in females, this may contain the right adnexa.[3]

Signs and Symptoms The clinical diagnosis of acute appendicitis based on a detailed history and physical examination may be unreliable. Women with the clinical diagnosis of acute appendicitis have normal appendixes 22% to 47% of the time.[4] The difficulty in diagnosis is often from the varied presentation of the symptoms. Varied symptoms may be due to pregnancy, atypical location of the appendix, and extremes of age.[5] Women older than 50 often have pathology-like diverticulitis or cancer that is unrelated to the appendix when right lower quadrant pain suggests appendicitis. Elderly patients who have appendicitis may present with vague pain or no pain at all, so the diagnosis may be delayed.[6] The symptoms of acute appendicitis may be similar to gynecologic pathology, so in the female patient, the differential diagnosis of right lower quadrant pain includes acute appendicitis, ovarian cyst rupture, adnexal torsion, ectopic pregnancy, endometriosis, pelvic inflammatory disease, and acute postpartum ovarian vein thrombosis.[4]

The classic symptom sequence is present in approximately 50% of patients.[2] Complaints include vague periumbilical abdominal pain that may localize to the right lower quadrant over McBurney point. This is followed by anorexia, then nausea and vomiting. Low-grade fever is associated with these symptoms.[7] If emesis occurs prior to the pain, the diagnosis of appendicitis may be in doubt.[3] The initial physical examination shows a low-grade fever (approximately 37.8°C [100.04°F]), mild tachycardia, hypoactive bowel sounds, and tenderness to palpation over McBurney point. The psoas, obturator, and Rovsing sign may or may not be present. The progression of inflammation to perforation usually takes 24 to 36 hours. A rigid abdomen with rebound and guarding may indicate a perforated appendix leading to peritonitis. Laboratory data may show a mildly elevated leukocytosis with a left shift.[2]

Imaging

The most frequently used radiographic techniques for the diagnosis of appendicitis include helical CT and ultrasound. Helical CT has a 90% to 100% sensitivity and a 91% to 99% specificity for the diagnosis of acute appendicitis.[5] The procedure is readily available, independent of operator error, and highly accurate. Intravenous contrast can better image a thickened appendix. Periappendiceal inflammation, present in 98% of cases with acute appendicitis, is demonstrated on the helical CT by periappendiceal fluid collection, fat stranding, fascial thickening, and a hazy change in the adjacent mesenteric fat. Appendicolith, periappendiceal phlegmon, or abscess on helical CT is highly suggestive of appendicitis. High-resolution ultrasound with posterior manual compression, color and power Doppler has sensitivity of 75% to 90% and specificity of 86% to 100% in the diagnosis of appendicitis. It is mobile, widely available, relatively inexpensive, and does not use ionizing radiation. Sonography is, however, operator dependent.[8]

Treatment The options for treatment of acute appendicitis include open appendectomy (OA), laparoscopic appendectomy (LA), and nonsurgical therapy. Nonsurgical therapy includes a combination of prolonged antibiotics and close monitoring. Of significance, 40% of patients treated with nonsurgical therapy eventually required surgical therapy.[2] **Consequently, the treatment of choice for acute appendicitis is surgery**. Antibiotic therapy with percutaneous drainage followed by interval appendectomy in 6 to 12 weeks has been used successfully in selected cases of appendiceal perforation and abscess formation.[2]

The choice of surgical approach to appendicitis may depend on the clinical presentation and surgeon's preference.[9] **LA is associated with a higher rate of normal appendices, less advanced appendicitis, and is used in cases where the diagnosis is uncertain.** Conversely, OA is associated with a higher rate of perforated appendicitis, more critically ill patients, and is used in cases of certain diagnosis of appendicitis.[10] Although these associations have been reported in retrospective reviews, randomized controlled trials and meta-analyses report that both LA and OA are effective in treating acute, gangrenous, and perforated appendicitis.[11] Conflicting evidence exists regarding the increased incidence of intra-abdominal abscess formation after LA is performed for a perforated appendix.[4] There is some concern that the pneumoperitoneum required for laparoscopy may spread infected material throughout the peritoneal cavity.[12] Advantages of LA include lower wound infection rates, decreased postoperative pain, and faster return to normal activity. This procedure is both diagnostic and therapeutic.[4,11] LA does increase operative costs and may increase the risk of postoperative abscess. Overall, pregnant women and obese patients seem to gain the most benefit from LA.[2]

LA Technique There are various techniques for performing an LA. The surgery is generally performed under general anesthesia. The patient is supine with both arms tucked close to the body (Figure 14–1). Women are positioned in a modified dorsal lithotomy position to allow for transvaginal uterine manipulation. The surgeon and the assistant stand on the left of the patient while the instrument nurse stands on the right. The video monitor is placed

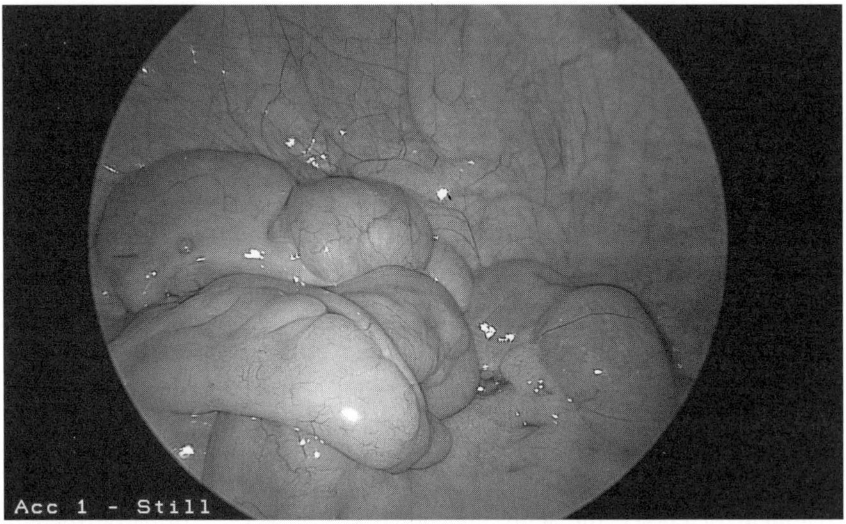

Figure 14–1. Laparoscopic identification of the appendix.

on the right near the patient's feet. The first cannula, 12 to 15 mm, is placed infraumbilically by either an open or closed technique. The abdomen is insufflated with carbon dioxide; the laparoscope is then inserted. After intra-abdominal access has been established, tilting the operating table 15 degrees to the left is usually helpful. A thorough examination of the entire peritoneal cavity is performed to confirm the diagnosis of appendicitis and to evaluate gynecologic pathology. Once the decision has been made to perform the appendectomy, two trocars, 5 and 10 mm, are placed in the right and left lower quadrants. If an additional trocar is needed, it is placed two finger breadths above the symphysis pubis. If fluid or abscess is noted around the cecum or the cul-de-sac, it should be aspirated and sent for Gram stain and culture. The appendix is retracted anteriorly and cephalad with an atraumatic grasper through the lower right trocar to place the mesoappendix on tension. The mesoappendix and the appendicular artery are coagulated from the tip of the appendix down to the base (see Figure 14–2). The base can be secured using various techniques. Two endoloops (1-0 or 2-0 chromic catgut) are used to secure the base of the appendix. The area distal to the ties is milked and the third endoloop is placed 2 to 4 mm distal to the other ties. The appendix is transected between the second and third loops, leaving the appendiceal stump doubly ligated. Staples, clips, stitches, and electrocautery are alternatives to endoloops. The appendix is then removed through the 10-mm trocar. If the appendix is thicker than 10 mm or perforated, a plastic bag is introduced into the abdominal cavity, and the appendix is placed inside it. The bag containing the appendix is removed through the umbilical port. The entire abdominal cavity should be irrigated. The base of the transected margin is

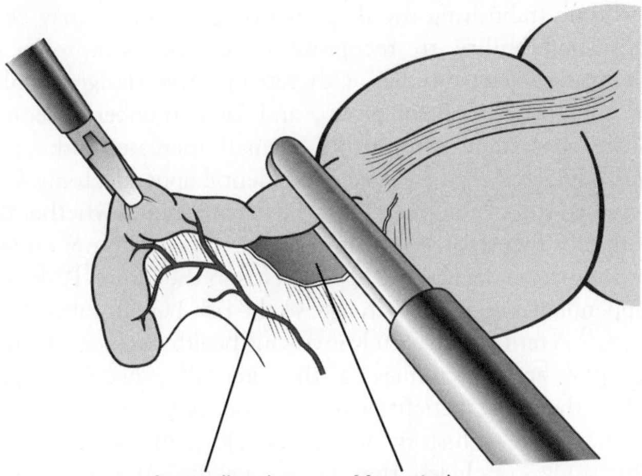

Figure 14–2. A mesenteric window is created, and an endoscopic stapler is used to ligate and divide the appendix.

inspected for hemostasis. Cauterization of the stump is not recommended because this can result in cecal fistula. Invagination of the stump is not necessary. Once satisfactory hemostasis has been achieved, the fascia at the 10-mm or larger trocar sites is reapproximated. All of the skin incisions are then closed. If an appendiceal mass or abscess is encountered, the surgeon must decide whether the appendectomy should continue via laparoscope or if the patient would benefit from conversion to an open appendectomy.[3,4] Contraindications to LA include inflammation of cecum with necrosis or phlegmon, perforation at the base of the appendix, and suspicion of appendiceal malignancy.[4] The pathology and need for antibiotics will determine the hospital stay. Hospitalization is not required for an unruptured appendix and an uncomplicated LA.

Incidental Appendectomy Elective coincidental appendectomy involves the removal of a normal appendix at the time of another surgery unrelated to the pathology of the appendix. Reasons to perform elective coincidental appendectomy are (a) to reduce the risk of mortality and morbidity from appendicitis in the future, including infertility resulting from a perforated appendix; (b) to eliminate undiagnosed incidental pathology in the appendix; and (c) to exclude the appendix from the differential diagnosis when the patient has abdominal or pelvic complaints.[3,13] Other groups that may benefit from this prophylactic procedure include women who may undergo pelvic or abdominal radiation or chemotherapy, women undergoing extensive pelvic or abdominal surgery after which extensive adhesions are anticipated, and patients in whom establishing the diagnosis of appendicitis may be difficult due to diminished ability to recognize or convey symptoms (eg, the developmentally disabled). Studies with retrospective design, small sample size, lack of appropriate control group, and large number of confounding factors indicate that there is probably a small increased risk of nonfatal complications associated with elective coincidental appendectomy. Given this small but increased risk of complications, the debate then is whether the added cost and morbidity incurred at the time of the appendectomy outweigh the cost and morbidity from developing appendicitis in the future. Risks associated with acute appendicitis increase with age, so the risk-benefit ratio change with the patient's age.[13] A retrospective study involving healthy women who underwent open coincidental appendectomies at the time of gynecologic procedures concluded that the most benefit was for patients younger than 35 years, especially if they have a history of PID, pelvic pain, or endometriosis.[3,13] However, the study concluded that under specific clinical circumstances, patients between the age of 35 and 50 may benefit from elective coincidental appendectomy. The data did not support elective coincidental appendectomy in patients older than 50 years. The decision to perform this prophylactic procedure should be based on specific clinical scenarios and after discussion of risks and benefits with the patient.[13]

Comprehension Questions

14.1 A 30-year-old woman presents with periumbilical pain that migrated to the right lower quadrant pain and nausea and vomiting. Which of the following symptoms occur most rarely in a patient with appendicitis?

A. Migration of pain
B. Presence of right lower quadrant pain
C. Nausea
D. Vomiting

14.2 A 44-year-old man is diagnosed with probable acute appendicitis. He is being counseled about the advantages of laparoscopic appendectomy. The patient has been researching about organ injuries with the laparoscope. In counseling the patient, which of the following is the most accurate statement regarding laparoscopic appendectomy?

A. More chance of wound infections
B. More chance of incisional hernia
C. More pain medication needed as outpatient
D. More chance of vascular injury

14.3 A 47-year-old woman undergoes a diagnostic laparoscopy for acute right lower quadrant pain. Upon examination of the abdominal cavity, the appendix appears edematous and there is a purulent collection of fluid in the cul-de-sac. In which of the following circumstances is a laparoscopic appendectomy advisable?

A. Purulent drainage is noted from the tip of the appendix
B. Purulent drainage is noted from the base of the appendix
C. A 3-cm mass is noted at the base of the appendix
D. The cecum is inflamed in appearance

ANSWERS

14.1 **A.** Frequency of common symptoms in appendicitis is abdominal pain approximately 100%, nausea 90%, vomiting 75%, and pain migration 50%.

14.2 **D.** Laparoscopy is associated with a higher risk of vascular injury as compared to open laparotomy due to the insertion of the instruments. Nevertheless, it is associated with decreased wound infection rates, shorter hospitalization, and less postoperative pain.

14.3 **A.** Contraindications to LA include inflammation of cecum with necrosis or phlegmon, perforation at the base of the appendix, and suspicion of appendiceal malignancy.

Clinical Pearls

See Table 1-2 for definition of level of evidence and strength of recommendation

- Only 50% of women will present with the classic symptom sequence: periumbilical pain migration to right lower quadrant pain, associated anorexia and nausea and vomiting, and low-grade fever (Level B).
- Helical CT is 90% to 100% sensitive for the diagnosis of appendicitis (Level B).
- Contraindications to LA include inflammation of cecum with necrosis or phlegmon, perforation at the base of the appendix, and suspicion of appendiceal malignancy (Level B).
- Elective coincidental appendectomy is highly beneficial for patients younger than 35 years and in selected cases for patients between the age of 35 and 50 (Level A).

REFERENCES

1. Flum D, Loepsell T. The clinical and economic correlates of misdiagnosed appendicitis: nationwide analysis. *Arch Surg.* 2002;137:799-804.
2. Shelton T, McKinlay R, Schwartz RW. Acute appendicitis: current diagnosis and treatment. *Curr Surg.* 2003;60(5):502-505.
3. Jarnigan BK. *The Vermiform Appendix in Relation to Gynecology in TeLinde's Operative Gynecology*. 9th ed. Philadelphia, PA: Lippincott, Williams & Wilkins.
4. Kumar R, Erian M, Sinnot S, Knoesen R, Kimble R. Laparoscopic appendectomy in modern gynecology. *J Am Assoc Gynecol Laparosc.* 2002;9(3):252-263.
5. Rao PM, Feltmake CM, Rhea JT, et al. Helical computed tomography in differentiating appendicitis and acute gynecologic conditions. *Obstet Gynecol.* 1999;93(2): 417-421.
6. Velanovich V, Harkabus M, Tapia F, et al. When it's not appendicitis. *Am Surg.* 1998;64:7-11.
7. Hardin DJ Jr. Acute appendicitis: review and update. *Am Fam Phys.* 1999;60: 2027-2034.
8. Birnbaum BA, Wison SR. Appendicitis at the millennium. *Radiology.* 2000;215: 337-348.
9. Cervini P, Smith LC, Urbach DR. The surgeon on call is a strong factor determining the use of a laparoscopic approach for appendectomy. *Surg Endosc.* 2002;16:1774-1777.
10. McGreevy JM, Finlayson SR, Alvarado R, et al. Laparoscopy may be lowering the threshold to operate on patients with suspected appendicitis. *Surg Endosc.* 2002;16:1046-1049.
11. Golub R, Siddiqui F, Pohl D. Laparoscopic versus open appendectomy: a meta-analysis. *J Am Coll Surg.* 1998;186:545-553.
12. Cuschieri A. Appendectomy—laparoscopy or open? *Surg Endosc.* 1997;11:319-320.
13. American College of Obstetricians and Gynecologists. Elective coincidental appendectomy. ACOG Committee Opinion No. 323, 2005.

Case 15

A 29-year-old G4P1021 Hispanic woman at 11 weeks' gestation presents to the ED with a complaint of abdominal pain and vaginal bleeding that began 4 hours ago. She has a past obstetrical history significant for pelvic inflammatory disorder 10 years prior (treated as an outpatient) and two spontaneous first-trimester miscarriages both treated with dilation and curettage of the uterus. The patient reports an uneventful spontaneous vaginal delivery of her son 18 months ago. She has not seen a physician yet for this pregnancy, but reports no abnormalities before this morning. The pain started this morning abruptly along with the vaginal bleeding. She reports dizziness, but denies syncope. Vaginal bleeding is the same as her menses. The vital signs taken at intake in the ED were BP 80/40 mm Hg and HR 110 beats/min. Her hemoglobin level was 6.7 g/dL and quantitative β human chorionic gonadotropin (β-hCG) level was 16,000 mIU/mL. Pelvic transvaginal ultrasound reveals an empty uterine cavity, possible chorionic sac near the cornual region of the uterus, and a moderate amount of free fluid in the cul-de-sac.

- What is the most likely diagnosis?
- What is your next step?
- What interventions are undertaken with this diagnosis?

ANSWER TO CASE 15: Ectopic Pregnancy—Laparotomy

Summary: This is a 29-year-old G4P1021 woman at 11 weeks' gestation with abdominal pain and vaginal bleeding. She is hypotensive, and has ultrasonographic and clinical evidence of an abnormal pregnancy and intra-abdominal hemorrhage.

➤ **Most likely diagnosis:** Ruptured interstitial pregnancy.

➤ **Next step:** Surgical intervention.

➤ **Interventions:** Exploratory laparotomy versus operative laparoscopy.

ANALYSIS

Objectives

1. Be able to diagnose an interstitial pregnancy.
2. Be familiar with management options for interstitial pregnancy.
3. Be familiar with the surgical techniques employed to treat this condition.

Considerations

This is a 29-year-old G4P1021 Hispanic woman at 11 weeks' gestation presents with a complaint of abdominal pain and vaginal bleeding. Suspicion of an abnormal pregnancy was confirmed by pelvic ultrasound. Ultrasound demonstrated an empty uterine cavity and a separate chorionic sac near the cornual region of the uterus. The patient's vital signs and ultrasound finding of free fluid in the posterior cul-de-sac suggest a ruptured ectopic pregnancy.

Initially, it is crucial for the physician to assess the hemodynamic stability of the patient. This is generally screened by orthostatic blood pressure readings, J-V distension, capillary refill time, skin turgor, and laboratory readings. In cases such as acute hemorrhage, the complete blood (cell) count (CBC) level of hemoglobin may not have equilibrated with the actual blood loss amount since the patient is bleeding whole blood. A normal hemoglobin in this patient may be falsely reassuring. Internal bleeding is suggested by the free fluid seen in the posterior cul-de-sac on ultrasound as well as the patient's stating that she feels light-headed. Abdominal examination may reveal tenderness to palpation and rebound tenderness suggestive of peritoneal irritation from blood in the abdominal cavity.

Identifying the location of the pregnancy in a patient presenting with abdominal complaints and a positive pregnancy test is essential. In the case of this patient, a pelvic ultrasound was performed. No intrauterine pregnancy was visualized, and a separate chorionic sac near the cornual region was seen. These findings suggest an abnormal pregnancy in the interstitial region. Ruptured interstitial (cornual) ectopic pregnancy in a patient who demonstrates hemodynamic instability necessitates operative management. The patient's wishes for future fertility must be addressed before proceeding with surgical management. Surgical options include laparoscopic management, but are reserved for the more stable patient and dependent on surgeon experience. Generally, in an unstable patient, time is of the essence and exploratory laparotomy is the method of choice.

APPROACH TO Ectopic Pregnancy—Laparotomy

DEFINITIONS

INTERSTITIAL PREGNANCY: Also known as cornual ectopic pregnancy. Pregnancy implantation within the tubal segment that penetrates the uterine wall.

INTERSTITIAL LINE SIGN: Ultrasonographic term used to describe the visualization of an echogenic line extending from the endometrial cavity into the cornual region and abutting the interstitial mass or gestational sac.

ANGULAR PREGNANCY: Embryo implantation in the lateral angle of the uterine cavity medial to the internal ostium of the fallopian tube.

CLINICAL APPROACH

Interstitial pregnancy (cornual ectopic pregnancy) is an implantation of a pregnancy within the tubal portion piercing the wall of the uterus. This form of ectopic pregnancy accounts for only 2% to 3% of all ectopic locations.[1] Overlooking this form of ectopic pregnancy due to the rarity is dangerous due to the rich arterial blood supply from the ovarian and uterine arteries at this location.

Differentiation between an interstitial and angular pregnancy must be determined. Angular pregnancy occurs when an embryo implants in the lateral angle of the uterine cavity medial to the internal ostium of the fallopian tube. Angular pregnancies may lead to asymmetric and symptomatic enlargement of the uterus that may be misinterpreted as a cornual ectopic pregnancy. Differentiation may further be clouded by a pregnancy in a septated or bicornuate uterus. Laparoscopy may be needed to further evaluate the anatomy.

As compared to other ectopic pregnancies, interstitial pregnancies are associated with a high maternal morbidity. This is largely because presentation of an interstitial pregnancy generally occurs later than a classic ectopic pregnancy, they are difficult to diagnose, and they frequently present with massive intraperitoneal hemorrhage when ruptured. The delayed rupture is due to the denser tissue (myometrium) surrounding the gestation in the interstitium as compared to the thinner tubal segment allowing greater distensibility. Thus, diagnosis generally occurs around 10 to 14 weeks. Rupture may not occur until 16 weeks. Because of the unfortunate location of the interstitial segment of the tube in a richly vascularized location, initial presentation may be profound shock. Vaginal bleeding may be a presenting symptom with or without abdominal pain in women presenting with an unruptured cornual ectopic pregnancy. Evidence of acute-onset abdominal pain combined with a positive pregnancy test necessitates an evaluation of the location of the pregnancy in most instances.[2,3]

Risk factors for interstitial pregnancies are generally the same as for all ectopic pregnancies. These include a history of PID, previous pelvic surgery, previous ectopic pregnancy, and the use of assisted reproductive technology (ART) (ovulation induction or in vitro fertilization). PID and prior pelvic surgery may damage the tubes and create areas of blockage or stricture that may predispose improper implantation.[2,3] A unique risk factor for interstitial implantation is ipsilateral salpingectomy. This occurs in 25% to 37.5% of patients with cornual ectopics.[4]

Diagnosis

Diagnosis of interstitial pregnancies is similar to that with other tubal ectopic pregnancies. Ultrasonographic evidence along with clinical clues often suggests the diagnosis. Symptoms seen include acute abdominal pain, intraperitoneal bleeding, low hematocrit, and a positive pregnancy test. Further testing includes pelvic ultrasound and quantitative β-hCG. Timor-Tritsch et al.[5] described the following transvaginal ultrasound criteria for interstitial pregnancy:

1. An empty uterine cavity
2. A chorionic sac seen separately and measuring less than 1 cm from the most lateral edge of the uterine cavity
3. A thick myometrial layer surrounding the chorionic sac

Specificity for these criteria was 88% to 93%, while sensitivity was only 40%. The "interstitial line sign" has been used by some in diagnosis of cornual ectopic and differentiation from angular pregnancies.[6] This term refers to the visualization of an echogenic line extending from the endometrial cavity into the cornual region and abutting the interstitial mass or gestational sac. Ackerman et al.[7] have claimed 80% sensitivity and 98% specificity, using the "interstitial line sign" in diagnosis of interstitial pregnancy. Tulandi and Al-Jaroudi[8] demonstrated diagnosis by ultrasound in 71.4% of patients.

Treatment Options

Treatment options include medical management and surgical resection (laparoscopic vs laparotomy). The patient's wishes for future childbearing and the amount of damage to the uterus must be taken into account when deciding on a treatment course. First reported by Tanaka et al.[9] and subsequently by Lau and Tulandi,[10] methotrexate has been utilized to treat unruptured interstitial pregnancies. Lau and Tulandi[10] reported an 83% success rate with this modality. Local administration via laparoscopic or hysteroscopic administration versus systemic administration of methotrexate have been described. Success with local administration is reported to be 91% versus 79% for systemic. Treatment with methotrexate also requires a compliant patient who will follow up in order to follow serum β-hCG levels.[11]

Medical management with methotrexate and laparoscopic surgical treatment options have a common variable of a hemodynamically stable patient. Moon et al.[12] demonstrated that vasopressin and electric cauterization methods for bleeding control and cornual incision, encircling suture before evacuation of the conceptus methods, and endoloop before evacuation of the conceptus method, were similar in effectiveness in treating both ruptured and unruptured cornual pregnancies via laparoscopy. Traditional laparoscopic procedures have used cornual excision or a combination of approaches to remove the interstitial pregnancy. Hemostasis may be achieved by ligating the ascending branches of the uterine vessels via intra- or extracorporeal suturing or the gastrointestinal anastomosis (GIA) stapler.

Surgical Therapy

Surgical management of the hemodynamically unstable patient generally requires laparotomy. Two large bore IVs, availability of blood products, and fluid resuscitation are critical. Cornual resection and repair of the defect by laparotomy is the standard conservative surgical procedure for the interstitial pregnancy with an unruptured uterus. Hysterectomy may be necessary if a large uterine rupture has occurred or if the interstitial pregnancy is very large. If the pregnancy is deemed to be so advanced that repair of the cornu would be technically difficult or medically dangerous, hysterectomy may be the only option.[13]

The classic technique for excision of the interstitial pregnancy is via cornual resection and salpingectomy via laparotomy (Figure 15–1). Patients with extensive rupture may require an emergency hysterectomy for definitive treatment. The classic cornual resection would be the treatment of choice in the patient described in the above case presentation. There are numerous ways to perform a cornual resection, but all follow similar principles:

1. The ipsilateral tube must be removed from the mesosalpinx attempting to spare the ovary if possible (see see Figure 15–1, the ectopic is too large and involving the ovary necessitating oophorectomy; in Figure 15–2 and 15–3, the ovary is spared).

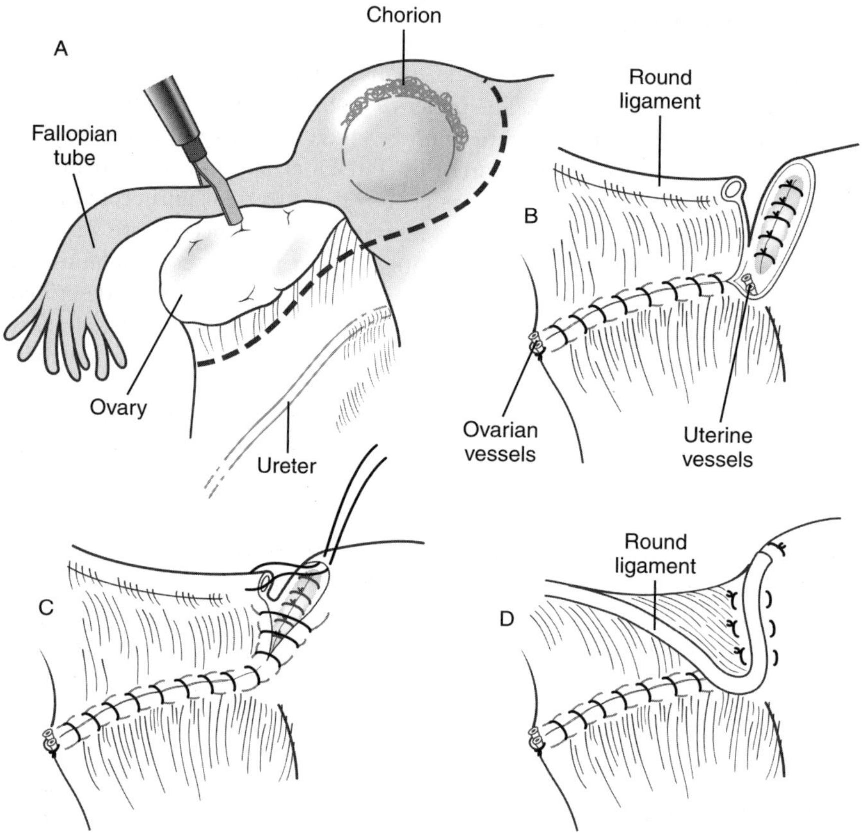

Figure 15–1. Salpingo-oophorectomy with resection of interstitial pregnancy.

2. Vasopressin may or may not be utilized to further help with hemostasis at the cornu.

   A mixture of 20 U of vasopressin with 30 mL of saline injected in the myometrial incision site may be performed.
3. The ascending uterine vessels are ligated nearest the cornu via a figure-of-eight suture (see Figure 15–1B).
4. In a V-shaped incision, the pregnancy is incised and the myometrium is approximated with a figure-of-eight closure utilizing an O delayed absorbable suture. Note the optional placement of a figure-of-eight suture below the cornual pregnancy prior to resection, allowing quick hemostasis when resection performed as suture is already present and only needs to be tied (Figure 15–3).[5] If necessary, the round ligament may be cut and resutured to the cornu and uterine serosa using interrupted sutures. Mattress

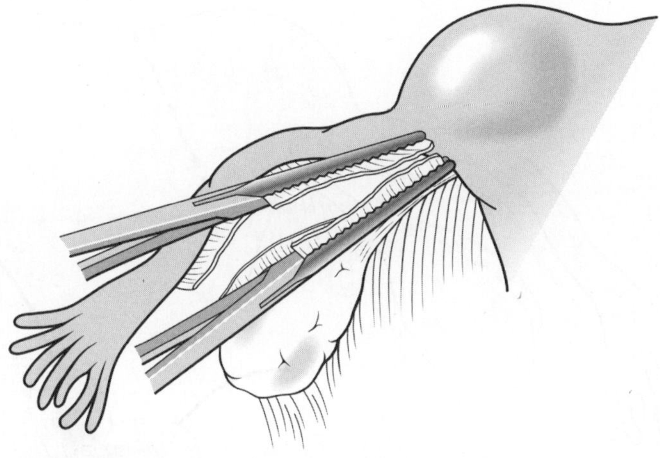

Figure 15–2. Resection tube from mesosalpinx.

sutures are utilized to bring the round and broad ligaments over the incision. Additional interrupted 2-O or 3-O delayed absorbable sutures are then utilized to secure the serosa of the round ligament to the serosa of the uterus. This last maneuver maintains the operative site in a permanent retroperitoneal position (see Figure 15–1C and D).

Uterine rupture is a possibility at the site of a prior interstitial pregnancy. The rates of rupture are currently not established. Maternal mortality rates attributed to cornual ectopic pregnancy are estimated at 2% to 2.5 % with the vast majority due to rupture and extensive hemorrhage. The risk of rupture with a subsequent pregnancy must be discussed with the patient when conservative (ie, nonhysterectomy) methods are employed.[13-15]

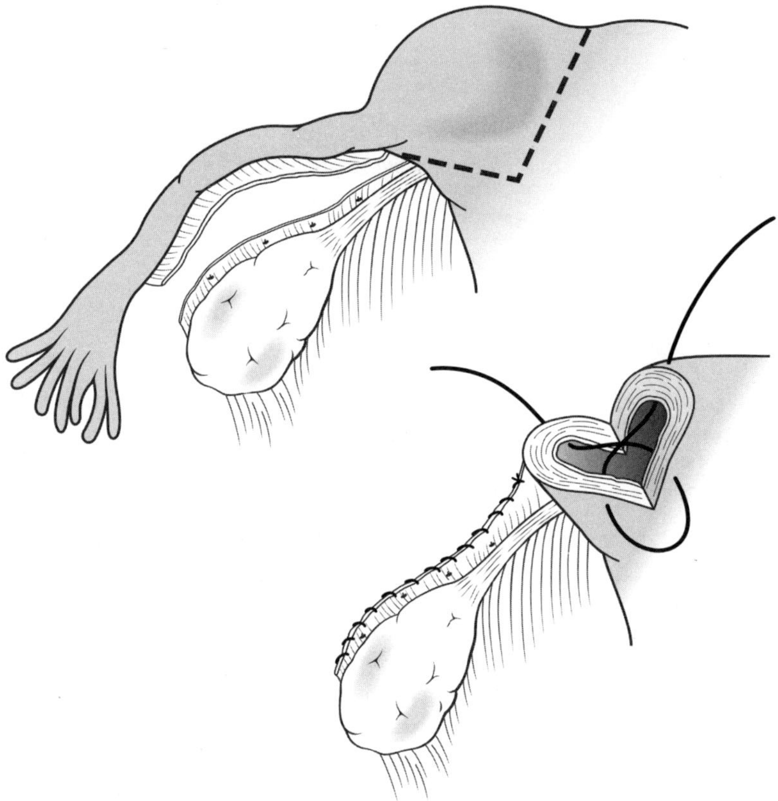

Figure 15–3. Cornual resection preserving the ovary.

Comprehension Questions

15.1 Which patient is most likely to have an interstitial pregnancy?

A. A 22-year-old African American G2P1001 woman at 6 weeks' gestation with a history of *Chlamydia* treated 3 years ago

B. A 30-year-old Hispanic G1P0 woman at 22 weeks' gestation with vaginal spotting

C. A 37-year-old Caucasian G2P1001 woman at 12 weeks' gestation who has undergone ART

D. A 19-year-old Hispanic G2P0101 woman at 15 weeks' gestation with a history of cocaine usage

15.2 A 30-year-old Caucasian G3P1102 woman at 8 weeks' gestation has a transvaginal ultrasound showing evidence of an interstitial pregnancy measuring less than 1.5 cm. She is hemodynamically stable. Which is the best treatment for this patient?
A. Methotrexate
B. Wedge resection of uterus
C. Hysterectomy
D. Diagnostic peritoneal lavage

15.3 In which patient would laparoscopic treatment be a viable option?
A. A 17-year-old G2P0010 woman with sonographic evidence of free fluid in the posterior cul-de-sac and BP of 80/40.
B. A hemodynamically stable 33-year-old G3P0020 woman at 12 weeks' gestation with no evidence of intrauterine pressure (IUP) on ultrasound and a 3-cm cornual gestational sac with a heartbeat.
C. An unstable 27-year-old G2P0100 woman at 10 weeks' gestation who presents with a complaint of syncope and abdominal pain.
D. A 25-year-old G3P1102 woman at 14 weeks' gestation with profuse vaginal bleeding, abdominal pain, and free fluid seen on ultrasound.

15.4 A hypotensive 38-year-old at woman 12 weeks' gestation who has undergone ART presents to the ED with complaints of severe abdominal pain and vaginal bleeding. Exploratory laparotomy shows evidence of rupture of the uterus and extensive hemorrhage. What intervention may be necessary in this patient?
A. Uterine artery embolization
B. Cornual wedge resection
C. Hysterectomy
D. B-Lynch stitch

ANSWERS

15.1 **C.** Assisted reproductive technology has been the latest risk factor for interstitial pregnancies. IVF as well as ovulation induction techniques have been associated with cornual pregnancies. The incidence of heterotopic pregnancy in the ART population has been estimated at 1 in 100. Though controversial, conservative medical and surgical management approaches have been used in small published series; Lau and Tulandi[10] followed nine cases conservatively resulting in two-thirds (six out of nine) of the intrauterine pregnancies delivering at term. Certainly, this should not be viewed as standard treatment, since massive hemorrhage has been described with these ectopic pregnancies. With increasing number of embryos transferred, the rate of interstitial heterotopic pregnancies climbs as well.

15.2 **A.** Methotrexate has been demonstrated as a viable option in the patient without evidence of uterine rupture. Systemic and direct administration via laparoscopy or hysteroscopy of methotrexate has been performed with an overall success rate of 83%. The patient must be counseled about the risks of uterine rupture with subsequent pregnancies if she opts for a conservative approach. Reliability of the patient must also be assessed. The patient must follow up for serial draws of β-hCG levels in order to monitor the response to methotrexate.

15.3 **B.** When choosing the correct surgical modality, the patient must be assessed as a whole. In each case an ectopic pregnancy is suspected. The patient in option B is hemodynamically stable and thus it would be a more suitable option for laparoscopic management. Uterine rupture is a relative contraindication to laparoscopic management. The extent of the rupture site is difficult to assess via ultrasound. Laparoscopic management has been described for cases of minimal rupture at the site of the cornual gestation. As with any surgical technique, the skill of the surgeon and the overall state of the patient must be fully taken into account before a modality is decided upon.

15.4 **C.** Conservative surgical management may be detrimental to the patient if a situation presents with severe uterine rupture. The rich blood supply to the uterus may necessitate removal of the uterus in order to achieve lifesaving hemostasis. The patient from question 15.4 has a uterine rupture and severe hemorrhage. The extent of damage to the uterus must be assessed as well as future childbearing wishes. Hysterectomy is viewed as a last resort, but may be necessary if bleeding is unable to be controlled via conservative efforts. The decision to proceed with laparotomy is the correct choice because of the hemodynamic instability.

Clinical Pearls

(See Table 1-2 for definition of level of evidence and strength of recommendation)

- Methotrexate is an option for management in the appropriately selected patient (Level B).
- Laparoscopic methods are viable options for treatment of both ruptured and unruptured interstitial pregnancies in the hemodynamically stable patient (Level B).
- Uterine rupture is a potential complication for subsequent pregnancies when conservative methods of treatment are utilized (Level C).

REFERENCES

1. Breen JL. A 21-year survey of 654 ectopic pregnancies. *Am J Obstet Gynecol.* 1970;106:1004.
2. Cunningham FG, Leveno KJ, Bloom SL, Gilstrap III LC, Wenstrum KD. Ectopic pregnancy. In: *Williams Obstetrics*. 22nd ed. New York, NY: McGraw-Hill; 2005:253-272.
3. Katz VL, Lentz GM, Lobo RA, Gershenson DM. Ectopic pregnancy. In: *Comprehensive Gynecology*. 5th ed. Philadelphia, PA: Mosby; 2007:389-415.
4. Society for Assisted Reproductive Technology and American Society for Reproductive Medicine. Assisted reproduction technology in the United States: 2000 results generated from the American Society for Reproductive Medicine/Society for Reproductive Technology Registry. *Fertil Steril.* 2004;81:1207.
5. Timor-Tritsch IE, Monteagudi A, Matera C, et al. Sonographic evolution of cornual pregnancies treated without surgery. *Obstet Gynecol.* 1992;79:1044-1049.
6. Auslender R, Arodi J, Pascal B, et al. Interstitial pregnancy: early diagnosis by ultrasonography. *Am J Obstet Gynecol.* 1983;146:717-718.
7. Ackerman TE, Levi CS, Dashfesky SM. Interstitial line: sonographic finding in interstitial (cornual) ectopic pregnancy. *Radiology*. 1993;189:83-87.
8. Tulandi T, Al-Jaroudi D. Interstitial pregnancy: results generated from the Society of Reproductive Surgeons registry. *Obstet Gynecol.* 2004;103:47-50.
9. Tanaka T, Hayashi J, Kutsuzawa T, et al. Treatment of interstitial ectopic pregnancy with methotrexate: report of a successful case. *Fertil Steril.* 1982;37:851-852.
10. Lau S, Tulandi T. Conservative medical and surgical management of interstitial ectopic pregnancy. *Fertil Steril.* 1999;72:207-215.
11. Weissman A, Fishman A. Uterine rupture following conservative surgery for interstitial pregnancy. *Eur J Obstet Gynecol Reprod Biol.* 1992;44:237-239.
12. Moon HS, Choi YJ, Park YH, et al. New simple endoscopic operations for interstitial pregnancies. *Am J Obstet Gynecol.* 2000;182:114-121.
13. Rock J, Jones H. Ectopic pregnancy. In: *Te Linde's Operative Gynecology*. 10th ed. Philadelphia, PA: Lippincott Williams & Wilkins; 2008:798-824.
14. Baggish MS, Karram MM. Surgical management of ectopic pregnancy. In: *Atlas of Pelvic Anatomy and Gynecologic Surgery*. 2nd ed. Philadelphia, PA: Elsevier Saunders; 2006:279-282.
15. Gilstrap III LC, Cunningham FG, Vandorsten JP. Ectopic pregnancy. In: *Operative Obstetrics*. 2nd ed. New York, NY: McGraw-Hill; 2002:355-378.

Case 16

Your patient for surgery is a 40-year-old obese black woman, G2P2002, with increasingly heavy, painful menses and pelvic pressure. She has a long history of symptomatic uterine fibroids which have been treated in the past with gonadotropin-releasing hormone agonists (GnRH-a) and myomectomy. She has also had two cesarean sections and a bilateral tubal ligation. On physical examination, her BMI is 35 kg/m^2. Her uterus was enlarged to 20 weeks' size, irregular, and there was a firm mass protruding into the left adnexa. Pelvic sonography confirmed your suspicion of multiple uterine leiomyomata, one of which is protruding into the left adnexal area.

You have decided to proceed with a total abdominal hysterectomy. A vertical midline incision is used to open the abdomen, and you immediately encounter extensive omental adhesions, involving the abdominal wall, uterus, and bowel. These structures are freed, the uterus is exposed, and a self-retaining retractor is used to provide adequate exposure. The round ligaments are located and transected to expose the retroperitoneal space. The right ureter is easily identified, and you are able to secure the right uterine vasculature without difficulty. The left ureter is more difficult to find and you are never sure it is positively identified because of limited exposure due to the protruding fibroid and increased bleeding on that side.

- ➤ What pre- or intraoperative strategies might have made the operation easier and safer?
- ➤ What can be done to confirm the presence or absence of ureteral injury?
- ➤ What complications could you anticipate in the postoperative period for this patient?

ANSWERS TO CASE 16: Total Abdominal Hysterectomy

Summary: A 40-year-old black woman with multiple abdominal surgeries in the past, a large fibroid uterus, and obesity is taken to the operating room for symptomatic uterine fibroids, which have failed medical management and myomectomy. A leiomyoma is protruding into the left adnexal region, and the left ureter is difficult to identify.

- ➤ **Preoperative strategies:** Pretreatment with GnRH-agonists or antagonists, aromatase inhibitors, or progesterone receptor modulators may be useful.
- ➤ **Intraoperative strategies:** Intraoperative myomectomy, midline vertical abdominal incision, and a large self-retaining retractor.
- ➤ **Strategies to safeguard ureter:** Preoperative placement of a ureteral stent, cystoscopy prior to the completion of the case.
- ➤ **Postoperative complications:** Wound infection, ileus, deep vein thrombosis, atelectasis, blood transfusion, neuropathies.

ANALYSIS

Objectives

1. Describe the common indications for hysterectomy.
2. Describe other surgical approaches to hysterectomy.
3. List the two most common complications of abdominal hysterectomy, and how to avoid them.

Considerations

Our case presents the gynecologic surgeon with several challenges. The size of the patient and the size of the uterus make the procedure more difficult. GnRH-agonists or antagonists, aromatase inhibitors, or progesterone receptor modulators have all been shown to shrink the size of most leiomyomas to some degree. Any decrease in uterine size should make the procedure less difficult and reduce blood loss. The next question would be how to access the abdominal cavity. Depending on the skill and experience of the surgeon, the laparoscopic approach may be feasible, and robotic surgery may be an option if those resources were available. An abdominal hysterectomy, however, would be the classic approach to this patient. A vertical midline incision allows for adequate exposure of the entire abdominal cavity and can easily be extended if necessary. This type of incision also makes lysis of adhesions somewhat easier.

In these cases with a large mass in an obese patient, exposure is critical. Several types of retractors are available to use, depending on the surgeon's preference. The Bookwalter retractor (Codman Raynham, MA) is a large retractor that allows for the placement of multiple blades in almost any position around the incision. This can be immensely helpful. Mobility of the uterus is the next issue that must be resolved. How easy will it be to visualize the structures necessary to successfully and safely complete the operation? At this point, the surgeon must decide whether to reduce the size of the uterus. There are multiple approaches to intraoperative myomectomy, again depending on the surgeon's skill and experience. Once the uterus is mobile enough to expose the pelvic sidewall, the broad ligament can be opened. This allows for entry into the retroperitoneal space, which then allows for identification of the ureter and the uterine blood supply. It also helps in freeing the bladder from the lower uterine segment, especially when the patient has had previous cesarean sections. Using sharp dissection with gentle "push-and-spread" blunt dissection reduces bladder injuries when the bladder is adherent to the lower uterine segment.

Identification of the ureter is essential and should not be too difficult if one has adequate exposure. Preoperative stenting of the ureter has been proposed as a way to help identify the ureter. Lighted stents are also available. There is debate about how useful the stents really are, and their use should be individualized. Opening the retroperitoneal space over the bifurcation of the iliac vessels higher in the pelvis is another way to identify the ureter, especially when dissection lower in the pelvis is difficult or obscured. Assuming that the ureter can be identified, the ovary can be removed if necessary and the uterine arteries skeletonized and ligated. Once the blood supply to the uterus is secured, amputation of the uterine fundus should be considered. This gives the surgeon much better access to the cervix if it is to be removed, or the procedure can be completed if the surgeon has decided to do a subtotal hysterectomy. In those instances of a deep pelvis and a long cervix, a subtotal procedure, if appropriate, can be a wise decision.

Intraoperative cystoscopy should be considered, especially if there is difficulty taking down the bladder flap and identifying the ureter, or there is concern that the ureter may have been injured. If a cystoscope is not available or if you do not routinely do cystoscopy, the dome of the bladder can be opened, the bladder inspected, and the ureters visualized. By giving the patient indigo carmine dye intravenously, you should clearly demonstrate bilateral ureteral patency within about 10 minutes. Two important considerations are to ensure that the patient's volume status is adequate; a patient who has had significant hemorrhage may have decreased urine production and delayed dye in the bladder. Additionally, the surgeon should be prepared to visualize the ureteral openings prior to infusion of the indigo carmine. Once the dye is in the bladder, further evaluation becomes complicated. In other words, the best time to assess ureteral patency is with the first spurts of dye. If ureteral patency is not demonstrated, reexploration of the retroperitoneal space and correction of the problem can be accomplished without having to return the patient to the operating room. The bladder can then be closed in two layers and a Foley catheter left in place for 7 to 10 days. There are several concerns postoperatively for this patient. Obesity puts our patient at increased risk of wound infection, deep vein thrombosis, and postoperative atelectasis. Her intra-abdominal adhesions increase her risk of a small bowel injury, and increased manipulation of the bowel with lysis of the adhesions increases her risk of a postoperative ileus. Her large, myomatous uterus and possible intraoperative myomectomy increase the risk of significant intraoperative blood loss, and may necessitate a blood transfusion. The use of surgical retractors may result in peripheral nerve injuries and subsequent neuropathies.

APPROACH TO
Total Abdominal Hysterectomy

DEFINITIONS

SUBTOTAL HYSTERECTOMY: Removal of the corpus of the uterus from the cervix at or below the level of the internal cervical os.

GNRH-AGONIST: Synthetic compounds which bind to the gonadotropin-releasing hormone receptor in the pituitary gland and cause receptor down-regulation. This suppresses the release of follicle-stimulating hormone (FSH) and luteinizing hormone (LH), thus creating reversible hypogonadism.

AROMATASE INHIBITOR: Compounds that inhibit the action of the aromatase enzyme which converts androgens into estrogens.

BOOKWALTER RETRACTOR: A large versatile self-retaining retractor for abdominal incisions that allows for the use of multiple blade applications.

CLINICAL APPROACH

Hysterectomy is the most common, nonobstetrical surgical procedure performed in the United States, but recently the rate has been declining. The rate has decreased from 5.38/1000 women-years in 2003 to 5.1/1000 women-years in 2004. In 2004, 67.9% of hysterectomies were done by the abdominal approach.[1] This rate varies in different regions of the country but has been fairly consistent for several years. This is in spite of many authors promoting vaginal surgery for the large uterus and advancements in laparoscopic instrumentation and robotics.

The traditional indications for hysterectomy include abnormal uterine bleeding unresponsive to medical management, large pelvic masses, dysmenorrhea unresponsive to conservative therapy, cancerous or precancerous conditions of the pelvic organs, and uterine prolapse. Certain causes of pelvic pain such as chronic pelvic inflammatory disease, pelvic endometriosis, or ectopic pregnancy may be appropriately treated with hysterectomy as well. Of course, other conditions may be present that warrant hysterectomy, thus making clinical judgment and experience important in the management of the individual patient. Uterine fibroids and their associated problems continue to be the most frequent indications for hysterectomy. Recently, there have been several new medical and surgical advances which are effective in treating many of these common gynecologic problems while preserving the uterus. GnRH-a (eg, Leuprolide) have been shown to shrink uterine fibroids and relieve the associated symptoms on a temporary basis.[2] Aromatase inhibitors (eg, letrozole) and progesterone receptor modulators (mifepristone) have also been found to have similar effects. Procedures such as uterine artery embolization, ultrasound myolysis, and hysteroscopic or laparoscopic myomectomy may be effective treatment modalities in selected cases. Patients, however, often request hysterectomy and see it as the permanent solution to their ongoing gynecologic problems. The combination of multiple symptoms, lack of symptom resolution with previous treatment, and a previous history of GnRH-a usage increase the likelihood of the patient eventually having a hysterectomy.[3]

Once the decision for an abdominal hysterectomy has been made, there are many options regarding surgical approach. The surgeon has a choice of the type and location of the abdominal incision. Whatever incision is chosen should allow for adequate exposure of the pelvis. The presence of lateral masses, broad ligament fibroids, or a deep pelvis is especially important to ascertain. In other words, during the preoperative physical examination, the surgeon should carefully assess the patient's pelvis for number, extent, and mobility of the uterus in the pelvis. All too often, the less experienced surgeon merely "traps" the uterus between the two hands to confirm an enlarged uterus. A systematic approach will be rewarded: during vaginal examination, palpation of the anterior lower uterine aspect and cervix for masses and tenderness, then laterally, and then finally posteriorly. A rectovaginal examination should then be performed correlating the findings from the vaginal examination. Mobility of the uterus and masses should be tested. The surgeon should make a mental note of feasibility of elevating the uterus, working around cervical fibroids, and ligating uterine vessels. Palpation of the bony pelvis to determine adequate room is likewise important. If there is no room between the uterus and the pelvic sidewall, assessment for hydronephrosis and possible ureteral compression should be suspected.

Another important consideration of the type of abdominal incision is the need for exposure of the upper abdomen. Any adhesions from the patient's previous surgeries can be addressed. The retroperitoneal space is easily accessible for visualization of the ureter, exposure of the uterine vessels, and development of the bladder flap; unless the patient has had prior extensive retroperitoneal surgery and/or malignancy, this space should be easily accessible. Adnexal or other unexpected abdominal pathology can be thoroughly evaluated and treated. Other gynecologic problems such as pelvic prolapse or stress urinary incontinence may be corrected at the same time. Prophylactic appendectomy or salpingo-oophorectomy is often combined with abdominal hysterectomies. Abdominal hysterectomy is associated with higher complication rates and longer recovery times for the patient.

Vaginal hysterectomy is an underutilized procedure. Many pelvic surgeons use the vaginal approach when the uterus is not too large, sufficiently mobile, and the pathology is benign and confined to the uterus. Difficulty comes with limited descent of the uterus, a small pelvis with limited visibility, or the suspicion of adnexal disease. Laparoscopically assisted vaginal hysterectomy has helped overcome many of these limitations. Vaginal hysterectomy has fewer complications, less blood loss, shorter hospital stays, and is well tolerated by the patient.[4]

The laparoscopic hysterectomy continues to gain favor among pelvic surgeons, and has recently increased in frequency. Improvement in instrumentation and the optics of the laparoscopic cameras, new energy sources, as well as robotic devices have dramatically enhanced the surgeon's armamentarium. This approach allows the pelvic surgeon to visualize the abdominal cavity, treat adnexal disease or other pelvic pathology, and accomplish difficult dissections while maintaining the advantages of minimally invasive surgery. As the skills of the laparoscopic surgeon advance, more hysterectomies that traditionally would have been done abdominally are now being done laparoscopically. In fact, the proportion of abdominal hysterectomies has decreased as a result of these minimally invasive procedures. While laparoscopic surgery is associated with shorter hospital stays and faster patient recovery, it is still more expensive (in most cases) and requires special training and equipment.

In recent years, the supracervical or subtotal hysterectomy is being performed more commonly. Advocates for preservation of the cervix assert that it improves sexual satisfaction and pelvic support. Studies have not shown substantial benefits.[5,6] Many debate the necessity of removing the cervix, especially as our knowledge and treatment of cervical disease changes. It is a valuable technique in difficult cases when there is limited visibility or accessibility to the cervix in a deep pelvis.

Technique

Once the surgeon has opened the abdomen and exposed the pelvic organs, the uterus should be elevated out of the pelvis. This is usually done by grasping the cornual area on each side with a Kocher or Kelly clamp. Care should be taken to use another technique when uterine leiomyomata may make the cornual regions less flexible and more prone to bleeding. The round ligaments are identified and suture ligated with a transfixing stitch. The round ligament is then transected which opens the broad ligament, opening the way into the

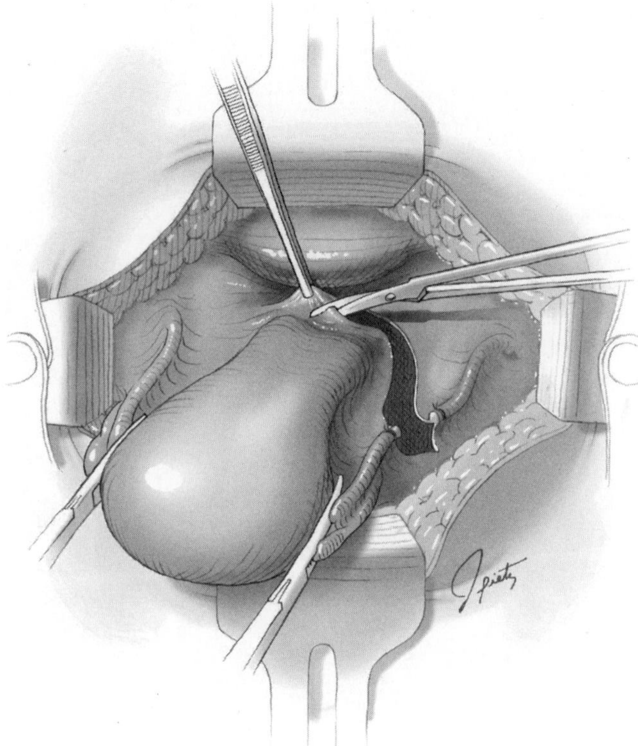

Figure 16–1. Round ligaments are ligated, divided, and anterior leaf of the broad ligament opened. *(Reproduced, with permission, from Schorge JO, Schaffer JI, Halvorson LM, et al.* Williams Gynecology. *New York: McGraw-Hill, 2008:906.)*

retroperitoneal space, and enabling the bladder to be dissected away from the uterus (Figures 16–1 to 16–3). Using Metzenbaum scissors, the anterior leaf of the broad ligament is opened in the direction of the lower uterine segment. Using sharp dissection, the bladder flap is taken off the lower uterine segment and pushed off the cervix. Care should be taken in patients with prior cesareans to avoid injury to the bladder. The posterior leaf of the broad ligament is opened parallel and lateral to the infundibulopelvic ligament. This incision may be extended cephalad as necessary. The retroperitoneal space can be exposed by using blunt and sharp dissection techniques. The ureter should be identified on the medial leaf of the broad ligament. Once the ureter is positively identified, the infundibulopelvic ligament can be isolated and ligated safely. With the retroperitoneal space open, the uterine arteries can be identified and extraneous connective tissue skeletonized of the vessels. Using a Heaney clamp, the uterine arteries are clamped at the junction of the body of the uterus and the cervix. This step is one of the most dangerous regarding possible ureteral injury, and thus, it is critical for the surgeon to have dissected the

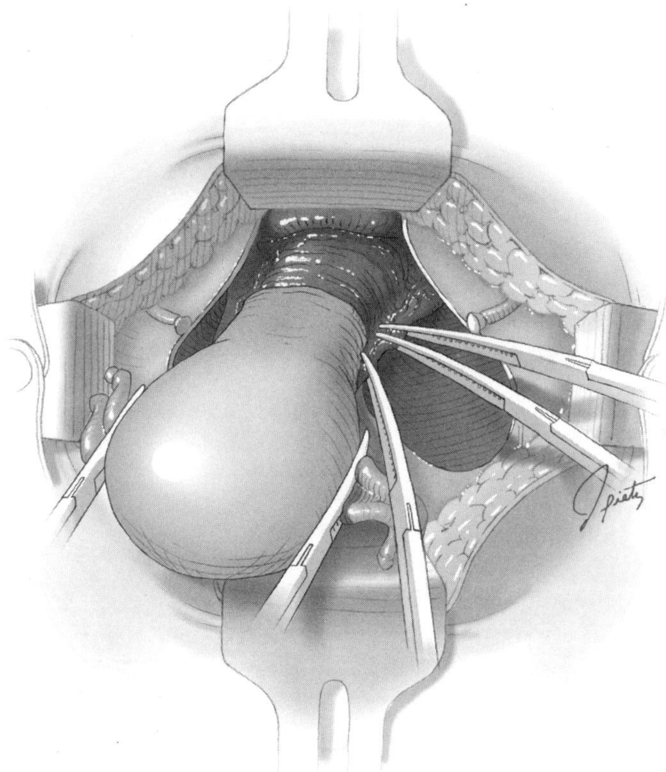

Figure 16–2. Uterine artery is ligated. *(Reproduced, with permission, from Schorge JO, Schaffer JI, Halvorson LM, et al.* Williams Gynecology. *New York: McGraw-Hill, 2008:908.)*

bladder anteriorly and the connective tissue laterally away from the uterus. Assuming that the cervix will be removed, the dissection is carried down the sides of the cervix being sure that the clamp "slides off" the cervix. Keeping the clamp as close to the uterus as possible also reduces the risk of ureteral injury. When the dissection reaches the tip of the cervix, a curved, heavy clamp is used to clamp the uterosacral ligament, any remaining paracervical tissue, and a small part of the upper vagina. Often, cutting this pedicle will open the top of the vagina. With the top of the vagina open, the cervix can be removed from the vagina by using curved Mayo or Jorgenson scissors. Care must be taken not to excise an excessive amount of vaginal tissue with the cervix. The vaginal cuff can then be closed or left open. If the cuff is being closed, this can be accomplished by using interrupted figure-of-eight sutures or a running suture. If the cuff will be left open, the edges of the cuff should be oversewn with a running, interlocking suture. All pedicles should be inspected and hemostasis ensured before closing the abdomen. The choice of suture to be used is probably best

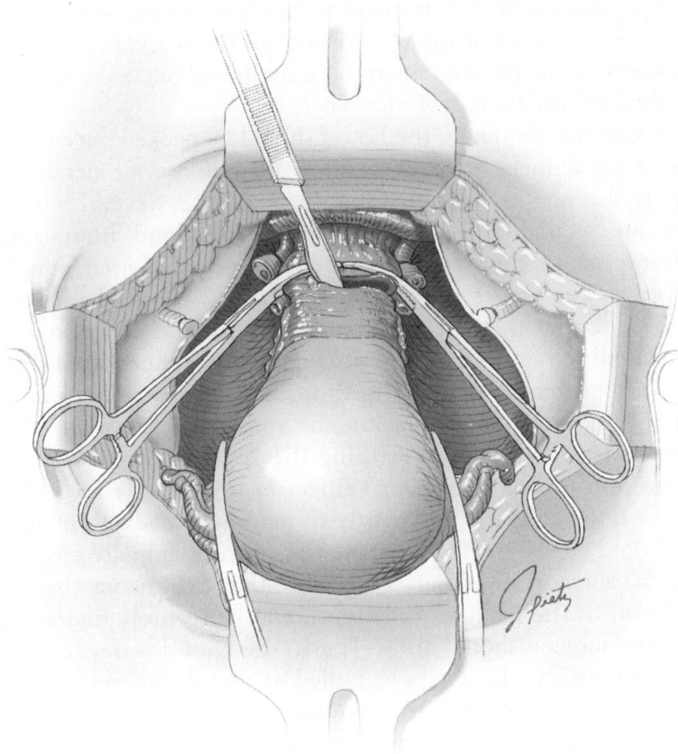

Figure 16–3. After curved clamps are placed on the vagina, the cervix is excised. *(Reproduced, with permission, from Schorge JO, Schaffer JI, Halvorson LM, et al.* Williams Gynecology. *New York: McGraw-Hill, 2008:909.)*

left to the preference of the surgeon. A 0- or 2-0–delayed absorbable suture is most commonly used. Most surgeons prefer to ligate vascular pedicles twice, once with a tie followed by a transfixing suture ligature. The abdominal wall closure can be done with a 0-delayed absorbable suture in an interrupted or running fashion. A locking-type stitch should not be used on the fascia as it may contribute to strangulating the tissue and diminishing the strength of the wound. The skin edges may be approximated with suture or clips.

Measures to Simplify the Surgery

All surgeries are easier when you operate with good assistants and a well-trained operating room team. If special instruments, retractors, suture, or energy sources may be needed, they should be requested prior to starting the operation. All instruments should be in good working order, and the operating room staff should know how to operate all special equipment and/or devices. Adequate exposure is mandatory, and the abdominal incision should provide adequate exposure for you to operate on the expected pathology. While cosmetic concerns are important, they should never compromise your ability to perform the right operation safely.

Once inside the abdomen, the bowel should be packed out of the pelvis. Large moist lap sponges are excellent for this purpose. Proper selection of retractors is also important in maintaining exposure. Several self-retaining retractors are available and each has strengths and limitations. The Bookwalter retractor, however, is an excellent retractor for large incisions in large patients. The blades of all retractors should be checked after placement to be sure that they are not pressing against the abdominal wall; for instance, lateral retractors may impinge on the femoral nerves of the patient leading to a nerve palsy. Also, moist sponges should be used to protect the edges of the incision before placing the retractor blades. All dissection should be done either sharply or using the "push-and-spread" technique. Blunt dissection using the surgeon's finger is a frequently used technique, but must be done carefully and gently to minimize inadvertent injury. All pedicles should be clamped so that the tips of the clamp are clearly visualized, and the surgeon should always be sure that extraneous tissue has not been included in the pedicle. Pedicles should be securely tied with square knots and the surgeon should always "push" the knot down with their index finger. The uterus should always be pulled up and deviated to the opposite side from the operating surgeon when dissecting or placing clamps. When clamping the uterine arteries, the clamp should be placed at a 90-degree angle to the uterus. The pedicle should be cut to the tip of the clamp, but not past.

When suturing these pedicles, the needle must be inserted at the tip of the clamp so that all of the tissue is included in the tie so as not to allow vascular deligation. Again, good hemostasis must be ensured before closing the abdomen. Filling the pelvis with normal saline, then slowly aspirating it out will often allow the surgeon to see small but actively bleeding vessels they might have otherwise missed.

Complications

Total abdominal hysterectomies are associated with more complications than the other routes of removing the uterus. This may be because the more difficult cases are often done abdominally (ie, malignancies). Urinary tract injuries and wound infections are the two most common complications of abdominal hysterectomy. Urinary tract injuries occur in up to 4.8% of cases.[7] Eighty percent of these injuries involve the bladder, especially if the patient has had previous surgery (ie, cesarean sections), radiation, or malignancy.[7] Ureteral injuries occur most commonly as the ureter crosses inferior to the uterine artery. Ureteral injuries are often unrecognized at the time of surgery and are frequently asymptomatic. Risk factors for ureteral injuries include an enlarged uterus, significant adnexal pathology, prior pelvic surgery, and pelvic prolapse. Routine cystoscopy prior to the completion of the procedure has dramatically increased the detection rate of both bladder and ureteral injuries.[8] Wound infections after abdominal hysterectomy occur in 3% to 8% of cases.[7] Risk factors include obesity, diabetes, and length of procedure. Prophylactic antibiotics have been shown to reduce this risk and are recommended for routine use.[9] The use of subcutaneous drains or closure of the subcutaneous space has not been shown to be particularly effective at reducing the rate of subsequent infection.[7,10] Bleeding problems, either intraoperatively or postoperatively, can be significant and may require transfusion. Less common problems arise with postoperative ileus, neuropathies related to the use of surgical retractors, deep vein thromboses (DVT), pulmonary embolus, and incisional hernias. Abdominal hysterectomy is not associated with an increased risk of new-onset urinary incontinence and does not adversely affect sexual satisfaction.[11,12] As mentioned, all patients should receive prophylactic antibiotics prior to the procedure. The patient, in this case, should be evaluated for her risk of DVT. Pelvic surgery is, by itself, a risk factor for DVT, and prophylaxis with graduated compression stockings, sequential compression devices, or medical therapy using either unfractionated heparin or low-molecular-weight heparin is indicated.[13] Other risk factors include obesity, age more than 40 years, smoking, diabetes, cancer, and known thrombophilias. Adequate postoperative pain management is imperative. Patient-controlled analgesia (PCA) pumps allow for more patient control, quicker relief, and less dependence on the nursing staff.

Comprehension Questions

16.1 A total abdominal hysterectomy is performed on a 44-year-old woman with a large uterine fibroid. Postoperatively, the patient complained of the inability to walk. On examination, she had weakness of the right leg and absent right patellar reflexes. Which of the following is the most likely etiology?

A. Ligation of the external iliac artery
B. Nerve compression at the right popliteal region
C. Right lateral retractor impinging on the femoral nerve
D. Injury to the right obturator nerve near the obturator foramen

16.2 A 39-year-old woman is taken to the operating room for an abdominal hysterectomy. The left retroperitoneal space is opened from the round ligament cephalad. Where should the surgeon look for the left ureter?

A. Adjacent to the left lateral pelvic side wall.
B. At the floor of the retroperitoneal space described.
C. Attached to the medial leaflet of the broad ligament.
D. The ureter is not found in this area, and the surgeon should advance the incision higher in the pelvis.

16.3 In performing a hysterectomy, the surgeon dissects the areolar tissue away from the uterine vessels (skeletonization) prior to performing ligation of the vasculature. Which of the following describes the main purpose of the skeletonization process?

A. Allows for less chance of bowel injury
B. Allows for less chance of urinary tract injury
C. Allows for less chance of vascular injury
D. Allows for less chance of nerve injury

ANSWERS

16.1 **C.** In laparotomy surgeries, especially with an abdominal hysterectomy, the lateral retractor blades may impinge on the femoral nerve and cause femoral nerve palsy. The symptoms include decreased strength of the quadriceps, absent patella reflex, and inability to walk. Prevention includes ensuring sufficient padding between the lateral retractor and the lateral side wall, especially with deep retractor blades.

16.2 **C.** The ureter is routinely found adherent to the medial leaflet of the broad ligament upon opening the retroperitoneal space cephalad to the round ligament. If the patient, however, has had prior surgery and the retroperitoneal space has been dissected previously, the ureter may be in other locations.

16.3 **B.** Although the skeletonization process serves multiple purposes, including ensuring a better ligation of the vessels, the main purpose is to release the ureter and bladder from the uterus, thus minimizing the clamps and ligation from injuring those urinary structures.

Clinical Pearls

See Table 1-2 for definition of level of evidence and strength of recommendation

- ➤ The preoperative use of GnRH-a to reduce the size of the uterus may make the surgical procedure easier to perform and reduce blood loss (Level B).
- ➤ The Bookwalter retractor is an excellent retractor to use for surgery on obese patients and large masses (Level C).
- ➤ If the ureter cannot be identified deeper in the pelvis, look for it as it crosses over the common iliac artery (Level C).
- ➤ Postoperative cystoscopy has increased the detection rates of unrecognized bladder and ureteral injuries (Level B).
- ➤ If you are not comfortable with cystoscopy, opening the dome of the bladder allows for visualization of the ureteral orifices with minimal risk to bladder function (Level C).
- ➤ Subtotal hysterectomy should be considered if removing the cervix is difficult (Level C).

REFERENCES

1. Whiteman MK, Hillis SD, Jamieson DJ, et al. Inpatient hysterectomy surveillance in the United States, 2000-2004. *Obstet Gynecol Surv.* 2008 May;63(5):304-305.
2. American College of Obstetricians and Gynecologists. ACOG Practice Bulletin. *Alternatives to Hysterectomy in the Management of Leiomyomas.* Washington, DC. No. 96, August 2008.
3. Learman LA, Kuppermann M, Gates E, Gregorich SE, Lewis J, Washington AE. Predictors of hysterectomy in women with common pelvic problems: a uterine survival analysis. *J Am Coll Surg.* 2007 Apr;204(4).
4. Nieboer TE, Johnson N, Lethaby A, et al. Surgical approach to hysterectomy for benign gynecological disease. *Cochrane Database Syst Rev.* 2006;(3):CD003677.
5. Learman LA, Summitt RL Jr, Varner RE, et al. Total or Supracervical Hysterectomy (TOSH) Research Group. A randomized comparison of total or supracervical hysterectomy: surgical complications and clinical outcomes. *Obstet Gynecol.* 2003 Sep;102(3):453-462.
6. Sokol AI, Green IC. Laparoscopic hysterectomy. *Clin Obstet Gynecol.* 2009 Sep;52(3):304-312.
7. Stany MP, Farley JH. Complications of gynecologic surgery. *Surg Clin North Am.* 2008 Apr;88(2).
8. Ibeanu OA, Chesson RR, Echols KT, Nieves M, Busangu F, Nolan TE. Urinary tract injury during hysterectomy based on universal cystoscopy. *Obstet Gynecol.* 2009 Jan;113(1):6-10.
9. Tanos V, Rojansky N. Prophylactic antibiotics in abdominal hysterectomy. *J Am Coll Surg.* 1994;179:593-600.

10. Cardosi RJ, Drake J, Holmes S, et al. Subcutaneous management of vertical incisions 3 or more centimeters of subcutaneous fat. *Am J Obstet Gynecol.* 2006;195(2):607-614.
11. Gustafsson C, Ekström A, Brismar S, Altman D. Urinary incontinence after hysterectomy—three-year observational study. *Urology*. 2006 Oct 1;68(4):769.
12. Mokate T, Wright C, Mander T. Hysterectomy and sexual function. *J Br Menopause Soc*. 2006 Dec;12(4):153-157.
13. American College of Obstetricians and Gynecologists. ACOG Practice Bulletin. *Prevention of Deep Vein Thrombosis and Pulmonary Embolism*. No. 84, August 2007.

Case 17

A 58-year-old G3P3 Caucasian woman presents to your office complaining that, "I look like I am 6 months pregnant." She gives a 6-month history of early satiety and increasing abdominal girth. She has lost 15 lb (6.8 kg) over the same time period and has noted a change in bowel habits with increasing constipation and diarrhea. She noticed some shortness of breath over the last few weeks. She reports no significant past medical history and has never had surgery. She has always had normal Papanicolaou (Pap) smears and underwent normal physiologic menopause without complications at age 52. She had a mammogram 2 years ago and has never had a colonoscopy. Her family history is noncontributory.

On physical examination, her abdomen is distended and no masses are palpable. She has a positive abdominal fluid wave. Pelvic examination reveals a normal appearing cervix and a palpable mass along the right adnexa that is more prominent on rectovaginal examination. Her stool guaiac is positive.

Her internist ordered a CT scan of the abdomen and pelvis. A large volume of ascites is noted. Additional findings include omental caking and an 8-cm complex mass partially compressing the sigmoid colon.

- What additional evaluation/treatment is needed prior to surgical intervention?
- What is your most likely diagnosis?
- What type of surgery should she undergo?

ANSWERS TO CASE 17: Ovarian Cancer Surgery

Summary: This is a 58-year-old G3P3 woman with a pelvic mass, ascites, weight loss, and bowel symptoms whose most likely diagnosis is ovarian cancer.

- **Additional preoperative evaluation/treatment:** Check complete blood count (CBC), comprehensive metabolic panel, chest x-ray, electrocardiogram (ECG), and cancer antigen 125 (CA-125). Given patient's age and CT findings, she should have a colonoscopy prior to surgical intervention.
- **Most likely diagnosis:** Ovarian cancer.
- **Type of surgery:** She should undergo exploratory laparotomy with the goal of optimal cytoreduction.

ANALYSIS

Objectives

1. Recognize the symptoms of ovarian cancer.
2. Be familiar with requirements of optimal cytoreduction and surgical staging in patients with early- and advanced-stage ovarian cancer.
3. Describe stage I cancer and fertility preservation.
4. Describe tumors of low malignant potential (LMP) and the possible need for staging.
5. Describe the management of adnexal masses during pregnancy.

Considerations

This is a 58-year-old Caucasian G3P3 woman with symptoms suggestive of ovarian cancer. Symptoms associated with ovarian cancer include **pelvic/abdominal pain, urinary urgency, increased abdominal size, and early satiety.**

In the preoperative evaluation, the physician should at a minimum, obtain a CBC, comprehensive metabolic panel, chest x-ray, and ECG for women older than 50 years. Thrombocytosis is seen in 22% of patients with ovarian cancer, which may be associated with advanced-stage disease. Serum electrolytes and liver function tests may identify underlying medical conditions which need correction prior to surgery. A chest x-ray should be performed preoperatively to evaluate for pulmonary metastases and pleural effusions. A screening colonoscopy is an important part of the preoperative evaluation if significant bowel complaints are noted, for example, change in stool caliber or an increase in constipation, or if the physical examination or CT scan suggests the possibility of a primary bowel carcinoma. A **CA-125 level** should be drawn preoperatively to serve as a **baseline** level for **follow-up** if ovarian carcinoma is found.

The goal of cytoreductive surgery is the removal of the maximum amount of tumor possible to enhance the effectiveness of subsequent chemotherapy. Current practice parameters suggest that **optimal cytoreduction** means that there is no residual disease greater than **1 cm (cumulative)**. Primary surgical cytoreduction typically includes a total abdominal hysterectomy, bilateral salpingo-oophorectomy, omentectomy, pelvic and para-aortic lymph node dissection, and resection of any metastatic foci. Cytoreduction surgery may commonly include splenectomy, bowel resection, resection of metastatic peritoneal and diaphragmatic implants, and, rarely, liver resection and cholecystectomy.[1-3] Optimal cytoreduction may not be feasible in patients with extra-abdominal metastases or with extensive disease in the hepatic parenchyma or porta hepatis, along the root of the small bowel mesentery, or in patients with bulky suprarenal lymphatic disease.[4] Preoperative imaging may assist in the decision to proceed with primary surgery or neoadjuvant chemotherapy.

APPROACH TO Suspected Ovarian Cancer

DEFINITIONS

CYTOREDUCTIVE SURGERY: The surgical process by which as much of the bulk of malignant tissue as possible is removed. Debulking is considered optimal when the largest residual tumor mass is less than 1 cm.

CANCER ANTIGEN 125: A protein that is found on the surface of most epithelial ovarian cancer cells, as well as peritoneal and fallopian tube carcinomas. An elevated serum level may indicate possible ovarian malignancy although in a premenopausal woman, there are conditions that can falsely elevate the CA-125 such as endometriosis, pregnancy, uterine fibroids, or pelvic inflammatory disease. A level exceeding 35 mcg/mL is considered elevated.

INTRAPERITONEAL CHEMOTHERAPY: Chemotherapy administered directly into the peritoneal cavity rather than intravenously.

NEOADJUVANT CHEMOTHERAPY: The use of chemotherapy prior to surgery to chemically debulk the cancer and make subsequent surgery less complicated and increase the chance of optimal cytoreduction. However, whether or not neoadjuvant chemotherapy improves overall survival is still controversial.

CLINICAL APPROACH

Most patients with ovarian cancer will present with advanced-stage disease, as currently, there is no proven way to detect early disease. Many patients present with pelvic or abdominal pain, early satiety, and increased abdominal girth for several months preceding diagnosis. A recent study showed that when affected women were carefully questioned, many of them reported having the above symptoms for at least 12 days out of each month during the 12 months prior to diagnosis: 60% of those with early-stage invasive disease and 79% of those with advanced-stage invasive disease. While all of these symptoms are nonspecific when they occur with increasing frequency and severity, they merit an evaluation for possible ovarian cancer.[5]

Etiology

Epidemiologic association with increased risk of ovarian cancer includes early menarche, late menopause, low parity, infertility, the use of perineal talc, and consumption of galactose. The use of oral contraceptives for at least 5 years and history of a tubal ligation are associated with a decreased risk. The use of fertility-enhancing medications has not been definitively associated with an increased risk.

Hereditary ovarian cancer is associated with *BRCA1* gene mutations, located on chromosome 17. The risk to develop ovarian cancer can be as high as 28% to 44% in patients from these high-risk families. Another gene, *BRCA2*, located on chromosome 13, is associated with a smaller proportion of ovarian cancers. The risk of development of ovarian cancer for *BRCA2* mutation carriers approaches 27%.[6] A third important syndrome is the Lynch syndrome, also known as hereditary nonpolyposis colon cancer syndrome (HNPCC). Patients with Lynch syndrome have a higher-than-expected risk to develop either endometrial and ovarian cancers or colon cancer. Thus, affected patients with a strong family history of ovarian or breast cancer should undergo genetic counseling and testing. Those found to have a deleterious mutation may choose to reduce their risk for developing cancer by undergoing prophylactic salpingo-oophorectomy after completion of childbearing. Patients who desire to retain their childbearing potential may opt to take birth control pills, which decreases the risk of ovarian cancer.

Diagnosis

The diagnosis of ovarian cancer is ideally made by obtaining tissue for histologic examination (see Figure 17–1 in a patient who presented with an adnexal mass undergoing laparoscopy). Although surgical evaluation for a persistent adnexal mass is preferred, there are clinical scenarios that may contraindicate surgery. For example, patients with multiple medical problems deemed unfit for cytoreduction surgery may opt to undergo needle biopsy for tissue diagnosis, thoracentesis, or paracentesis for cytologic diagnosis. Subsequently, these patients may be considered for neoadjuvant chemotherapy if cancer is diagnosed.

Patients diagnosed with apparent **Stage I (no obvious metastatic cancer outside of the ovary)** invasive ovarian carcinoma need **comprehensive surgical staging** as the risk of undetected metastatic disease is high. Comprehensive surgical staging includes hysterectomy with bilateral salpingo-oophorectomy,

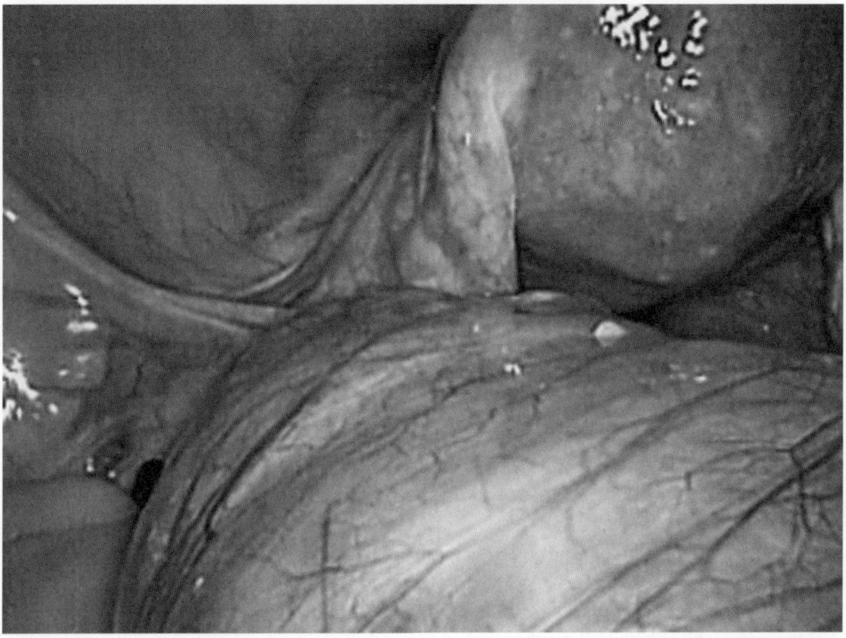

Figure 17–1. A large cystic ovarian mass is noted on laparoscopy. *(Courtesy of Dr. Cristo Papasakelariou.)*

omentectomy, and pelvic and para-aortic lymphadenectomy. A biopsy is done to evaluate any clinically suspicious area in the abdominal cavity. If no abnormality is readily visible, random biopsies are taken **from the bladder peritoneum, bilateral pelvic sidewall, posterior cul-de-sac, bilateral paracolic gutters, and from each side of the undersurface of the diaphragm**. Collection of peritoneal washings for cytologic examination is also done.

Early Cancer in Women Desiring Fertility Patients with early-stage ovarian cancer who desire future fertility present a unique group of patients for the gynecologic oncologist. A conservative approach, preserving the uterus and contralateral ovary, may be used if the likelihood of cure is not compromised while preserving reproductive potential. Comprehensive surgical staging in this group of patients is of utmost import. As a definitive diagnosis based on frozen section diagnosis may be difficult, these patients accept the risk that further surgical procedures may be necessary based on final histologic diagnosis. Generally, these patients may opt to undergo hysterectomy and removal of the contralateral ovary at the completion of childbearing.[7,8]

Low Malignant Potential Patients with a low malignant potential (LMP) or borderline tumor have a much better prognosis than patients with invasive ovarian cancers. Surgical staging is important for these patients because **5% of patients with borderline tumors diagnosed on frozen section analysis**

Table 17–1 FIGO STAGING FOR PRIMARY OVARIAN CANCER

Stage I: Limited to ovaries

Stage IA: Limited to one ovary, no tumor on external surface, capsule intact.

Stage IB: Limited to both ovaries, no tumor on external surface, capsule intact.

Stage IC: Tumor stage IA or IB but with tumor on the surface of one or both ovaries or capsule rupture or ascites positive for malignancy or with positive peritoneal washings.

Stage II: Involving one or both ovaries, limited to pelvis

Stage IIA: Extension or metastases to uterus and/or fallopian tubes.

Stage IIB: Extension to other pelvic tissue.

Stage IIC: Tumor either stage IIA or IIB but with tumor on the surface of one or both ovaries or capsule rupture or ascites positive for malignancy or with positive peritoneal washings.

Stage III: Extension beyond true pelvis

Stage IIIA: Involving one or both ovaries grossly limited to pelvis with negative nodes but histologically confirmed microscopic seeding of abdominal peritoneal surfaces. Negative nodes.

Stage IIIB: Involving one or both ovaries with histologically confirmed implants of abdominal peritoneal surfaces, none greater than 2 cm. Negative nodes.

Stage IIIC: Abdominal implants greater than 2 cm in diameter and/or positive retroperitoneal or inguinal nodes.

Stage IV: Distant metastases

If pleural effusion is present, cytologic diagnosis is necessary for a patient to be staged as having stage IV disease. Parenchymal disease is also allotted to this stage. Extraperitoneal disease is also included in stage IV.

Abbreviation: FIGO, International Federation of Gynecology and Obstetrics.

may have true invasive carcinoma upon final pathologic diagnosis. However, patients who have a final pathologic diagnosis of low malignant potential have an excellent 5-year survival rate of 99% for stage I and 92% for stages II and III (see Table 17–1 for ovarian cancer staging). Even for patients with advanced-stage disease, adjuvant therapy is not recommended because it has not been shown to improve survival. Approximately 10% of patients will develop recurrent disease, which is often managed by repeat surgical removal of recurrent lesions with careful pathologic evaluation for progression to invasive carcinoma.[9,10]

Ovarian Cancer in Pregnancy Patients diagnosed during the first trimester of pregnancy with an adnexal mass, measuring 6 cm or greater, merit close observation. Most of these masses will resolve by the second trimester. However, up to 28% of patients with a persistent mass may develop acute symptoms, necessitating emergent surgery. Thus, a reasonable management schema is to surgically evaluate persistent masses between 15 and 19 weeks' of gestation. Among patients who undergo surgery during pregnancy, common findings are a dermoid cyst or serous cystadenoma; the chance of finding a malignant tumor is low, usually less than 5%. Waiting beyond 23 weeks increases the risk of adverse pregnancy outcomes, including preterm delivery. The decision to perform either laparoscopic or open surgery during pregnancy depends on the individual patient's clinical situation and the ability of her surgeon.[11]

Treatment

The initial treatment for ovarian cancer is optimal cytoreduction as survival is clearly improved with lower volume of residual disease. This step cannot be overemphasized, and meticulous care and sufficient time should be devoted to the removal of cancer to maximize the patient's outcome. After maximal cytoreduction, adjuvant chemotherapy with a platinum-based regimen is the standard. **Intraperitoneal chemotherapy** has recently been shown to improve median overall survival when compared to intravenous chemotherapy in advanced-stage ovarian cancer patients. In this trial conducted by the Gynecologic Oncology Group (2006), patients received IV paclitaxel (135 mg/m^2) over 24 hours, then intraperitoneal cisplatin (100 mg/m^2) on day 2 and intraperitoneal paclitaxel (60 mg/m^2) on day 8 every 3 weeks for six cycles. Although only 42% of patients were able to complete all six cycles of intraperitoneal chemotherapy due to complications, the intraperitoneal chemotherapy group had a 16-month increase in median overall survival. Patients undergoing intraperitoneal therapy reported a decreased quality of life when compared to patients undergoing conventional intravenous chemotherapy, but these differences equalized at 1 year following treatment. For patients who are not ideal candidates for intraperitoneal chemotherapy, chemotherapy with intravenous carboplatin (starting dose area under the curve [AUC] = 5-6 mg/mL • min) and paclitaxel (175 mg/m^2) every 3 weeks for six cycles is given.[12]

Surgical Approach

Surgery for ovarian cancer is almost universally approached through a vertical skin incision, whose length may be extended as the need arises. After entry into the abdomen, peritoneal washings are obtained and sent for cytologic evaluation. If ascites is present, this is collected and sent in lieu of washings. Systematic exploration of the abdominal cavity is performed to evaluate the extent of disease and the plan for resection of disease. Careful assessment is important for prognostic purposes, plan for the surgical resection, and later consideration for adjuvant therapy. In addition to evaluation of the pelvic organs, particular attention is paid to the surfaces of the diaphragm bilaterally, the mesentery of the small bowel, and the retroperitoneal lymphatic nodes.

For patients not interested in future fertility, surgery includes removal of the uterus, bilateral tubes and ovaries, omentum, and pelvic and para-aortic lymph nodes. For patients with widespread peritoneal metastases, removal of metastatic disease is achieved to enable optimal cytoreduction (largest residual disease < 1 cm). Commonly, the sigmoid colon and ovarian masses are coalesced into one large tumor mass for which surgical planes are not found. In this case, a retroperitoneal approach to remove en bloc all affected organs is taken as the planes of dissection are often still preserved in this area despite massive intra-abdominal disease.

The omentum is often infiltrated and thickened with tumor. This "omental cake" can be dissected from the underlying transverse colon and stomach and removed. Bowel resection and reanastomosis are done to enable optimal cytoreduction. Disease on peritoneal surfaces may be removed by a technique referred to as "peritoneal stripping." This stripping technique may be done also for tumor plaques on the diaphragm in which case inadvertent entry into the thoracic cavity and resultant pneumothorax is an uncommon, but not rare, complication.

Lymphadenectomy is performed for staging from the level of the renal veins, past the bifurcation of the aorta and iliac vessels and until the circumflex vein as the vessels enter the inguinal canal. Enlarged nodes are removed as part of cytoreduction. Often, identifying the avascular areas of the pelvis, for example, the pararectal and paravesical spaces, makes surgery easier. Identifying the course of the ureter is important to avoid injury, especially when there is significant disease distorting pelvic anatomy.

At the end of the surgery, the abdomen is closed using a mass closure, such as the Smead-Jones technique or its various modifications. The strength of the closure is critical due to the patient likely having recurrence of ascites, and possible delayed wound healing such as due to malnutrition. Good technique is important to prevent infectious or dehiscence wound complications that may delay adjuvant chemotherapy.

Complications

When operating in the deep pelvis, injury to vascular structures and massive blood loss are possible. In anticipation of blood loss and need for transfusion, a type and cross match should be done prior to surgery. The planned procedure is discussed with the anesthesiologist so that adequate lines and monitoring equipment are available for emergent use. Intraoperatively, if a vessel injury occurs, pressure is quickly applied with either a sponge stick or the surgeon's hand. Subsequently, a clamp may be used to obtain hemostasis and the vessel repaired.

Entry into the intestinal tract is a common occurrence, either intentionally or inadvertently, as part of surgery for ovarian cancer. Prompt recognition of inadvertent entry is the key to prevention of further complications, including abscess and fistula formation. Serosal tears and small luminal entry are easily repaired with sutures. Occasionally, larger injury may necessitate resection and reanastomosis of the normal bowel segments.

Ureteral injury is best avoided by tracing the normal course of the ureters in the retroperitoneal space within the medial leaf of the broad ligament. For patients with distorted retroperitoneal anatomy (eg, patients with previous retroperitoneal dissection, severe endometriosis, or renal anomalies), preoperative ureteral stenting may assist the surgeon by allowing intraoperative palpation of the course of the ureters when visualization is impossible. Obvious injury is repaired intraoperatively. However, simple ureteral stenting will allow most small injuries to heal spontaneously. Occasionally, late injury due to devascularization of the ureters may not present until more than 1 week after surgery.

The risk of postoperative complications increases with the extent of surgery and the comorbidities of the patient. Fever and ileus are frequent occurrences, as are urinary tract and wound complications. Anemia is common, both from the disease process and surgical blood loss. Blood loss greater than 1 L occurs in as many as 20% of patients.

Thromboembolic disease is a common complication of surgery. Postoperative ovarian cancer patients have all three characteristics identified as Virchow triad: hypercoagulability due to the cancer, vessel wall injury, and stasis from the surgical procedure itself. Pre- and postoperative DVT prophylaxis is critically important. There are many published guidelines for the use of sequential compression devices and heparin, both unfractionated and low-molecular weight. For the postoperative cancer patients, heparin in the immediate postoperative period is preferred. Extended thromboprophylaxis after hospital discharge is recommended in selected high-risk patients, for example, those with past history of DVT or a hypercoagulable state.[13]

Splenectomy is often part of cytoreduction for disease in the upper abdomen. Complications include pancreatic injury and pancreatic pseudocyst formation as the spleen lies in proximity to the pancreas. Most patients will also have a transient leukocytosis and thrombocytosis. Ideally, 14 days prior to a planned splenectomy, the patient will undergo preoperative immunization for *Haemophilus influenzae*, *Streptococcus pneumoniae*, and *Neisseria meningitidis* as asplenic patients have increased risk of infection from these encapsulated organisms. Postoperative immunization may also be done 14 days after surgery.[14]

Comprehension Questions

17.1 A 25-year-old nulligravida woman undergoes exploratory laparotomy and left salpingo-oophorectomy for an adnexal mass. Frozen section analysis shows a borderline serous tumor. The rest of the abdomen and pelvis is grossly normal. Which of the following is an appropriate intraoperative management?

A. Close the abdomen as she is interested in fertility and await final histologic diagnosis.
B. Proceed with total abdominal hysterectomy and remove the contralateral tube and ovary.
C. Proceed with surgical staging without removing the uterus and contralateral ovary.
D. Biopsy the contralateral ovary and remove the ovary if abnormal.

17.2 Which of the following statements is correct for a patient who has a *BRCA1* mutation?

A. Prophylactic bilateral salpingo-oophorectomy is indicated after completion of childbearing.
B. The patient has an 80% lifetime risk of developing ovarian cancer.
C. If the patient is interested in delaying future fertility, oral contraceptive usage may increase her risk of developing ovarian cancer.
D. She has a mutation on chromosome 11.

17.3 A 21-year-old at 9 weeks' of gestation presents for her first prenatal examination. You diagnose an adnexal mass measuring 6 cm with complex features. She is completely asymptomatic. Which of the following is an appropriate management for this patient?

A. Expectant management with serial ultrasounds.
B. Immediate laparotomy and unilateral salpingo-oophorectomy.
C. No further evaluation; the adnexal mass is most likely a corpus luteum and should resolve.
D. Immediate laparoscopic evaluation with plans for conversion to laparotomy if a cancer is suspected.

17.4 A 22-year-old G0 woman recently had surgery for a left adnexal mass and underwent a unilateral salpingo-oophorectomy. The other ovary appeared normal during the case. Final pathology revealed a serous tumor of low malignant potential. What is the next management step?

A. Immediate exploratory laparotomy and staging.
B. Immediate operative laparoscopy with staging.
C. Observation and close follow-up.
D. Immediate exploratory laparotomy with a total abdominal hysterectomy and removal of contralateral adnexa.

ANSWERS

17.1 **C.** Surgical staging is appropriate as a frozen section diagnosis of a borderline (LMP) tumor carries approximately 5% risk of upstaging to an invasive carcinoma on final histologic examination. Random biopsy of a grossly normal contralateral ovary is not indicated because it is unlikely to find microscopic foci of tumor, but may lead to complications such as bleeding, necessitating removal of a normal ovary. Removal of the uterus or the remaining ovary is not indicated if the patient is interested in future fertility.

17.2 **B.** The *BRCA1* mutation is an autosomal dominant mutation located on chromosome 17. This mutation confers up to an 80% lifetime risk of development of breast cancer and a 28% to 44% lifetime risk of developing ovarian cancer. Current recommendations include the use of oral contraceptives for women who are interested in future fertility to decrease the risk of developing ovarian cancer, and prophylactic bilateral salpingo-oophorectomy after completion of childbearing. Other recommendations for carriers include increased breast surveillance and gynecologic surveillance of the ovaries with serial ultrasounds and measurement of CA-125. Even after prophylactic oophorectomy, there is a risk of developing peritoneal carcinoma; thus, continued gynecologic surveillance is mandatory.

17.3 **A.** A pregnant patient with an asymptomatic adnexal mass needs follow-up. This is most easily done with serial ultrasounds. Immediate surgical evaluation is not indicated unless the patient is symptomatic. If the mass persists at 15 to 19 weeks' gestation, surgical evaluation either with laparoscopy or laparotomy for a mass greater than 6 cm is reasonable even if the patient is asymptomatic. With a large mass, there is a risk of torsion and acute pain later in pregnancy, which may lead to adverse pregnancy outcomes.

17.4 **C.** Recent studies have shown that survival and outcome for patients with low malignant potential tumors of the ovary are not dependent on surgical staging. As she has not completed childbearing, she needs observation and close follow-up but does not require repeat surgery for staging.

Clinical Pearls

See Table 1-2 for definition of level of evidence and strength of recommendation

- Patients who have a strong family history of breast and/or ovarian cancer should undergo genetic counseling and possible testing for *BRCA1* and *BRCA2*. Risk-reducing salpingo-oophorectomy should be offered to these patients once they have completed childbearing (Level A).
- The goal of surgical staging is to leave minimal disease residual. Optimal cytoreduction means that there is no residual cancer mass of larger than 1 cm (Level A).
- Adjuvant therapy with intraperitoneal chemotherapy has recently been shown to increase survival in patients with ovarian cancer (Level A).
- Patients who present with less than a 1-year history of pelvic/abdominal pain, urinary urgency, and early satiety occurring more than 12 d/mo merit an evaluation for ovarian cancer (Level B).
- Consider surgery for pregnant patients with growing or persistent adnexal masses of larger than 6 cm at 15 to 19 weeks (Level C).

REFERENCES

1. Chen LM, Leuchter RS, Lagasse LD. Splenectomy and surgical cytoreduction for ovarian cancer. *Gynecol Oncol.* 2000;77:362-368.
2. Eisenhauer EL, Abu-Rustum NR, Sonoda Y, et al. The addition of extensive upper abdominal surgery to achieve optimal cytoreduction improves survival in patients with Stage IIIC-IV epithelial ovarian cancer. *Gynecol Oncol.* 2006;103:1083-1090.
3. Eisenkop SM, Spirtos NM, Lin WC. Splenectomy in the context of primary cytoreductive operations for advanced epithelial ovarian cancer. *Gynecol Oncol.* 2006;100:344-348.
4. Chi DS, Eisenhauer DL, Lang J, et al. What is the optimal goal of primary cytoreductive surgery for bulky stage IIIC epithelial ovarian carcinoma? *Gynecol Oncol.* 2006;103:559-564.
5. Goff BA, Mandel LS, Drescher CW, et al. Development of an ovarian cancer symptom index: possibilities for earlier detection. *Cancer.* 2007;109:221-227.
6. King MC, Marks JH, Mandell JB for the New York Breast Cancer Study Group. Breast and ovarian cancer risks due to inherited mutations in BRCA1 and BRCA2. *Science.* 2003;302:643-646.
7. Rao GG, Skinner EN, Gehrig PA, Duska LR, Miller DS, Schorge JO. Fertility-sparing surgery for ovarian low malignant potential tumors. *Gynecol Oncol.* 2005;98:263-266.
8. Schilder JM, Thompson AM, DePriest PD, et al. Outcome of reproductive age women with Stage IA or IC invasive epithelial ovarian cancer treated with fertility-sparing therapy. *Gynecol Oncol.* 2002;87:1-877.
9. Ayhan A, Guven ESG, Guven S, Kucukali T. Recurrence and prognostic factors in borderline ovarian tumors. *Gynecol Oncol.* 2005;98:439-445.

10. Wingo SN, Knowles LM, Carrick KS, Miller DS, Schorge JO. Retrospective cohort study of surgical staging for ovarian low malignant potential tumors. *Am J Obstet Gynecol.* 2006;194:20-22.
11. Stany MP, Elkas JC. Laparoscopy for adnexal masses in pregnancy? *Contemporary OB/Gyn.* 2007;52:44-49.
12. Armstrong DK, Bundy B, Wenzel L, et al. Intraperitoneal cisplatin and paclitaxel in ovarian cancer. *N Engl J Med.* 2006;354:34-43.
13. Kakkar AK. Prevention of venous thromboembolism in the cancer surgical patient. *J Clin Oncol.* 2009;27:4881-4884.
14. http://www.cdc.gov/mmwr/preview/mmwrhtml/mm5753a6.htm. Accessed December 17, 2009.

Case 18

A 32-year-old G3P3 Latin American woman presents to your clinic and reports several episodes of postcoital bleeding and a foul-smelling discharge for the last few months. She had her last Papanicolaou (Pap) smear 4 years ago after the birth of her last child but has not seen a physician since then. She has no history of medical problems. She has no history of abnormal Pap smears or sexually transmitted diseases. She had a tubal ligation at the time of her last delivery but no other surgeries. She smokes one pack of cigarettes daily. She first had intercourse at 15 years of age and has had five lifetime partners. She has been married to her current partner for 7 years.

On physical examination, she does not have a clinically visible lesion. Rectovaginal examination reveals that the cervix is approximately 4 cm in size and that the cervix is freely mobile. Supraclavicular and groin nodes are not palpable. You perform a Pap smear that is positive for a high-grade lesion. Colposcopy of the cervix shows areas of acetowhite epithelium and abnormal vessels. Pathological examination of the cervical biopsy reveals invasive squamous cell carcinoma approximately 2 mm below the basement membrane.

- ➤ What is your next step?
- ➤ What are your potential options for treatment?
- ➤ Would your management change if pathology revealed adenocarcinoma?
- ➤ What would you do if she were pregnant at 28 weeks' gestation?

ANSWERS TO CASE 18: Radical Hysterectomy

Summary: A 32-year-old G3P3 woman presents with postcoital bleeding. She does not have a clinically visible lesion. The Pap smear shows a high-grade lesion. She is diagnosed on colposcopically directed biopsy to have at least a microinvasive squamous cell carcinoma in that specimen.

- **The next step:** Cervical conization.
- **Potential options for treatment:**
  - Stage IA1: Extrafascial (simple) abdominal or vaginal hysterectomy or cervical conization with clear margins. A patient with Stage IA1 cancer and lymphovascular space invasion (LVSI) diagnosed on conization specimen will need treatment with radical hysterectomy and pelvic lymphadenectomy. Radiation therapy with chemotherapy may also be considered for patients who are not surgical candidates.
  - Stages IA2 to IIA: Radical hysterectomy with pelvic lymphadenectomy or primary radiation therapy and concurrent cisplatin-based chemotherapy.
  - Stage IIB and beyond: Primary radiotherapy with concurrent cisplatin-based chemotherapy.
- **If adenocarcinoma was found:** Patients with cervical adenocarcinoma are usually treated in a similar manner as patients with the more common histology of squamous carcinoma. For patients with early-stage squamous cell carcinoma, there does not appear to be a survival advantage whether a patient is treated primarily with surgery or concurrent chemoradiation therapy. However, one study suggests that patients with primary adenocarcinoma may have an improved outcome if surgery is done, even if subsequent adjuvant radiotherapy is needed.
- **If she were pregnant:** As she has no clinically apparent cervical lesion, she needs to undergo cervical conization to determine the depth of invasion. This will determine her clinical stage. Therapy will depend on the stage of disease, the gestational age of the fetus, and the patient's desires either for immediate treatment. Considerations include possible poor outcome for the pregnancy or for delayed therapy until the fetus reaches viability.

ANALYSIS

Objectives

1. Describe how to make the diagnosis of cervical cancer.
2. Describe how to stage cervical cancer.
3. Understand the options for treatment of cervical cancer, depending on the clinical stage.

4. List the pathologic indicators for adjuvant therapy after surgical treatment for cervical cancer.
5. Learn the options for management of a pregnant patient with cervical cancer.

Considerations

This is a 32-year-old G3P3 woman who presents to your clinic with worrisome symptoms of post-coital spotting and malodorous vaginal discharge, but has no obvious cervical lesion. Any patient who presents with unexplained postcoital bleeding requires an in-depth evaluation. Evaluation with a Pap smear is mandatory. If no visible cervical or vaginal lesions are seen, further evaluation is necessary which may include colposcopy with endocervical curettage. In this case, a cervical biopsy diagnosed invasive carcinoma of 2 mm below the basement membrane in the one area that was sampled. It is critical that the surgeon understand that the depth of this biopsy may not represent the worse invasion. The next step is cervical conization to determine the extent of the depth of invasion as this is difficult to determine the full extent on a small cervical biopsy specimen. If a cone biopsy reveals **microinvasion less than 3 mm** with clear margins (stage IA1) and no LVSI, the conization alone is adequate therapy if future fertility is desired. For patients with stage IA1 disease who are not interested in future fertility, simple hysterectomy is indicated. A lymph node dissection is unnecessary as the incidence of lymph node metastases in this clinical scenario is very low.

APPROACH TO Radical Hysterectomy

DEFINITIONS

RADICAL HYSTERECTOMY: A type of hysterectomy in which the uterus, upper-third vagina, cervix, and parametrial tissues are removed. The ureters are also dissected to ureterovesical junction (Class III hysterectomy).

EXTRAFASCIAL HYSTERECTOMY: A hysterectomy performed that develops the pubocervical fascia to allow total removal of uterus and cervix (Class I hysterectomy).

LYMPH-VASCULAR SPACE INVASION (LVSI): Small lymphatic and capillaries within the cervical stroma which can be seen on histologic sections. The presence of tumor near these vessels increases the risk of metastasis and leads to a poorer prognosis.

PARAMETRIUM: The tissue within the broad ligament and lateral to uterus and cervix.

CLINICAL APPROACH

Etiology

Epidemiologic risk factors for cervical cancer include early age at first coitus, multiple sexual partners, tobacco usage, low socioeconomic status, and immunosuppressive states (ie, transplant patients or patients with HIV). Human papillomaviruses 16 and 18 are most commonly associated with cervical dysplastic lesions and cervical carcinomas. However, not all infections of type 16 or 18 will progress to cervical cancer.

Clinical Presentation

The most common presenting symptom of invasive carcinoma of the cervix is abnormal vaginal bleeding or watery vaginal discharge. Among sexually active women, postcoital bleeding is usually a presenting symptom, but intermenstrual or postmenopausal bleeding may also occur. In some cases, symptoms of cervical cancer may not be recognized until the disease becomes advanced. As tumors grow, they can become infected and present with a malodorous vaginal discharge instead of vaginal bleeding. With very advanced disease, patients may present with pelvic or sciatic nerve pain or even with symptoms of a vesicovaginal or rectovaginal fistula.

Diagnosis

Any visible cervical lesion should be biopsied. The **false-negative rate for Pap smears in patients with invasive carcinoma may be as high as 50% due to the presence of necrosis limiting the cytologic diagnosis**. If a definitive diagnosis cannot be made on the basis of office colposcopic–guided biopsies, a diagnostic cervical conization may be required.

Staging of cervical cancer is clinical and International Federation of Gynecology and Obstetrics (FIGO) standards limit radiographic evaluation to chest radiography, intravenous pyelography, and barium enema (see Table 18–1). An examination under anesthesia is occasionally helpful if a good examination is not possible with the patient awake. A rectovaginal examination with emphasis on the presence of tumor in the parametrial tissue or the uterosacral ligament is mandatory. Under anesthesia, cystoscopy or proctoscopy is indicated if the patient has symptoms that are worrisome for either bladder or rectal involvement (hematuria or passage of stool per vagina). The FIGO classification system is not altered by lymph nodal involvement that is diagnosed radiographically. Computed tomography (CT), magnetic resonance imaging (MRI), or positron emission tomography (PET) scans are not acceptable for formalized staging purposes although these tests are routinely ordered to assist in treatment planning.[1]

Table 18–1 FIGO STAGING FOR CERVICAL CANCER

Stage I	The carcinoma is strictly confined to the cervix (extension to the corpus would be disregarded)
IA	Invasive carcinoma which can be diagnosed only by microscopy, with deepest invasion ≤5 mm and largest extension ≥7 mm
IA1	Measured stromal invasion of ≤3.0 mm in depth and extension of ≤7.0 mm
IA2	Measured stromal invasion of N3.0 mm and not N5.0 mm with an extension of not N7.0 mm
IB	Clinically visible lesions limited to the cervix uteri or pre-clinical cancers greater than stage IA *
IB1	Clinically visible lesion ≤4.0 cm in greatest dimension
IB2	Clinically visible lesion N4.0 cm in greatest dimension
Stage II	Cervical carcinoma invades beyond the uterus, but not to the pelvicwall or to the lower third of the vagina
IIA	Without parametrial invasion
IIA1	Clinically visible lesion ≤4.0 cm in greatest dimension
IIA2	Clinically visible lesion N4 cm in greatest dimension
IIB	With obvious parametrial invasion
Stage III	The tumor extends to the pelvic wall and/or involves lower third of the vagina and/or causes hydronephrosis or non-functioning kidney **
IIIA	Tumor involves lower third of the vagina, with no extension to the pelvicwall
IIIB	Extension to the pelvic wall and/or hydronephrosis or non-functioning kidney
Stage IV	The carcinoma has extended beyond the true pelvis or has involved (biopsy proven) the mucosa of the bladder or rectum. A bullous edema, as such, does not permit a case to be allotted to Stage IV
IVA	Spread of the growth to adjacent organs
IVB	Spread to distant organs

Abbreviations: CIN, cervical intraepithelial neoplasia; FIGO, International Federation of Gynecology and Obstetrics.

Fifteen to thirty percent of patients with advanced cervical cancer may have metastatic disease to para-aortic lymph nodes. PET scans have recently been shown to have a high sensitivity (75%-86%) to diagnose para-aortic metastases among patients with advanced disease. However, PET scans have a much lower sensitivity (50% for para-aortic metastases and 10%-53% for pelvic metastases) in diagnosing metastatic disease in patients with early-stage disease. Combination PET-CT scans may have an improved diagnostic yield over each modality individually.[1]

Treatment

Depending on clinical staging, surgery or chemoradiation will be offered to patients. The **outcome of patients with stage IA2 or IIA who receive radical hysterectomy or primary radiotherapy is similar, with overall survival ranging from 75% to 92%.** Therapeutic decisions are made after a thorough discussion of morbidities associated with each treatment type.[2,3]

Surgical management offers distinct advantages and disadvantages. Advantages include surgical staging, removal of bulky lymph nodes, ovarian conservation with transposition in younger patients, and preservation of vaginal function. The most common complication among patients undergoing radical hysterectomy is bladder dysfunction in the postoperative period, resulting in prolonged bladder catheterization or the need for intermittent self-catheterization. This is most likely due to injury to the sensory and motor nerve supply of the bladder. Pulmonary embolism, lymphocyst formation, and febrile morbidity from atelectasis and wound complications are less common, but not rare complications from surgery. Vesicovaginal or ureterovaginal fistulas occur in about 1% of cases.[4]

Some studies have also reported increased sexual dysfunction, including reduced arousal, decreased vaginal lubrication, and dyspareunia, among patients treated by radical hysterectomy.[5] Lymphedema may occur in patients who undergo pelvic lymphadenectomy, particularly if they need postoperative radiation therapy. Radiation therapy after radical pelvic surgery also increases the risk of developing bowel obstruction or fistulas.

Primary chemoradiation may be offered to patients at high risk for intraoperative complications to avoid surgical morbidity and mortality. However, radiation therapy may lead to vaginal shortening as well as a decrease in lubrication and worsened sexual functioning. Other morbidities associated with radiation therapy include bowel obstruction, fistula formation, chronic radiation cystitis and proctitis, and ovarian failure. Complications from radiation therapy tend to occur more distant from treatment and are usually chronic, whereas complications from surgery usually occur in the immediate postoperative period and do not usually persist.[6-8]

Patients with stage IB2 lesions (> 4 cm) are candidates for either surgery or primary chemoradiation. In a randomized trial of primary surgery versus radiation, **84% of patients with stage IB2 to IIA disease who underwent radical hysterectomy required postoperative adjuvant radiation therapy with more than 25% of patients experiencing severe morbidity**. Based on these results, many centers counsel patients with stage IB2 or more advanced lesions to have primary chemoradiation.

Patients who undergo surgery may need postoperative chemoradiation if certain high-risk features are present. If any of the following features are present, **positive pelvic lymph nodes, positive parametria, or positive margins**, patients should undergo **concurrent radiation and cisplatin chemotherapy**.

Approximately 25% of patients with stage IB1 disease will need adjuvant radiation therapy due to the presence of certain **intermediate risk factors (deep stromal invasion, LVSI, or lesion size > 4 cm)**. In a trial randomizing patients with these risk factors between no further therapy and pelvic radiation, patients who received radiation therapy had a 46% decreased risk of recurrence (18% among patients receiving radiation therapy vs 31% in patients with no further treatment).[9]

Surgical Therapy

For patients with stage IA1 with LVSI, IA2, IB, and IIA cervical cancer, radical hysterectomy and pelvic lymph node dissection is the surgical treatment option. In a modified radical hysterectomy (type II), the uterine artery is ligated as it crosses the ureter. The medial half of the cardinal ligaments and proximal uterosacral ligaments are resected. A more extensive dissection is done during a radical hysterectomy (type III). In the type III radical hysterectomy, the uterine artery is ligated at its point of origin at the superior vesical artery and the entire cardinal ligament is removed. The uterosacral ligament is resected from the attachment to the posterior pelvis. In clinical practice, aspects of both types II and III radical hysterectomies are done during each surgical case. More extensive radical hysterectomy options have been described, involving resection of the superior vesical artery, portions of the ureter, or the bladder. These operations are rarely done today to treat cervical cancer as patients with larger cervical lesions are treated primarily with chemoradiation therapy.

Specific anatomic spaces are opened during the radical hysterectomy. The **paravesical space** is bordered by the pubic symphysis anteriorly, the cardinal ligament posteriorly, the obliterated umbilical artery medially, and the obturator internus muscles laterally. The **pararectal space** is bordered by the cardinal ligament anteriorly, the sacrum posteriorly, the rectum medially, and the hypogastric artery laterally. The **rectovaginal space** is developed by opening the peritoneum at the pouch of Douglas and gently opening the space between the vagina and rectum with blunt dissection.

A **pelvic lymphadenectomy** is performed to remove lymphatic tissue within the following landmarks: lateral to the ureter, medial to the psoas muscle, inferior to the middle of the common iliac artery, and superior to the deep circumflex vein. The **obturator space** is opened by retracting the external artery and vein and identifying the obturator nerve. All lymphatic and fatty tissue is then removed out of the obturator space.

For patients with larger stage IB lesions (> 4 cm) and patients with stage IIA disease who opted for radical hysterectomy, there is an 80% chance that adjuvant radiation therapy will be recommended based on operative findings. Adjuvant radiation therapy, often with concurrent chemotherapy, is offered when patients have positive margins on the radical hysterectomy specimen, or metastatic disease in the lymph nodes. Adjuvant therapy is also considered when there are poor prognostic factors, for example, lymphovascular space invasion, large primary tumor size, or deep cervical stromal invasion, noted on the radical hysterectomy specimen.

Complications of a Radical Hysterectomy Urinary tract complications are frequently encountered after radical hysterectomy. It has been reported that up to 50% of radical hysterectomy cases have bladder dysfunction. The extensive dissection required for the surgery often results in denervation of the bladder and upper urethra. The majority of patients have normal bladder function within a year of the surgery. However, some patients require prolonged catheterization until bladder function returns. The use of either a suprapubic or transurethral catheter as well as intermittent self-catheterization have been described. Ureteral injury and fistula formation are not as common as bladder dysfunction and can be minimized by careful surgical technique.

The risk of infection is no different than in the case of a traditional hysterectomy. Preoperative single-agent broad-spectrum antibiotic is all that is necessary for infection prophylaxis. Depending on the length of surgery and blood loss, an additional dose of antibiotics may be required.

Venous thrombosis and pulmonary embolus are a particular concern to the surgeon. Given the extensive surgery, trauma to vein wall with lymphadenectomy, and immobility, these patients are at particularly high risk for venous thrombosis formation. Patients should receive intermittent pneumatic calf compression in the operating room, which is continued postoperatively until the patient is full ambulatory. High-risk patients may benefit from medical prophylaxis with either heparin or low-molecular-weight heparin.

Despite careful surgical technique, intraoperative hemorrhage may occur, and the surgeon must be prepared to deal with this complication. Blood products should be readily available at the time of surgery in the event that excessive bleeding occurs. The most frequent site of hemorrhage is venous bleeding from the pararectal fossa, presacral, and para-aortic regions. Unfortunately, as compared to arterial bleeding, venous bleeding is difficult to identify and is seldom improved with hypogastric artery ligation. A good understanding of anatomy is essential to try and minimize risk of hemorrhage.

Thankfully, nerve injury is not a frequent complication of a radical hysterectomy and rarely permanent. The obturator nerve is most likely nerve to be injured and results in inability to adduct lower extremities. Obturator nerve injury can occur with removal of obturator nodes and retractor use. Most nerve injuries can be minimized with proper patient placement/positioning, careful use of self-retaining retractors, careful surgical technique in dissection with good understanding of pelvic anatomy, and maintaining hemostasis.[10]

Radical Trachelectomy Patients with stage IA2 and IB1 (< 4 cm tumor size) lesions who desire future fertility may elect to undergo **a radical trachelectomy with pelvic lymphadenectomy**. A complete lymphadenectomy is first performed to evaluate for the presence of metastatic disease. Subsequently, radical trachelectomy may be done to remove the cervix and the parametrial tissue. The procedure may be done abdominally, laparoscopically, or with a combined laparoscopic and vaginal portion. Often a cervical cerclage is placed in the newly formed exocervix, which is now located approximately 1 cm below the lower uterine segment.[11]

Primary Radiation Therapy with Concurrent Chemotherapy For patients with stage IIB disease or higher, the treatment is concurrent radiation and chemotherapy. This modality is also used for earlier-stage disease when the patient is not a surgical candidate. Typically, the patient receives external beam radiation to the pelvis followed by vaginal brachytherapy with tandem and ovoids placement. During radiation therapy, the patient will also receive concurrent platinum-based chemotherapy. **Ideally, all radiation therapy is completed within a span of 56 days, as delays in treatment are associated with a decreased overall survival.**

When counseling a patient with early-stage disease who is a candidate for either chemoradiation therapy or primary surgery, arguments in favor of primary surgery usually include better preservation of vaginal length and the avoidance of long-term risk of radiation (enteritis, bowel obstruction, etc), whereas the proponent of primary chemoradiation therapy cites the usual tolerability of treatment by most patients and the avoidance of surgery with its attendant risks. However, stage for stage, in those with early disease (<4 cm), neither modality has been shown to have a survival advantage over the other.

Patients with Adenocarcinoma In general, cervical adenocarcinoma is treated similarly, stage for stage, as squamous carcinoma. However, in one study of patients with stage IB to IIA cervical cancer randomized to primary radical surgery versus radiation therapy, those **patients with adenocarcinoma who underwent primary surgery had improved progression-free and overall survival rates**.

Pregnant Patients with Newly Diagnosed Cervical Cancer **Delayed diagnosis** of cervical cancer in pregnancy is common because symptoms of **postcoital bleeding, vaginal discharge, vaginal bleeding, and pelvic pain** are frequently associated with pregnancy. Most patients receive a Pap smear early on entry into prenatal care. If an abnormal Pap smear is found and the patient has no visible lesion, colposcopy **without** endocervical curettage is done. If the colposcopy is adequate and a biopsy reveals cervical intraepithelial neoplasia (CIN), the patient may undergo a vaginal delivery. Further evaluation and treatment are done at 6 weeks after delivery.

If the colposcopy is inadequate or the biopsy reveals microinvasion or possible carcinoma, cervical conization is needed in a similar manner as if the patient were not pregnant. Ideally, conizations are performed during the **second trimester** because the risk of fetal loss is less than 10%. If performed in the first trimester, the rate of fetal loss may be as high as 24%. In the third trimester, the risk of loss is less, but the risk of hemorrhage is significant.

A **cervical conization in pregnancy** should be performed only if necessary to diagnose or stage a cervical cancer due to the high risk of potential complications, including **premature labor, spontaneous abortion, infection, and hemorrhage**. Pregnant patients may safely undergo MRI to determine tumor volume, nodal enlargement, and potential metastasis.[12] Consultation with gynecologic oncologists and maternal-fetal medicine specialists is highly recommended to help manage these difficult patients.

Careful counseling with the patient and her family must be undertaken for the management of any patient diagnosed with cervical cancer during pregnancy as the treatment is dependent on the stage of disease and the wishes of the mother. Patients with stage IA1 cervical cancer diagnosed by conization may be safely followed throughout pregnancy.[13] Patients at less than 20 weeks' gestation who have more advanced lesions and do not desire continuation of the pregnancy may **undergo radical surgery or radiation therapy with cisplatin as definitive treatment.** Patients who have pregnancies exceeding 20 weeks' gestation can generally be expectantly managed to await fetal maturity. While the number of patients reported in the literature is small, the current data suggest that delaying treatment for stage I disease during pregnancy does not decrease survival as compared to undergoing immediate therapy.

Because patients with cervical cancer are at higher risk for hemorrhage or failure to dilate, some advocate for cesarean section delivery. Among patients with advanced-stage disease, radiation therapy is the preferred treatment modality. Definitive data are not available regarding delays in treatment and potential effects on advanced disease.

Comprehension Questions

18.1 A 39-year-old woman is noted to have an exophytic cervical lesion, which on biopsy reveals invasive squamous cell carcinoma. Which of the following diagnostic aids is used in staging cervical cancer?

A. MRI
B. PET scan
C. Chest x-ray
D. CT scan of the abdomen and pelvis

18.2 A patient has a biopsy of a 5-cm cervical lesion showing squamous carcinoma. A rectovaginal examination shows obvious evidence of parametrial involvement on the left, but no sidewall involvement. The lesion invades the mucosa of the left vaginal fornix. A CT scan shows pathologically enlarged pelvic and para-aortic lymph nodes. Which of the following is her cancer stage?

A. Stage IIA
B. Stage IIAB
C. Stage IIIA
D. Stage IVB

18.3 Which of the following is the most common complication of radical hysterectomy?

A. Bladder atony
B. Pulmonary embolism
C. Massive blood loss
D. Lymphedema
E. Small bowel obstruction

18.4 For which of the following cervical cancer patients is a radical hysterectomy and lymphadenectomy the most appropriate treatment?

A. A 46-year-old woman with a conization specimen showing 2-mm stromal invasion

B. A 25-year-old nulligravida woman with a 5-cm cervical lesion with vaginal or parametrial involvement

C. A 23-year-old nulligravida woman with a cervical conization showing 5-mm stromal invasion

D. A 25-year-old G1P1 woman with a cervical conization showing 3-mm stromal invasion and no lymphovascular space invasion

ANSWERS

18.1 **C.** FIGO staging of cervical cancer is clinical and relies on a good pelvic examination. Radiographic evaluation is limited to chest radiography, barium enema, and intravenous pyelogram. In current practice, a CT scan, a PET scan, or combination PET-CT scan are often done. Information obtained on these tests is included in the treatment planning for the patient; however, it does not influence the stage of the patient.

18.2 **B.** The patient has a cervical cancer that involves the upper vagina (IIA), but also parametria but not to the side wall (IIB). Thus, she has stage IIB disease. The information obtained on the CT scan may influence treatment planning. In this case, she is a candidate for extended-field radiation therapy for the enlarged para-aortic lymph node.

18.3 **A.** The most common complication of radical hysterectomy is bladder atony. This is most likely due to bladder denervation from the extensive dissection.

18.4 **C.** Radical hysterectomy and lymph node dissection are appropriate therapies for patients with stages IA2 to IIA cervical cancer. Patients with stage IA1 disease who have lymphovascular space invasion also need radical hysterectomy with lymph node dissection as there is a risk of lymph node metastasis. A patient with 3-mm or less cervical stromal invasion without lymphovascular space invasion is adequately treated with cervical conization with negative margins or simple hysterectomy.

Clinical Pearls

See Table 1-2 for definition of level of evidence and strength of recommendation

- After radical hysterectomy, adjuvant radiation therapy is given if the patient has certain risk factors, including tumor size larger than 4 cm, the presence of lymphovascular space invasion, or deep stromal invasion (Level A).
- The survival data for patients undergoing radical hysterectomy versus patients undergoing radiation therapy are similar in patients with stages IB to IIA disease. Patients with stage IIB or higher disease are treated with primary chemoradiation therapy (Level A).
- Fifteen percent of patients with early disease will have lymphatic spread diagnosed after radical hysterectomy and pelvic lymphadenectomy (Level B).
- Patients who present with symptoms of postcoital bleeding should undergo complete evaluation, including Pap smear, endocervical curettage, and colposcopy (Level C).
- All visible cervical lesion needs to be biopsied. A Pap smear is inadequate to rule out invasive carcinoma of the cervix (Level C).

REFERENCES

1. Gold M. PET in cervical cancer—implications for "staging," treatment planning, assessment of prognosis and prediction of response. *J Natl Compr Canc Netw*. 2008;6:37-45.
2. Holtz D, Dunton C. Traditional management of invasive cervical cancer. *Obstet Gynecol Clin North Am*. 2002;29:645-657.
3. Landoni F, Maneo A, Colombo A, et al. Randomized study of radical surgery versus radiotherapy for stage IB-IIA cervical cancer. *Lancet*. 1997;350:535-540.
4. Covens A, Rosen B, Gibbons A, et al. Differences in the morbidity of radical hysterectomy between gynecologic oncologists. *Gynecol Oncol*. 1993;51:39-45.
5. Bergmark K, Avall-Lundquist E, Dickman P, Hennignsohn L, Steineck G. Vaginal function and sexuality in women with a history of cervical cancer. *N Engl J Med*. 1999;340:1383-1389.
6. Gray H. Primary management of early stage cervical cancer (IA1-IB) and appropriate selection of adjuvant therapy. *J Natl Compr Canc Netw*. 2008;6:47-51.
7. Delgado G, Bundy B, Zaino R, Sevin B, Creasman W, Major F. Prospective surgical-pathological study of disease-free interval in patients with stage IB cervical cancer after radical hysterectomy and bilateral pelvic lymphadenectomy. *Gynecol Oncol*. 1990;38:352-357.
8. Sedlis A, Bundy B, Rotman M, Lentz S, Muderspach L, Zaino R. A randomized trial of pelvic radiation therapy versus no further therapy in selected patients with stage IB carcinoma of the cervix after radical hysterectomy and pelvic lymphadenectomy: a Gynecologic Oncology Group Study. *Gynecol Oncol*. 1999;73:177-183.

9. Rose P, Bundy B, Watkins E, et al. Concurrent cisplatin-based radiotherapy and chemotherapy for locally advanced cervical cancer. *N Engl J Med.* 1999;340:1144-1153.
10. Rock J, Jones H. Cancer of the cervix. In: *Te Linde's Operative Gynecology*. 10th ed. Philadelphia, PA: Lippincott Williams & Wilkins; 2008:1277-1281.
11. Plante, M. Radical vaginal trachelectomy: a fertility preserving option for young women in early stage cervical cancer. *Gynecol Oncol.* 2005;99:S143-S146.
12. Zanetta G, Pellegrino A, Vanzulli A, DiLelio A, Milani R, Mangioni C. Magnetic resonance imaging of cervical cancer in pregnancy. *Int J Gynecol Cancer.* 1998;8:265-269.
13. Hannigan E, Whitehouse H, Atkinson W, Becker S. Cone biopsy during pregnancy. *Obstet and Gynecol.* 1982;60:450-455.

Case 19

A 33-year-old African American G1P0010 woman complains about increasing pelvic pressure and urinary frequency for the past 6 months. She reports that her menses have increased from lasting 5 days to now 12 days in duration with heavier flow and quarter-size clots. She denies any dizziness, shortness of breath, or constipation. She has no chronic medical conditions. She has no children, and she and her husband would like to have a child.

On examination, she is noted to be afebrile with normal vital signs. Her abdominal examination reveals an irregular mass in the midline approximately 16 weeks in size and nontender. Pelvic examination reveals a mobile, irregular mass in midline approximately 16 weeks in size and nontender. She has no adnexal tenderness, and no masses are palpated. A CBC reveals that she is anemic with hemoglobin of 6.8 g/dL. Her urine culture was negative.

- ➤ What is the most likely diagnosis?
- ➤ What is your diagnostic workup for this patient?
- ➤ What is the best therapy for this patient?
- ➤ What complications can result from the treatment?

ANSWERS TO CASE 19: Myomectomy

Summary: This is a 33-year-old woman, nulliparous, with menorrhagia, and a pelvic mass suggestive of leiomyomata.

- **Most likely diagnosis:** Uterine leiomyoma
- **Diagnostic workup:** CBC, endometrial biopsy, prolactin, thyroid-stimulating hormone (TSH), follicle-stimulating hormone (FSH), pregnancy test, pelvic ultrasound
- **Best treatment:** Myomectomy
- **Complications:** Hysterectomy, recurrence, adhesions, longer hospitalization, continued infertility

ANALYSIS

Objectives

1. List indications for myomectomy.
2. Describe several routes for myomectomy.
3. List possible complications resulting from myomectomy.

Considerations

This is a 33-year-old nulliparous woman whose symptoms and physical findings are consistent with uterine fibroids. She complains of menorrhagia (with resultant anemia) and urinary frequency. Her symptoms include both menorrhagia (with resultant anemia) and urinary frequency. Because of her asymptomatic anemia, the patient is a candidate for medical therapy and iron supplementation. Medical therapy options include the use of medroxyprogesterone acetate depot (Depo-Provera), oral contraceptive pills, and GnRH-a. Of the options listed, GnRH-agonist would be the most effective treatment for her uterine fibroids. However, because of limited duration of GnRH usage (6 months) and likely recurrence after treatment, medical management would not be the best management option at this time. Given her age, desired fertility, and symptoms, the patient is a candidate for a myomectomy. Alternative treatments for fibroids including uterine artery embolization and ultrasonography-focused ablation are not options for this patient given her desired fertility.

APPROACH TO
Myomectomy

CLINICAL APPROACH

Leiomyomas (also fibroids or myomas) are benign monoclonal tumors originating from a single smooth muscle cell that has undergone a chromosomal mutation. They are a bundle of smooth muscle cells and fibrous tissue surrounded by a fibrous capsule. The leiomyomas are symptomatic in 25% to 50% of women, but upon pathological review of hysterectomy specimen, the prevalence may be as high as 80%. Risk factors for the development of leiomyoma include increasing age, early menarche, low parity, tamoxifen use, obesity, and some studies show high-fat diet. Myomas tend to grow and become more symptomatic in nulliparous women. African American women have the highest incidence of fibroids. Hispanic, Asian, and Caucasian women have similar rates for the development of leiomyoma. There is a familial tendency to develop fibroids. Smoking has been associated with a decrease in incidence of leiomyoma. Leiomyomas can grow in any part of the body that has smooth muscle; the uterus is the most common organ in the pelvis to develop fibroids. Leiomyoms can be found in the fallopian tubes, round ligament, and about 5% of the time on the cervix.

Uterine leiomyoma can be diagnosed with 95% certainty with physical examination alone. On palpation, a uterus feels enlarged, firm, and irregular. Myomas can grow laterally and may inhibit the palpation of the adnexa. Ultrasound is recommended when the patient is obese and/or when adnexal pathology cannot be ruled out with physical examination alone.

Most leiomyoms are asymptomatic and do not require treatment. The number, size, and location of the myoma can produce different symptoms. Symptoms include pelvic pressure, dysmenorrhea, menorrhagia, urinary frequency, and constipation. Fibroids can cause hydroureter or hydronephrosis and have been linked to infertility. Therapeutic options include medical management with progestins (norethindrone, medrogestone, medroxyprogesterone acetate), antiprogestins (mifepristone), and gonadotropin-releasing hormone analogues. Surgical procedures include myomectomy and hysterectomy. Other methods for treatment of fibroids include uterine artery embolization, high-frequency ultrasonography, laser treatment, cryotherapy, and thermoablation. Approximately 30% of hysterectomies list symptomatic uterine fibroids as the primary indication. The choice of the treatment method should be based on various medical and social characteristics of the patient. These factors include age, parity, desire for childbearing, severity of symptoms, size and number of leiomyoms, location of the myoma, other medical conditions, suspicion of malignancy, proximity of menopause, and desire to preserve uterus.[1]

In the presence of leiomyoms, myomectomy may be the management option if the patient desires to retain her uterus, if there is a single pedunculated myoma, or if the presence of myoma is thought to be the cause of infertility or repeated pregnancy losses. Women with symptomatic uterine fibroids who no longer desire to bear children may be best treated with a hysterectomy, the definitive treatment for uterine leiomyoma. For women who desire future childbearing or who want to preserve their uterus, myomectomy may be the best management.

Myomectomy only removes the portion of the myoma that is visible and accessible. Occasionally, small myoma may be retained intentionally. If myomectomy is the chosen therapy, the myoma can be removed via an abdominal incision, laparoscopy, or hysteroscopy. Before proceeding with the removal of the myoma, appropriate evaluation must be done for the presence of a pelvic mass and abnormal uterine bleeding. Anemia may be treated with GnRH-a and iron supplementation prior to the myomectomy. GnRH-a can also decrease the size of the leiomyoma, but the enucleation of the myoma is more difficult due to a less distinct plane between the myoma and the normal uterus. Myomectomy is associated with more adhesions and longer hospital stays than a hysterectomy. Hysterectomy is associated with more urinary tract injuries. Contraindications to a myomectomy include pregnancy, advanced adnexal disease, malignancy, and the situation where removal of the myoma would result in the significant reduction of the endometrial surface causing the uterus not to be functional.[2-9]

Abdominal Myomectomy

An abdominal myomectomy is the route of choice when there are numerous myomas in multiple locations (subserosal, intramural, submucosal). Multiple myomectomy is usually more difficult and time consuming than a hysterectomy. Intraoperative blood loss for myomectomy correlates with the uterine size prior to surgery, total weight of the myomas removed, and operating time. Resolution of menorrhagia and pelvic pressure is overall 81%. Several studies show that the morbidity of the two procedures is similar. The risk of unexpected hysterectomy when performing a myomectomy is less than 1%. The hysterectomy can result from leiomyomatosis or from complications of the myomectomy. Recurrence of myomas is of concern after myomectomy. Studies using transvaginal ultrasound show recurrence of approximately 51% at 5 years. Other studies show that clinically significant myoma recurrence is 10% at 5 years, with one-third of those patients eventually undergoing a hysterectomy. The rate of recurrence of myomas depends on the number of myomas removed. The recurrence risk is 11% for a single myoma and 26% for multiple myomas. When myomectomy is performed in patients desiring fertility, pelvic adhesions, and dissection in the area of the interstitial portion of the fallopian may result in postoperative infertility.[10-12]

A careful pelvic examination while the patient is under anesthesia will allow for a better idea of which type of skin incision to make. After the appropriate skin incision is made and peritoneum entered, the uterus and adjacent adnexal structures are to be evaluated. When multiple fibroids are noted, the uterine incision should be the one that allows the exposure to multiple fibroids minimizing the number of uterine incisions. To decrease intraoperative blood loss, uterine tourniquets or injectable intrauterine vasoconstrictive agents can be used. Multiple studies have demonstrated the effectiveness of vasoconstrictive agents in decreasing the need for blood transfusion[13] and decreasing intraoperative blood loss.[14] When comparing mechanical occlusion and injection of vasoconstrictive agents, Ginsberg et al.[15] found no significant differences in blood loss or transfusion requirements between the groups. A linear or elliptic incision is then made on the uterus and carried down to underlying myoma. The myoma can then be grasped and the cleavage plane between the myoma and surrounding myometrium can be easily identified (Figure 19–1). After the myoma is removed, the dead space can be

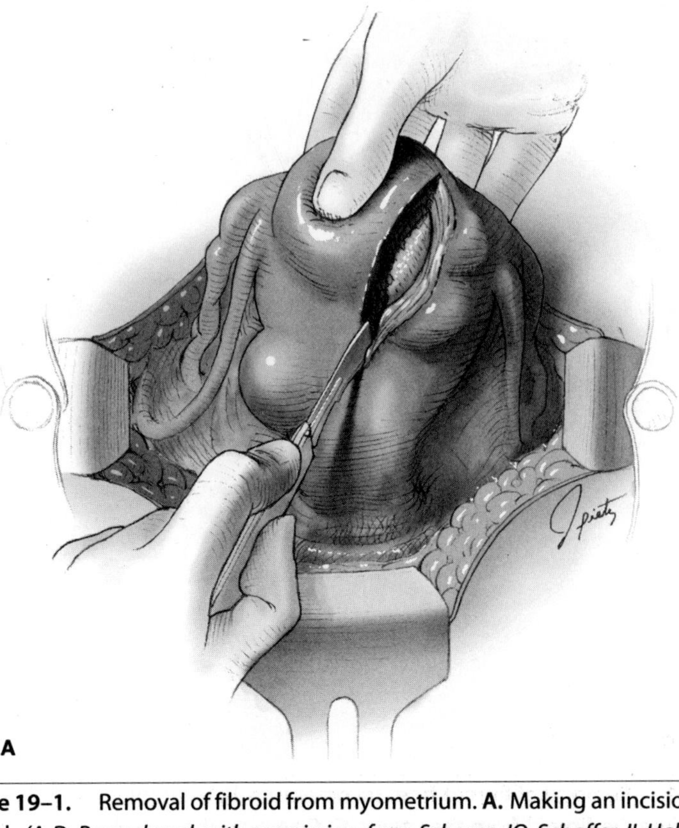

A

Figure 19–1. Removal of fibroid from myometrium. **A.** Making an incision over the fibroid. *(A-D: Reproduced, with permission, from Schorge JO, Schaffer JI, Halvorson LM, et al.* Williams Gynecology. *New York: McGraw-Hill, 2008: 901-904.)*

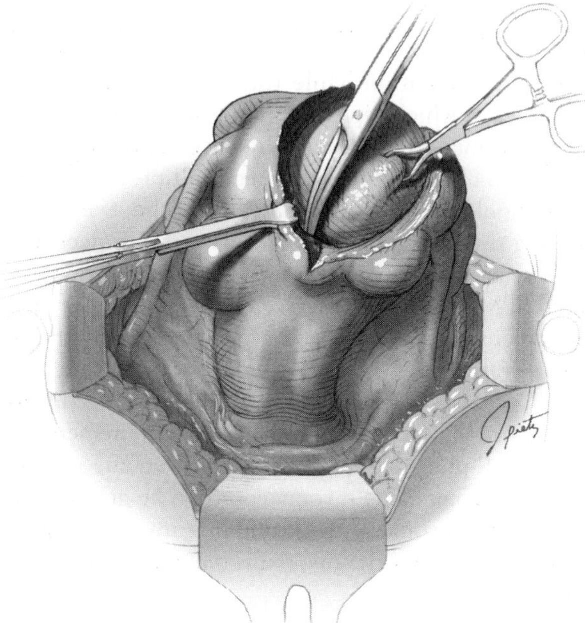

B

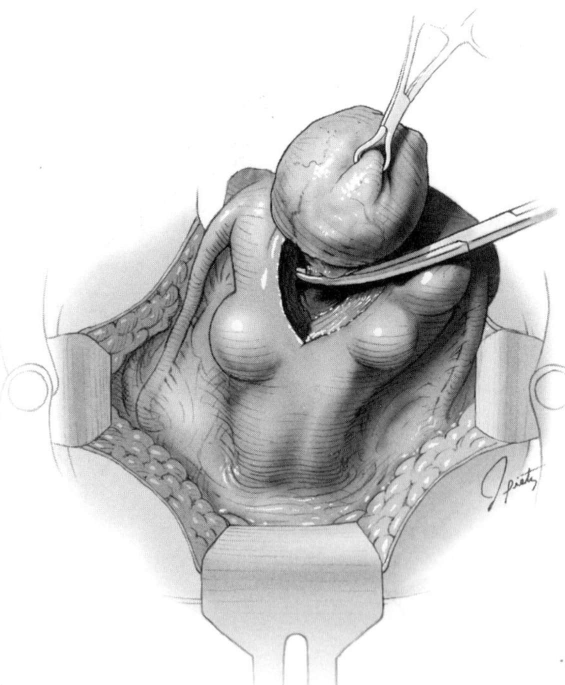

C

Figure 19–1. Removal of fibroid from myometrium. **B.** Using blunt and sharp dissection to free the fibroid from the uterus. **C.** Clamping the vascular pedicle to the fibroid to prepare for ligature.

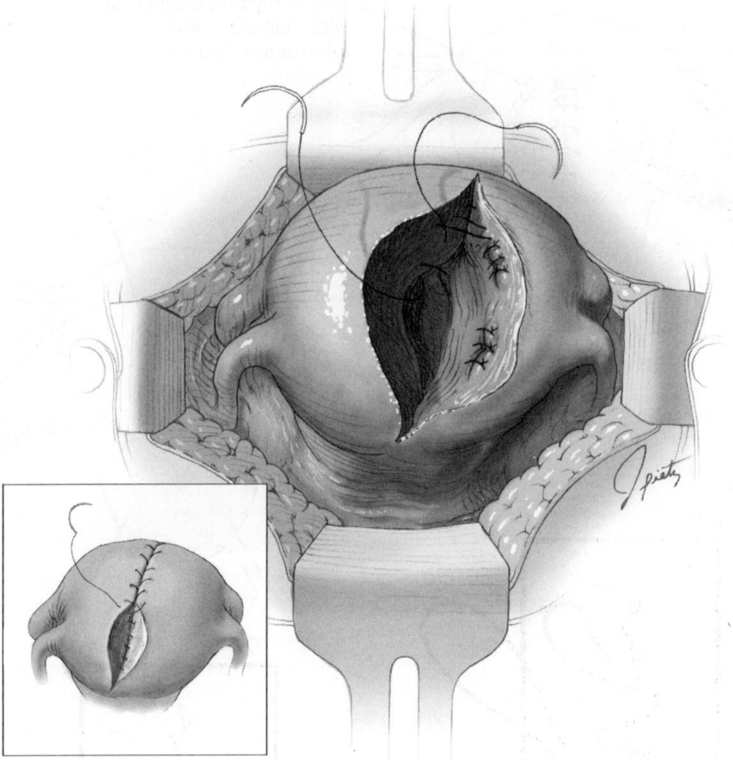

D

Figure 19–1. Removal of fibroid from myometrium. **D.** The uterue defect is repaired in layers.

obliterated with interrupted sutures. The serosal edge can be reapproximated with a "baseball" stitch (Figure 19–2). The risk of adhesive disease can be minimized with meticulous surgical technique and possibly with the use of absorbable or nonabsorbable barriers.[16]

Laparoscopic Myomectomy

A laparoscopic myomectomy can be considered if the myomas are subserosal or pedunculated and easily accessible. Benefits for a laparoscopic approach include decreased postoperative morbidity and faster recovery.[17] The myoma can be excised and removed from the peritoneal cavity via a colpotomy incision or after morcellation via the laparoscopic cannula. A laparotomy is recommended for myomas that are larger than 8 cm, multiple leiomyoms, or with deep intramural myomas. There is a 2% to 8% rate of converting to an open procedure. There is also a recurrence rate of 33% at 27 months, which is higher than that of an open myomectomy. Cases of uterine rupture in pregnancies following laparoscopic myomectomy have been reported. This may be

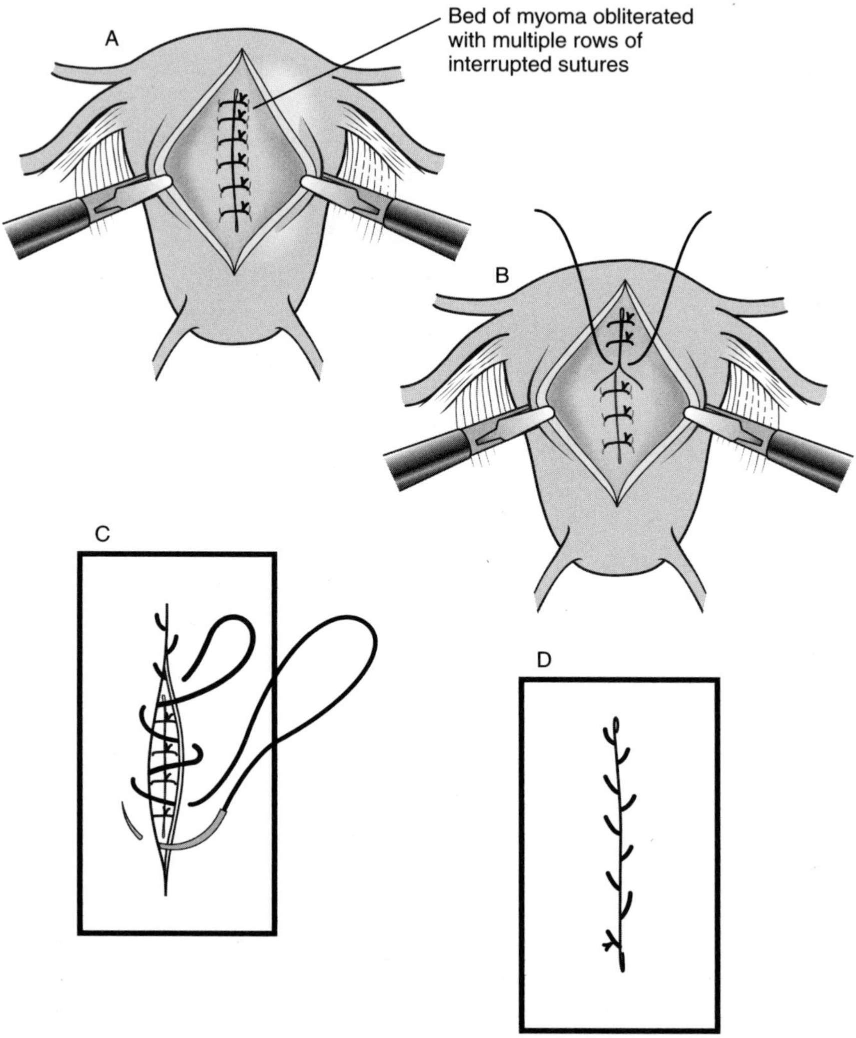

Figure 19–2. Uterine closure after myomectomy. A large uterine defect is in three separate layers using interrupted sutures for the first two layers, and a "baseball stitch" for the last layer.

due to inadequate reconstruction of the myometrium at the time of the myomectomy.[18-20]

The use of robotics to perform myomectomies has had mixed results. Most studies have demonstrated a quicker recovery, shorter length of stay, and less intraoperative blood loss. However, the costs and operative times were significantly higher in the robotic group and conversion rate to laparotomy was 8.6%.[21,22] It appears the same limitations of traditional laparoscopy hold true for robotic myomectomy—difficult enucleation of myoma without tactile feedback.[23]

Hysteroscopic Myomectomy

Hysteroscopy is used to remove submucosal leiomyoms. Indications for hysteroscopic myomectomy include abnormal bleeding, history of pregnancy loss, infertility, and pain. Contraindications include endometrial cancer, pelvic infection, inability to distend the uterine cavity, inability to go around the lesion, and the extension of the myoma deep into the myometrium. Fertility rates after hysteroscopic myomectomy are good; 59% of patients conceived after resection of the submucosal fibroids. Approximately 20% of patients who underwent hysteroscopic myomectomy will need additional treatment after 5 to 10 years. Symptomatic myoma after the initial surgery can result from the growth of new myoma or recurrence from incompletely excised myoma.

To minimize the risk of uterine perforation, the submucosal fibroid should be evaluated closely for myometrial involvement. When the fibroid invades the myometrium, there is a greater risk of uterine perforation and a simultaneous laparoscopy/hysteroscopy can be performed. After the appropriate operative hysteroscopic distending medium (sorbitol, Hyskon [dextran, high molecular weight]) is infused, the endometrial cavity can be evaluated for the extent of myoma involvement. Using the resectoscope and a cutting current of 60 to 80 W, the myoma can be sequentially resected. Care must be taken to only apply current when resectoscope loop is being withdrawn from the fundus (never toward fundus due to increased perforation risk). Careful attention must be paid to distending media in/out and deficits.

Many authors recommend a hysterosalpingogram 4 months after a myomectomy to evaluate the uterine cavity and the fallopian tubes and a delay of 4 to 6 months after surgery before attempting to conceive. Previously, a cesarean delivery was recommended only if the endometrium was entered during the myomectomy. However, if extensive dissection of the myometrium is carried out in the process of a myomectomy, even if the endometrium in not disturbed, a cesarean delivery is usually advised following a pregnancy. Cesarean delivery is not recommended after the removal of a pedunculated fibroid or after small hysteroscopic resection.[24]

Comprehension Questions

19.1 A 43-year-old white G3P3 woman has symptoms of pelvic pressure and abnormal uterine bleeding. A pelvic examination reveals a 16-week-size irregular uterus. An ultrasound shows a 10-cm pedunculated leiomyoma from the fundus of the uterus. No adnexal masses were noted. Which of the following should be the next step?

A. Endometrial biopsy
B. Hysterectomy
C. Abdominal myomectomy
D. Laparoscopic myomectomy

19.2 Which of the following cases has a higher chance of recurrence of leiomyoma?

A. A 32-year-old woman who underwent hysteroscopic myomectomy for a single pedunculated fibroid
B. A 44-year-old woman who underwent a laparoscopic resection of a 5-cm subserosal fibroid
C. A 32-year-old woman who underwent an abdominal myomectomy for an 8-cm myometrial fibroid
D. A 44-year-old woman who underwent an abdominal myomectomy for five uterine fibroids

19.3 Which of the following points is most important to be emphasized in counseling a patient undergoing myomectomy for infertility?

A. Complications of myomectomy can lead to a hysterectomy.
B. Adhesions caused by the myomectomy surgery usually can be prevented.
C. Patients with infertility are usually cured after a myomectomy.
D. The location of fibroid and its resection do not affect fertility.

ANSWERS

19.1 **A.** Before any therapeutic measures are taken, it is critical to complete a full diagnostic evaluation. It is possible that the abnormal uterine bleeding is caused by leiomyoma; however, endometrial pathology must be ruled out in this patient who is older than 35 years with abnormal uterine bleeding. This patient's symptoms as well as physical examination are consistent with uterine leiomyoms. If she did not wish to retain her uterus, hysterectomy would be the definitive treatment of choice. If she desired future children, myomectomy would be the best option. Since this is a pedunculated fibroid, laparoscopic removal can be considered.

19.2 **D.** The recurrence rate of leiomyoma depends on the number of myomas removed at the initial myomectomy. There is 11% recurrence after one myoma is removed. There is 26% recurrence rate after multiple myomas are removed.

19.3 **A.** Submucosal leiomyoms are most often associated with infertility and recurrent pregnancy losses. Myomectomy can improve fertility rates if all other causes of infertility have been ruled out. Risk of myomectomy includes formation of adhesions and blockage of the fallopian tube. A conservative surgery for uterine preservation can lead to a definitive hysterectomy.

Clinical Pearls

See Table 1-2 for definition of level of evidence and strength of recommendation

- Improvement in menorrhagia, pelvic pressure, and infertility has been noted after myomectomy (Level A).
- Hysterectomy is the only definitive cure for leiomyoms. Myomectomy has the risk of recurrence (Level B).
- The risks of myomectomy include possible hysterectomy, recurrence, adhesions, longer hospitalization, and continued infertility (Level B).
- After significant disturbance of the myometrium during a myomectomy, a cesarean delivery should be offered in the event of a pregnancy even if the endometrium was not disturbed (Level C).
- Myomectomy should be performed if the patient desires to retain her uterus or childbearing function (Level C).
- Laparoscopic and hysteroscopic myomectomy should be carried out only by experienced surgeons (Level C).

REFERENCES

1. Buttran VC, Reiter RC. Uterine leiomyomata: etiology, symptomatology, and management. *Fertil Steril.* 1981;36:433-445.
2. Acien P, Quereda F. Abdominal myomectomy: results of a simple operative technique. *Fertil Steril.* 1996;65:41-51.
3. American College of Obstetricians and Gynecologists. *Surgical Alternatives to Hysterectomy in the Management of Leiomyomas.* ACOG Practice Bulletin No. 16, May 2000. Washington DC.
4. Cramer SF, Patel A. The frequency of uterine leiomyomas. *Am J Clin Pathol.* 1990;94:435-438.
5. Ecker JL, Foster JT, Friedman AJ. Abdominal hysterectomy or abdominal myomectomy for symptomatic leiomyoma: a comparison of preoperative demography and postoperative morbidity. *J Gynecol Surg.* 1995;1:11-18.
6. Hillis SD, Marchbanks PA, Peterson HB. Uterine size and risk of complications among women undergoing abdominal hysterectomy for leiomyomas. *Obstet Gynecol.* 1996;87:539-543.
7. Iverson RE Jr, Chelmow D, Strohbehn K, Waldman L, Evantash EG. Relative morbidity of abdominal hysterectomy and myomectomy for management of uterine leiomyomas. *Obstet Gynecol.* 1996;88:415-419.
8. Katz VL, Lentz GM, Lobo RA, Gershenson DM. Benign gynecologic lesions. In: *Comprehensive Gynecology.* 5th ed. Philadelphia, PA: Mosby; 2007:441-450.
9. Wallach EE, Vlahos NF. Uterine myomas: an overview of development, clinical features, and management. *Obstet Gynecol.* 2004;104:393-406.
10. Fedele L, Parazzini F, Luchini L, Mezzopane R, Tozzi L, Villa L. Recurrence of fibroids after myomectomy: a transvaginal ultrasonographic study. *Hum Reprod.* 1995;10:1795-1796.

11. Fauconnier A, Chapron C, Babaki-Fard K, Dubuisson JB. Recurrence of leiomyomata after myomectomy. *Hum Reprod Update*. 2000;6:595-602.
12. Nezhat FR, Roemisch M, Nezhat Ch, Seidman DS, Nezhat CR. Recurrence rate after laparoscopic myomectomy. *J Am Assoc Gynecol Laparosc*. 1998;5:237-240.
13. Dillon T. Control of blood loss during gynecologic surgery. *Obstet Gynecol*. 1962;19:428.
14. Frederick J, Fletcher A, Simeon D, et al. Intramyometrial vasopressin as a hemostatic agent. *BJOG*. 1994;101:435.
15. Ginsberg E, Benson C, Garfield J, et al. The effect of operative technique and uterine size on blood loss during myomectomy: a prospective randomized study. *Fertil Steril*. 1993;60:956.
16. Rock J, Jones H. Leiomyomata uteri and myomectomy. In: *Te Linde's Operative Gynecology*. 10th ed. Philadelphia, PA: Lippincott Williams & Wilkins; 2008:707-721.
17. Mais V, Ajossa S, Guerrriero S, Mascia M, Solla E, Melis GB. Laparoscopic versus abdominal myomectomy: a prospective, randomized trial to evaluate benefits in early outcome. *Am J Obstet Gynecol*. 2005;174:654-658.
18. Rock J, Jones H. Diagnostic and operative laparoscopy. In: *Te Linde's Operative Gynecology*. 10th ed. Philadelphia, PA: Lippincott Williams & Wilkins; 2008:330-331.
19. Chu J, Hu Y, Xia-Chan C, et al. Laparoscopy versus open myomectomy—a meta-analysis of randomized controlled trials. *Eur J Obstet Gynecol Reprod Biol*. 2009;145:14-21.
20. Seinera P, Arisio R, Decko A, Farina C, Crana F. Laparoscopic myomectomy: indications, surgical technique and complication. *Hum Reprod*. 1997;12:1927-1930.
21. Advincula AP, Xu X, Goudeau S, Ransom SB. Robotic-assisted laparoscopic myomectomy versus abdominal myomectomy: a comparison of short-term surgical outcomes and immediate costs. *J Minim Invasive Gynecol*. 2007;14:698-705.
22. Advincula AP, Song A, Burke W, Reynolds RK. Preliminary experience with robot assisted laparoscopic myomectomy. *J Am Assoc Gynecol Laparosc*. 2004;11:511-518.
23. Visco AG, Advincula AP. Robotic gynecologic surgery. *Obstet Gynecol*. 2008; 112:1369-1384.
24. Ubaldi F, Tournaye H, Camus M, Van der Pas H, Gepts E, Devroey P. Fertility after hysteroscopic myomectomy. *Hum Reprod Update*. 1995;1:81-90.

Case 20

A 46-year-old G3P3 woman is coming into the office for follow-up for menorrhagia. She originally presented to her gynecologist 2 months previously with complaints of heavy vaginal bleeding for several years, and the loss of a moderate amount of urine with Valsalva and cough; the loss of urine was reported as bothersome to her and limited her activities. She denied dysuria and urgency symptoms. She required the use of a sanitary pad to protect her clothing from her incontinence. On examination, she was found to have an enlarged uterus (18 cm in size) with multiple fibroids. A cotton tip applicator in the urethra moved 70 degrees with Valsalva, and the patient was noted to have a small cystocele and loss of urine with Valsalva. An endometrial biopsy was performed and revealed benign secretory endometrium; aa urine culture was negative for growth. Medical therapy with oral contraceptive pills had been initiated for her menorrhagia, and she was instructed on pelvic floor exercises. The patient reported that she complied with both the OCP's and pelvic floor exercises, which provided no relief of symptoms. She is mildly anemic (hemoglobin 11.5 g/dL) requiring oral iron supplements. A urodynamic study is performed and reveals genuine stress incontinence. Because of the size of her uterus, a total abdominal hysterectomy is planned for definitive therapy. The patient is also counseled about a surgery for treatment of her urinary stress incontinence.

➤ What are two urethropexy surgical therapies that could be performed for her urinary incontinence at the time of her abdominal hysterectomy?

➤ What is the main difference between the two most common urethropexy surgeries?

ANSWERS TO CASE 20: Urethropexy

Summary: This is a 46-year-old woman with symptomatic uterine fibroids not responsive to medical therapy desiring definitive therapy with a total abdominal hysterectomy. She also has stress urinary incontinence, for which she desires surgical therapy at the same time as the hysterectomy.

- **Urethropexy procedures:** Marshall-Marchetti-Krantz (MMK) and Burch procedures. Additionally, midurethral sling procedures could also be done.
- **Difference between MMK and Burch:** The primary difference between the MMK and Burch procedure is the points of attachment of the periurethral endopelvic fascia. The MMK was the first retropubic urethropexy procedure described and involves attachment of endopelvic fascia to the periosteum of the pubic symphysis. The Burch procedure attaches the endopelvic fascia to Cooper ligament.

ANALYSIS

Objectives

1. Describe the surgical principles of both the MMK and Burch procedures.
2. Become familiar with the important anatomical landmarks for both procedures.
3. Describe the strategies to prevent and recognize intraoperative complications.

Considerations

This is a 46-year-old woman with problems of urinary stress incontinence and symptomatic uterine fibroids. There are multiple surgical procedures to address stress urinary incontinence, which can be performed via an abdominal or vaginal approach. Recently, midurethral sling procedures have gained popularity, either via the transobturator route or transvaginal route. The gold standard surgical treatment of stress urinary incontinence in patient with a hypermobile bladder neck is via a retropubic approach with MMK or Burch procedures. In this patient, because an abdominal hysterectomy is being planned, a retropubic urethropexy can be easily performed through an abdominal incision. Given the small cystocele, a Burch procedure would likely be the ideal surgery as it may help correct the small cystocele.

APPROACH TO
Urinary Incontinence

DEFINITIONS

OSTEITIS PUBIS: Inflammation of the pubic bone's periosteum which can occur after suprapubic suspension procedures like the MMK.

URODYAMIC STRESS INCONTINENCE: Involuntary loss of urine when the intravesicular pressure exceeds the urethral closure pressure.

SPACE OF RETZIUS: Retropubic space where a retropubic urethropexy is performed.

CLINICAL APPROACH

Proper patient selection and surgeon expertise determine the success of any surgical procedure. In general, there are two primary surgical treatments for stress urinary incontinence: retropubic urethropexy and sling procedures. In order to select the proper surgery, many factors need to be weighed. Some factors to consider are the age/health of the patient, presence of other pelvic disease, degree of pelvic organ prolapse, physician expertise, and patient preferences. In this case, the patient has uterine pathology requiring a laparotomy with no evidence of significant pelvic organ prolapse. A retropubic urethropexy after the hysterectomy through the abdominal incision makes the most sense. Tension-free vaginal sling procedures would be best suited for patients desiring or requiring shorter operative and postoperative recovery times, having evidence of intrinsic sphincter deficiency, or undergoing concurrent vaginal surgery.

Published studies indicate that the 5- to 10-year cure rate is as high as 82% for both MMK and Burch procedures when properly performed.[1] This is comparable to success rates published for most sling procedures. Long-term (10-20 years) cure rate after a Burch procedure is reported as 69%. Most studies that have compared laparoscopic Burch procedures to the open procedure have shown similar cure rates (one study in 2004 demonstrated improved cure rates with open technique). Removal of the uterus, in the absence of uterine pathology or prolapse, does not improve the efficacy of the urethropexy procedure. Hysterectomy may increase operative blood loss, operative/postoperative time, and the possibility of vaginal prolapse in the future.[2-5]

A large multicenter randomized trial compared the Burch procedure with tension-free vaginal tape (TVT) procedures and demonstrated no significant difference in objective short-term (< 10 years) cure rates.[6] Bladder injuries were seen more often in TVT procedures, but Burch procedures had a higher incidence of delayed voiding and longer operative and postoperative recovery times.[7]

APPROACH TO
Retropubic Urethropexy

The two most common abdominal retropubic urethropexy procedures are the MMK and Burch procedures. Both procedures elevate and stabilize the anterior vaginal wall which, in turn, elevates the urethrovesical angle and proximal urethra into more of an intra-abdominal position. Either procedure can be performed by itself or in conjunction with another intra-abdominal procedure (abdominal hysterectomy). With the bladder neck in the intra-abdominal position, increased intra-abdominal pressure is equally distributed to both the urethra and bladder favoring continence.[3]

In the operating room, the patient is placed in dorsal supine position with legs in stirrups (Allen Universal Stirrups for example). A 16- to 18-Fr sterile Foley catheter is placed in the bladder with 30 cc of fluid in Foley bulb. A low transverse or low vertical incision is then made and carried down to the retropubic space.

The retropubic space, also known as "the space of Retzius," is a potential space lying outside the peritoneal cavity (Figure 20–1). It must be entered and dissected prior to proceeding with either an MMK or Burch procedure. The retropubic space is bounded by the anterior pubic bones and symphysis pubis anteriorly and bladder, urethra, and vagina posteriorly. The space is filled with loose areolar connective tissue, fat, and many blood vessels. If the patient has not had previous surgery in this space, the area can be opened with careful and gentle blunt dissection. Patients with previous surgery in the retropubic space, usually require sharp dissection due to dense adhesion formation. The urethra is palpated easily with the aid of the Foley catheter, and the inferior edge of the bladder is identified with the aid of the large Foley bulb and is seen as a rounded midline structure. If the bladder anatomy is not easily seen, a cystotomy can be performed in the dome of the bladder to aid in identifying the limits of the bladder.

Once the limits of the bladder have been determined, the endopelvic fascia is identified. Permanent (or at least delayed absorbable) sutures are then placed through the endopelvic fascia while a finger in the vagina elevates the endopelvic fascia. The use of a sterile thimble can be used on finger elevating the endopelvic fascia to minimize risk of needle stick injuries. The suture should be placed so that the needle is directed upward and toward the midline to avoid vessel injury. Two endopelvic fascia sutures are placed on each side of the urethra and tied. If an MMK is performed, the endopelvic fascia is suspended to the periosteum of the pubic symphysis. In contrast, the endopelvic fascia is suspended to Cooper ligament during the Burch procedure (see Figure 20–2). The suspension should be without significant tension

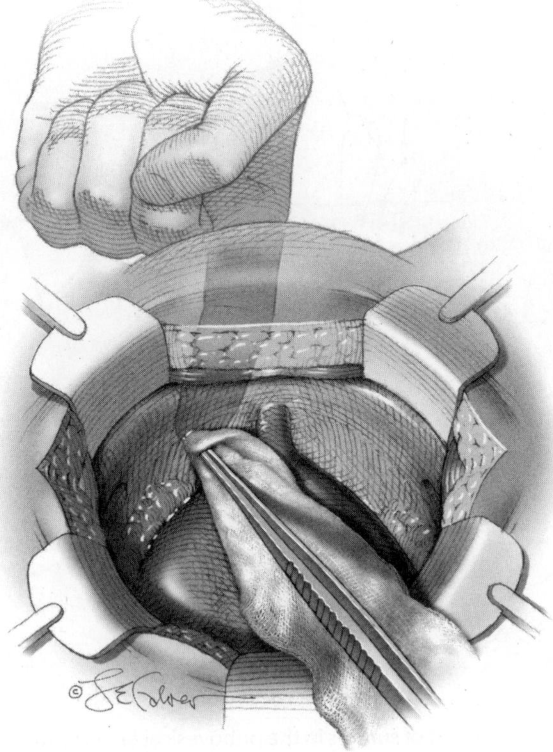

Figure 20–1. Dissecting the space of Retzius. *(Reproduced, with permission, from Schorge JO, Schaffer JI, Halvorson LM, et al.* Williams Gynecology. *New York: McGraw-Hill, 2008:978.)*

and that allows a finger between the endopelvic fascia and permanent attachment.[8-14]

Advantages of the Burch over the MMK include its ability to correct for a cystocele, firmer point of fixation, and the absence of osteitis pubis risk. The potential complication of hemorrhage exists for both procedures. Hemorrhage can occur from the vascular network of the rich thin-walled vessels located in the retropubic space or the longitudinal venous plexus that courses outside each anterior lateral vaginal fornix. Bleeding can be prevented by careful dissection and cauterization of blood vessels. If hemorrhage ensues, the gloved finger in the vagina, used for elevation of the endopelvic fascia, can be elevated to diminish bleeding until the source of the bleeding is identified and ligated. A surgical drain may be needed if excessive bleeding is noted in the retropubic space.[12]

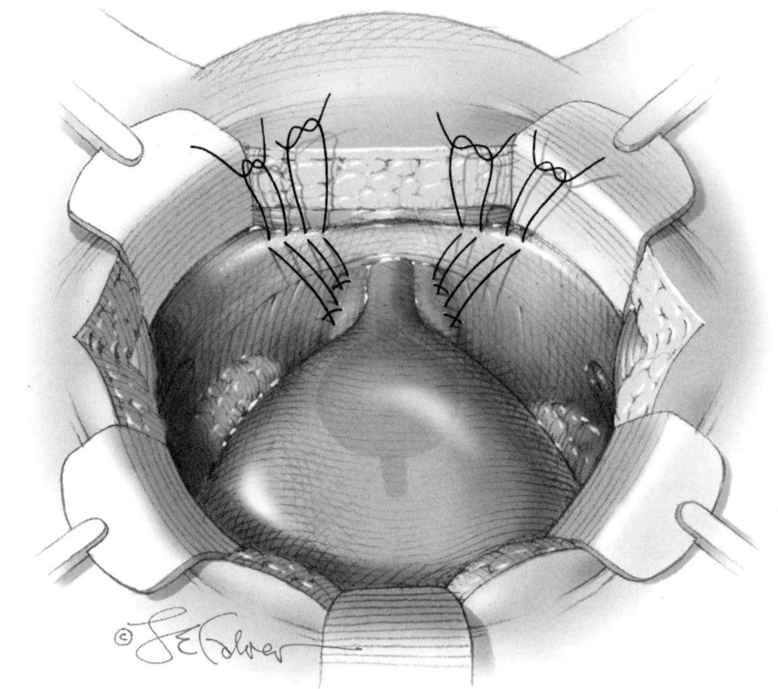

Figure 20–2. Placement of sutures in the pubovesical fascia to the Cooper ligament. *(Reproduced, with permission, from Schorge JO, Schaffer JI, Halvorson LM, et al.* Williams Gynecology. *New York: McGraw-Hill, 2008:979.)*

Postsurgical voiding dysfunction can be seen with either procedure. The development of detrusor instability occurs in 10% to 15% of patients[15,16] and once infection has been ruled out, should be addressed. Some degree of urinary retention is seen in 15% to 20% of patients. This often can be managed with prolonged bladder drainage and rarely with removal of suspension sutures. The incidence of urinary retention can be reduced intraoperatively by allowing a space (1-2 cm) between the suspended endopelvic fascia and fixation point.[2]

Osteitis pubis is a rare complication of the MMK procedure occurring in 1% to 2% of all patients.[15] This painful condition is caused by an inflammatory reaction (noninfectious) in the periosteum of the pubic bone, resulting in pain (osteomyelitis is the infectious form). When supportive care is not sufficient, the suspension sutures may need removal.

Comprehension Questions

20.1 A third-year resident is being instructed in the surgical management of a patient with urinary incontinence. How many total sutures (both sides added together) should be placed in the endopelvic fascia during a Burch or MMK procedure?

A. One
B. Two
C. Four
D. As many as possible

20.2 A 35-year-old woman underwent an MMK urethropexy procedure and developed symptoms consistent with osteitis pubis. Which of the following about osteitis pubis is most accurate?

A. Often occurs after a Burch Procedure.
B. Occurs in the immediate postoperative period.
C. Is a delayed complication (> 2 months).
D. Pain symptoms are constant with no aggravating or alleviating factors.

20.3 While performing a Burch procedure, a significant amount of bleeding is encountered in the space of Retzius. The area has blood pooling and it is difficult to detect the origin of the bleeding. What is your first course of action?

A. Place a surgical drain.
B. Elevate the endopelvic fascia with your finger in the vagina.
C. Place a suture in the general area of the bleeding.
D. Obtain vascular surgeon intraoperative consultation.

ANSWERS

20.1 C. Two to three sutures are recommended through the endopelvic fascia on each side of the urethra (total of four). A higher failure rate has been observed with one suture compared to two sutures. The placement of too many sutures can lead to urinary retention.

20.2 C. A patient with osteitis pubis usually presents with pubic pain and a "waddling" gate 2 months after an MMK. The pain is usually abrupt in nature, may radiate down the inner aspect of the thigh, and is aggravated by activity. In the absence of an infection, the patient is treated with bedrest, steroids, and analgesics. If symptomatic treatment is insufficient, the suspension sutures may need removal.

20.3 **B**. When entering the space of Retzius, careful meticulous dissection is required to avoid substantial bleeding. However, if hemorrhage ensues after stitch is placed in the endopelvic fascia or with dissection, the endopelvic fascia with finger in the vagina should be gently elevated. This maneuver usually decreases the bleeding and allows for better visibility. Once the vessel is identified, it can be suture-ligated or cauterized under direct visualization. Blindly placing sutures in the space of Retzius can lead to injury to the bladder or urethra.

Clinical Pearls

See Table 1-2 for definition of level of evidence and strength of recommendation

- Short-term outcomes of midurethral slings are similar to the traditional retropubic approach (Level A).
- The development of de novo detrusor instability occurs in about 15% of patients after a retropubic urethropexy (Level B).
- The placement of two to three permanent sutures in the endopelvic fascia during a Burch procedure has been shown to be superior to the placement of just one (Level B).
- In the event of hemorrhage in space of Retzius, elevation of the endopelvic fascia decreases the amount of bleeding so that the injured vessels can be visualized and ligated (Level C).

REFERENCES

1. Feyereisl J, Dreher E, Haenggi W, et al. Long-term results after Burch colposuspension. *AM J Obstet Gynecol.* 1994;171:647.
2. American College of Obstetricians and Gynecologists. *Urinary Incontinence in Women.* ACOG Practice Bulletin No. 63. Washington DC; 2005.
3. Katz VL, Lentz GM, Lobo RA, Gershenson DM. Urogynecology. In: *Comprehensive Gynecology*. 5th ed. Philadelphia, PA: Mosby; 2007:537-563.
4. Langer R, Ron-El R, Neuman N, Herman A, Bukovsky I, Caspi E. The value of simultaneous hysterectomy during Burch colposuspension for urinary incontinence. *Obstet Gynecol.* 1988;72:866-869.
5. Lapitan MC, Cody DJ, Grant AM. Open retropubic colposuspension for urinary incontinence in women. *Cochrane Database Syst Rev.* 2003;(1):CD009212. [DOI: 10.1002/14651858. CD002912].
6. Ward K, Hilton P. Prospective multicentre randomized trial of tension-free vaginal tape and colposuspension as primary treatment for stress incontinence. United Kingdom and Ireland Tension-Free Vaginal Tape Trial Group. *BMJ*. 2002;325:67-70.
7. Alcaly M, Monga A, Stanton SL. Burch colposuspension: a 10-20 year follow up [published erratum appears in *Br J Obstet Gynaecol.* 1996;103:290]. *Br J Obstet Gynaecol.* 1995;102:740-745.

8. Ankardal M, Ekerydh A, Crafoord K, Milsom I, Stjerndahl JH, Engh ME. A randomized trial comparing open Burch colposuspension using sutures with laparoscopic colposuspension using mesh and staples in women with stress urinary incontinence. *BJOG*. 2004;111:974-981.
9. Baggish M, Karram M. Operative setup and entry into the retropubic space and retropubic urethropexy for stress incontinence. In: *Atlas of Pelvic Anatomy and Gynecologic Surgery*. 2nd ed. Philadelphia, PA: Elsevier Mosby; 2006:333-338.
10. Hurt G. Retropubic urethropexy or colposuspension. In: *Urogynecologic Surgery*. 2nd ed. Baltimore: Lippincott Williams & Wilkins; 2000:80-92.
11. Moehrer B, Carey M, Wilson D. Laparoscopic colposuspension: a systematic review. *BJOG*. 2003;110:230-235.
12. Ostergard DR, Bent AE, Cundiff GW, Swift SE. Surgical correction of stress urinary incontinence. In: *Ostergard's Urogynecology and Pelvic Floor Dysfunction*. 5th ed. Philadelphia, PA: Lippincott Williams & Wilkins; 2003:455-467.
13. Rock J, Jones H. Urinary stress incontinence. In: *Te Linde's Operative Gynecology*. 10th ed. Philadelphia, PA: Lippincott Williams & Wilkins; 2008:936-955.
14. Wheeless CR. Retropubic urethropexy: Marshall-Marchetti-Krantz and Burch operations. In: *Atlas of Pelvic Surgery*. 3rd ed. Baltimore, MD: Williams & Wilkins; 1997:139-143.
15. Mainprize T, Drutz H. The Marshall-Marchetti-Krantz procedure: a critical review. *Obstet Gynecol Surv*. 1988;43:724-729.
16. Jarvis GJ. Surgery for genuine stress incontinence. *Br J Obstet Gynaecol*. 1994;101:371-374.

Case 21

A 19-year-old G1P0 Hispanic woman presents at 41 weeks' gestation for induction of labor. Her pregnancy was complicated by A1 gestational diabetes. Her estimated fetal weight was 9 lb (4 kg) by Leopold maneuver. The patient has a favorable cervix and adequate pelvis, and thus induction was begun with oxytocin (Pitocin). The patient progressed with a protracted labor course. An epidural anesthesia was placed after the patient reached 4 cm dilation. The nurse commented that the oxytocin was at 40 mU/min for greater than 8 hours even before the patient completed the first stage of labor. Oxytocin was continued at the same rate throughout the second stage of labor which lasted 2.5 hours.

An infant weighing 10 lb 3 oz (4.54 kg) was delivered via spontaneous vaginal vertex delivery over a third-degree midline laceration. The laceration was repaired while awaiting placental detachment. The placenta was delivered spontaneously and was intact. Immediately after the placental delivery, significant vaginal bleeding was noted. Attempts at uterine massage and intravenous dilute Pitocin administration were employed without success. The patient received methylergonine (Methergine) and prostagladin $F_{2\alpha}$ (Hemabate) that were also utilized to no avail. Estimated blood loss was nearly 2000 mL at this point. She is complaining dizziness/light-headedness and is found to have a pulse of 128 beats/min and BP of 86/42 mm Hg.

➤ What is the most likely diagnosis?

➤ What is your next step?

➤ What techniques may be utilized?

ANSWERS TO CASE 21: Surgical Management of Postpartum Hemorrhage

Summary: This is 19-year-old woman G1P0 at 41 weeks' gestation status post a spontaneous vaginal vertex delivery complicated by postpartum hemorrhage. Medical management for this condition has failed.

- **Most likely diagnosis:** Postpartum hemorrhage most likely secondary to uterine atony.
- **Next step:** Operative management.
- **Techniques utilized:** Arterial embolization, hypogastric artery ligation, B-lynch stitch, G stitch, packing of uterus, Logothetopulos pack (umbrella pack), SOS Bakri balloon tamponade (Cook Medical Inc., Bloomington, IN).

ANALYSIS

Objectives

1. Describe the symptoms and signs of postpartum hemorrhage.
2. List the management of the medical and surgical options for management of postpartum hemorrhage.
3. Be familiar with the techniques available for surgical management.

Considerations

This is a 19-year-old G1P0 Hispanic woman presenting at 41 weeks' gestation with a pregnancy complicated by gestational diabetes. Suspicion of a macrosomic infant was encountered at intake of the patient. The patient progress along a protracted first stage approached the upper limits of normal. Throughout her labor course oxytocin augmentation was continued at the upper level of normal as well. The delivered infant was indeed macrosomic. Bleeding persisted after the delivery of the placenta and after initial routine postdelivery protocols (oxytocin and uterine massage). Uterine atony was immediately suspected as it is the number one cause of postpartum hemorrhage. Of low suspicion were retained placental parts. This could be initially ruled out by inspection of delivered placenta and (if necessary) manual exploration of the uterus.

Given the patient's vital signs (mean arterial pressure of 50 mmHg) and symptoms, the patient is in advanced trauma life support (ATLS)-classified class 3 hypovolemic shock. The administration of fluids and IV access are imperative. Blood should be typed/crossed if possible and ready for transfusion. The patient needs to be monitored closely for the development of disseminated intravascular coagulation (DIC). Once the etiology of the hemorrhage is confirmed to be atony, multiple different medications can be given, including prostaglandins (prostaglandin E1 [PGE_1] analogue [misoprostol per rectum] and $F_{2\alpha}$ [Hemabate] and semisynthetic ergot alkaloids [methylergonine]). Because of the patient's clinical condition and the fact that medical management has failed, surgical intervention is necessary. Given the young age and future fertility desires of the patient, a more conservative surgical course must be considered. Options available include B-lynch stitch, G-stitch, various methods of compression via endometrial tamponade, and ligature of the uterine vasculature. These efforts must be considered in this patient as long as she is stable, before hysterectomy is deemed necessary.

APPROACH TO Postpartum Hemorrhage

DEFINITIONS

POSTPARTUM HEMORRHAGE: Hemorrhage following delivery from excessive bleeding from the placental implantation site, trauma to the genital tract and adjacent structures, or both. Loss of 500 mL of blood or more after completion of third stage of labor of a vaginal delivery or loss of 1000 mL of blood or more during a cesarean delivery. Significant bleeding that may result in hemodynamic instability if unabated.

UTERINE ATONY: Lack of myometrial contraction, clinically manifested by a boggy uterus.

HYPOGASTRIC ARTERY: Also known as the internal iliac artery. Posterior division branches: iliolumbar artery, lateral sacral arteries, superior gluteal artery. Anterior division: inferior gluteal artery, umbilical artery, superior vesical artery, uterine artery (females) or deferential artery (males), vaginal artery (females, can also arise from uterine artery), inferior vesical artery, middle rectal artery, internal pudendal artery.

B- AND G-LYNCH STITCH: Suturing techniques that result in uterine compression when uterine atony is encountered.

CLINICAL APPROACH

Assessment of the etiology of postpartum hemorrhage is paramount to the correct management of the situation. The classic definitions are exceeding 500-mL after vaginal delivery, or exceeding 1000 mL for a cesarean delivery, but these amounts not easily measured. Studies have found that about 5% of women delivering vaginally lost more than 1000 mL of blood and they also observed that the estimated blood loss (EBL) is commonly only half the actual loss. The substantial amount of blood loss that is deemed "routine EBL" is tolerated due to the initial hypervolemia that the pregnant patient develops during pregnancy. Increase of 1500 to 2000 mL of blood volume or 30% to 60% rise is encountered. The mother can encounter a great deal of blood loss before shock ensues.[1]

Efforts to minimize the amount of blood loss include medical and surgical management options. Medical management begins with routine oxytocin administration either during or immediately after the third stage of labor. Gentle uterine fundal massage is also employed. Further management entails the use of either prostaglandin $F_{2\alpha}$ (Hemabate) and/or semisynthetic ergot alkaloid (Methergine). Misoprostol, a PGE_1 analogue, has also been used rectally to induce uterine contraction. Medical management's approach is aimed at correcting the underlying basis of uterine atony, by promoting myometrial contraction.

When medical management measures fail, surgery must be considered. Hysterectomy is the most definitive and rapid approach to alleviating the bleeding, but of course, prevents future children. More conservative measures may be considered if the patient is stable and desires future fertility. These measures include methods that mechanically contract the uterus (B-lynch and G-stitch), or involve interruption of the vascular flow to the uterus. The focus of the remaining discussion will be on one such vascular interruption.

Bilateral hypogastric artery ligation has been described as a method to conservatively manage severe pelvic hemorrhage. One of the first documented accounts of this procedure was documented in 1893 at Johns Hopkins Hospital when Howard Kelly performed ligation of bilateral hypogastric arteries to control hemorrhage during hysterectomy for uterine cancer.[1]

Ligation of the hypogastric artery is associated with a 77% decrease in the pulse pressure just distal to the point of the suture. Bilateral ligation decreases pulse pressure by 85%.[2] The decreased pulse pressure allows for clot formation at the site of vascular injury. Blood flow is only decreased by 48% in vessels distal to the point of ligature. By ligating the anterior division of the hypogastric artery, it allows isolation of the collateral arterial circulation from the pelvis and reduced pulse pressure in the bleeding artery.

The technical execution of hypogastric artery ligation may be difficult at the time of severe hemorrhage; great precision must be employed to ensure proper anatomical identification to avoid vascular or ureteral injury. The peritoneum is opened on the lateral side of the common iliac near its bifurcation. The ureter is left attached to the medial peritoneal reflection to avoid disruption of its blood supply. It is important to ligate the anterior division of the hypogastric artery distal to the posterior parietal branch. The posterior division must be identified before the anterior division is ligated. The anterior division is dissected from the underlying hypogastric vein. Nonabsorbable suture is passed around the artery generally using a right-angle clamp and tied. The second free-tie suture is placed distal to the first ligature. Transection is not to be employed; in other words, the artery is ligated with suture but the artery is not divided. Ligation of the uterine artery may be performed at this point if it is able to be identified. In matters of postpartum hemorrhage, this may prove to be a valuable addendum to traditional hypogastric artery ligation techniques. The uterine artery is the first branch of the anterior division of the hypogastric artery and may be ligated at that location.[3-8]

Postpartum hemorrhage involves more than just the uterine artery as the source of blood flow to the uterus. The ovarian artery is an important collateral communication of the aorta to the uterine vasculature; thus, interruption of this large source of blood is beneficial in cases of postpartum hemorrhage. The lateral peritoneal incision is extended above the pelvic brim and the bifurcation of the common iliac artery. Ligation of both the ovarian artery and vein is acceptable if difficulty is encountered, identifying the artery from the vein. Bilateral ovarian arteries are dissected free from the retroperitoneal position at or above the pelvic brim and free-tied. One ligature is utilized and the artery is not to be transected. As with any procedure in this portion of the pelvis, care must be taken to avoid ureteral injury.

Cruikshank and Stoelk[9] describe an alternative method to ligation of the ovarian artery in the infundibulopelvic ligament. Instead, the artery is ligated at the point of anastomosis with the uterine artery in the medial mesosalpinx (preserving blood flow to the tube and ovary while decreasing flow to the uterus).

Fehrman goes as far to say that bilateral uterine artery ligation is a more effective treatment for life-threatening uterine hemorrhage than is bilateral hypogastric artery ligation. If this measure is not sufficient, then supplementary ligation of the round ligament and the ovarian ligaments at their junction with the uterine corpus may be employed.

Full-term delivery has been described after hypogastric artery ligation with and without ovarian artery ligation. Collateral blood supply develops over time. These collateral pathways provide enough blood flow to support a developing intrauterine pregnancy.

Morbidity is decreased with hypogastric artery ligation methods compared to hysterectomy as well as a preservation of fertility. Blood loss has been demonstrated to be substantially higher in women undergoing bilateral hypogastric artery ligation and a subsequent hysterectomy secondary to failure than in women who had a hysterectomy without attempts at artery ligation (5125 vs 3209 mL, respectively).[1]

Vascular complications are generally forgiving due to the rich pelvic anastomoses that are present. Potential complications arise when these collateral pathways are damaged. Several of the complications related to surgical interventions have been described. Complications include sterility, gangrene of the bladder, urinary tract injury and genitourinary fistula, bowel injury and genitointestinal fistula, vascular injury, pelvic hematoma, and sepsis. Ultrasound of the kidneys following complicated emergency pelvic surgery in order to exclude ureteric obstruction should be considered. Division of the posterior branch of the hypogastric artery has resulted in necrosis of the ipsilateral gluteal muscles. Major intraoperative complications arise from excessive blood loss and the management of shock and fluid replacement. A potential complication may arise if future embolization of bleeding arterial branches is attempted, and may be impossible to perform.[10]

Hypogastric artery ligation has been described as an option for management of postpartum hemorrhage in the properly selected patient. Fertility is preserved in the great majority of successful outcomes from this effort. Other surgical options in postpartum hemorrhage due to uterine atony include uterine artery ligation (Figure 21–1), B- and G-lynch suturing techniques (Figure 21–2), and ultimately hysterectomy. Uterine artery

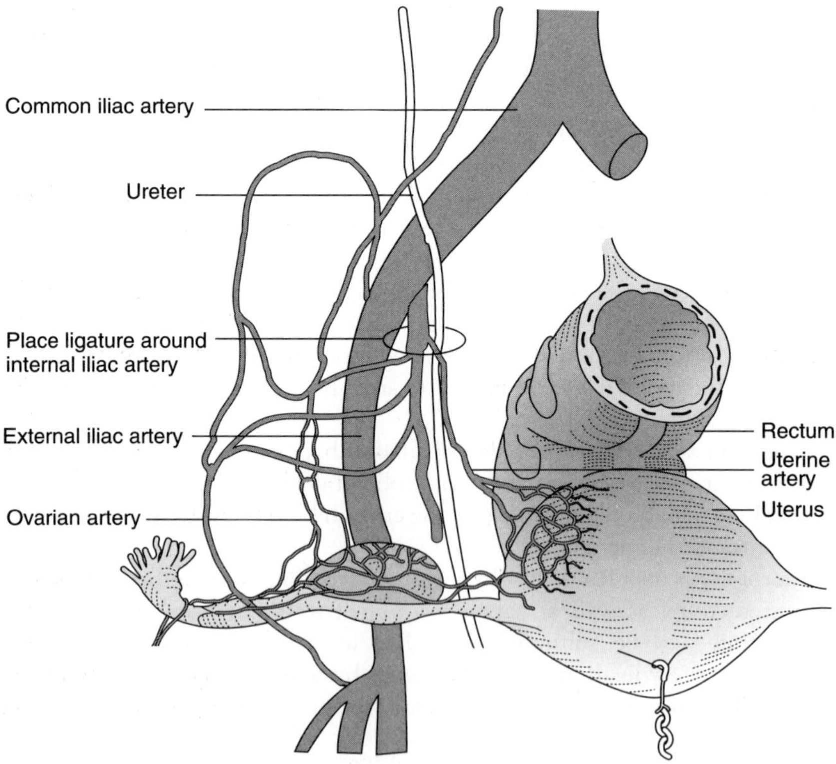

Figure 21–1. Internal iliac artery ligation should be distal to posterior trunk, and not incorporate the ureter. *(Reproduced, with permission, from DeCherney AH, Nathan L, Goodwin TM, et al.* Current Diagnosis & Treatment: Obstetrics & Gynecology, *10th ed. New York: McGraw-Hill, 2007:482.)*

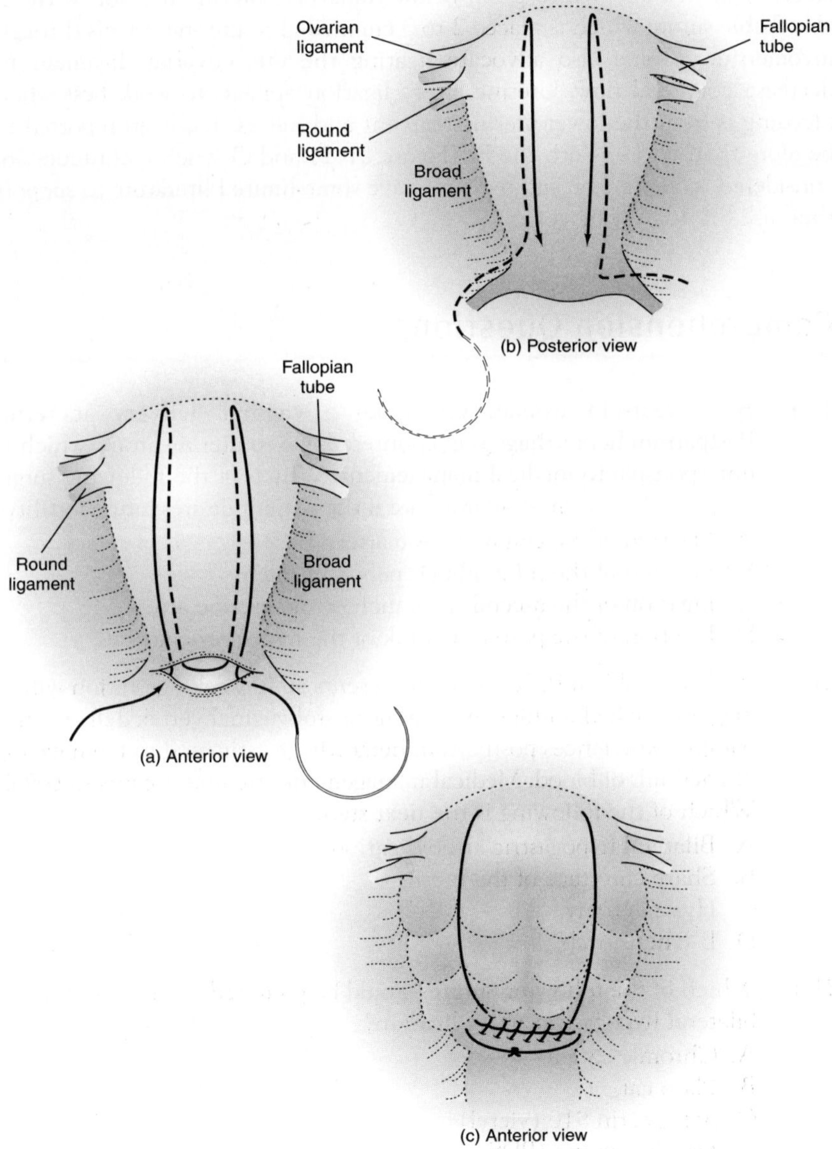

Figure 21–2. B-lynch suture is used as an external compression to the uterus. (*Reproduced, with permission, from DeCherney AH, Nathan L, Goodwin TM, et al.* Current Diagnosis & Treatment: Obstetrics & Gynecology, *10th ed. New York: McGraw-Hill, 2007:483.*)

ligation can be performed by most obstetricians in a safe manner. The uterine artery is ligated about 2 to 3 cm below transverse uterine incision with an absorbable suture which is placed 2 to 3 cm medial to uterine vessels through myometrium. Some also advocate ligating the utero-ovarian ligament to decrease collateral flow. Uterine artery ligation appears to work best when bleeding is from the lower uterine segment and success has been reported to be more than 95%.[11] Both the B- (Figure 21–2) and G-lynch techniques are considered "compression sutures" and have some limited literature to support their use.[1,12-14]

Comprehension Questions

21.1 A 21-year-old woman undergoes a vaginal delivery at term. Postpartum hemorrhage is encountered due to uterine atony, which is unresponsive to medical management. Which of the following surgical procedures is most appropriate if the patient desires future fertility?

A. Ligation of the common iliac artery
B. Ligation of the infundibular pelvic ligament
C. Ligation of the ascending branch of the uterine artery
D. Ligation of the posterior trunk of the hypogastric artery

21.2 A 37-year-old G6P5005 woman presents at 40 weeks' gestation with a diagnosis of hydramnios. After a successful vaginal vertex delivery, the patient experiences postpartum hemorrhage estimated to be in excess of 2500 mL of blood. Medical management attempts are unsuccessful. Which of the following is the next step?

A. Bilateral hypogastric artery ligation
B. Sharp curettage of the uterus
C. Hysterectomy
D. B-lynch stitch

21.3 Which of the following sutures would be preferred when performing a bilateral hypogastric artery ligation?

A. Chromic catgut
B. Plain catgut
C. polyglactin 910 (vicryl)
D. Polydioxanone (PDS

ANSWERS

21.1 C. In a patient with uterine bleeding, decreasing the arterial perfusion is one of the primary therapeutic strategies. Ligation of the ascending branch of the uterine artery bilaterally is effective and allows for fertility. Ligation of the infundibular pelvic ligament means sacrificing both ovaries which will lead to an infertile and castrated patient. Ligation of the common iliac artery should never be performed due to disruption of the arterial supply to the lower extremity. Ligation of the posterior trunk of the hypogastric artery leads to ischemia of the gluteal region.

21.2 C. Careful selection of patients for attempts at conservative management of hemorrhage is crucial to the morbidity of the patient. In this case a multiparous patient with a number of risk factors for postpartum hemorrhage was encountered (high parity, hydramnios). The patient is multiparous and has an excessive blood loss secondary to uterine atony. Given these factors, hysterectomy would be the most appropriate measure. Sharp dilation and curettage of the uterus is an option for patients experiencing postpartum hemorrhage secondary to retained products of conception. The B-lynch stitch is a suture that manually compresses the uterus. The suture has been effective in some cases, although there are limited published data comparing its effectiveness to that of hysterectomy.

21.3 C. Nonabsorbable suture (silk) and delayed absorbable suture (Vicryl) have been utilized in bilateral ligation of the hypogastric artery. PDS has a tendency to cut through the tissue when tying and thus would be contraindicated. The premise of the technique is to ligate the vessel and not to transect. Chromic is absorbable suture.

Clinical Pearls

See Table 1-2 for definition of level of evidence and strength of recommendation

- The most common cause of postpartum hemorrhage is uterine atony (Level B).
- Arterial embolization of uterine vasculature may be impossible to perform after bilateral hypogastric artery ligation (Level B).
- Fertility may be preserved with bilateral hypogastric artery ligation (Level B).
- Conservative surgical management is a possibility in the properly selected patient (Level C).
- Ureteral damage is a complication with bilateral hypogastric artery ligation and must be ruled out if clinically suspected at time of operation or postoperatively (Level C).

REFERENCES

1. Cunningham FG, Leveno KJ, Bloom SL, Hauth JC, Gilstrap LC III, Wenstrom KD. Obstetrical hemorrhage. In: *Williams Obstetrics*. 22nd ed. New York, NY: McGraw-Hill; 2005:809-854.
2. Burchell RC. Physiology of internal iliac artery ligation. *J Obstet Gynaecol Br Commonw*. 1969;57:642.
3. Evans S, McShane P. The efficacy of internal iliac artery ligation in obstetric hemorrhage. *Surg Gynecol Obstet*. 1985;160:250.
4. Fahmy K. Internal iliac artery ligation and its efficacy in controlling pelvic hemorrhage. *Int Surg*. 1969;51:244.
5. Reich WJ, Nechtow MJ. Ligation of the internal iliac (hypogastric) arteries: a life-saving procedure for uncontrollable gynecologic and obstetric hemorrhage. *J Int Coll Surg*. 1961;36:157.
6. Rock JA, Jones HW III. Control of pelvic hemorrhage. In: *Te Linde's Operative Gynecology*. 10th ed. Philadelphia, PA: Lippincott Williams & Wilkins; 2008:385-387.
7. Siegel P, Mengert WF. Internal iliac artery ligation in obstetrics and gynecology. *JAMA*. 1961;178:1059.
8. Slate WG. Internal iliac ligation. *Am J Obstet Gynecol*. 1966;95:326.
9. Cruikshank SH, Stoelk EM. Surgical control of pelvic hemorrhage: bilateral hypogastric artery ligation and method of ovarian artery ligation. *South Med J*. 1985;78:539.
10. Given FT, Gates HS, Morgan BE. Pregnancy following bilateral ligation of the internal iliac (hypogastric) arteries. *Am J Obstet Gynecol*. 1964;89:1078.

11 O'Leary JA. Uterine artery ligation in the control of postcesarean hemorrhage. *J Reprod Med.* 1995;40:189.

12. B-Lynch CB. Coker A, Laval AH, Abu J, Cowen MJ. The B-lynch surgical technique for control of massive postpartum hemorrhage: an alternative to hysterectomy? Five cases reported. *Br J Obstet Gynaecol.* 1997;104:372.

13. Hayman RG, Arulkumaran S, Steer PJ. Uterine compression sutures: surgical management of postpartum hemorrhage. *Obstet Gynecol.* 2002;99:502.

14. Rock JA, Jones HW III. Obstetric problems. In: *Te Linde's Operative Gynecology.* 10th ed. Philadelphia, PA: Lippincott Williams & Wilkins; 2008:827-829.

Case 22

A 45-year-old G4P4004 Caucasian woman presents with a 6-month history of increasing "pelvic heaviness." She had a postpartum bilateral tubal ligation following delivery of her last child. She relates that she had a forceps delivery with her first child, and that she stands at work most of the day as a surgical scrub tech. She has also noticed increasing dyspareunia, stating that, "It feels like my partner is hitting something when we have intercourse." She denies stress urinary incontinence, recurrent urinary tract infection, or difficulty with defecation. Her Pap smears have been normal throughout her life, and there has been no change in her menstrual pattern. She relates that 6 months of intensive Kegel exercises have not changed her symptoms. On pelvic examination, she has normal external genitalia. The vaginal mucosa demonstrates good estrogen effect, and there is adequate support of both the anterior and posterior vaginal walls. The parous cervix descends to within 1 cm of the vaginal introitus with a Valsalva maneuver. The uterus is nontender, and not enlarged, and the adnexa are not palpable. The rectal examination is unremarkable.

➤ What is the most likely diagnosis?

➤ What should be your next step?

ANSWERS TO CASE 22: Vaginal Hysterectomy

Summary: A 45-year-old woman presents with pelvic heaviness and dyspareunia. The pelvic examination reveals that her cervix descends to the vaginal introitus with Valsalva. According to the pelvic organ prolapse quantification (POP-Q) scoring system, this is stage II pelvic organ prolapse.[1]

➤ **Most likely diagnosis:** Uterine prolapse.

➤ **Next step:** Vaginal hysterectomy.

ANALYSIS

Objectives

1. Understand that most benign uterine pathology requiring hysterectomy is amenable to the vaginal approach.
2. Learn the indications, advantages, and disadvantages of vaginal hysterectomy compared to abdominal or laparoscopically assisted vaginal hysterectomy.

Considerations

Uterine prolapse to the extent described in this case is a common problem for parous women, and operative vaginal delivery is increasingly felt to be a risk factor for the later development of pelvic organ prolapse. For a healthy patient who is not desirous of having any more children, vaginal hysterectomy is the procedure of choice. It is difficult to say with certainty whether a given patient's prolapse will worsen, but it is not likely to improve over time. **In comparison to total abdominal hysterectomy (TAH) or laparoscopic hysterectomy (LH), vaginal hysterectomy (VH) is faster, cheaper, safer, less painful, and most cosmetically and sexually satisfying to the patient. For benign disease, almost all types of uterine or pelvic pathology, which require hysterectomy as the therapy of choice, can be accomplished vaginally.**[2] The goal of this chapter is to delineate the reasons why vaginal hysterectomy should usually be the hysterectomy route of first choice for most benign gynecologic conditions requiring uterine removal.

APPROACH TO
Vaginal Hysterectomy

DEFINITIONS

VAGINAL HYSTERECTOMY: Removal of the entire uterus through the vagina. When appropriate, this is often combined with **unilateral or bilateral salpingo-oophorectomy**, removing one or both fallopian tubes and ovaries vaginally coincident with the hysterectomy.

TOTAL ABDOMINAL HYSTERECTOMY: Removal of the entire uterus via a laparotomy incision, whether through a vertical or transverse incision. Can likewise include removal of tubes and ovaries as above.

LAPAROSCOPIC HYSTERECTOMY: This operation has three possible variants. LAVH is aided by the laparoscope, but not to include uterine artery ligation; LH, where the laparoscope is used to ligate the uterine arteries; and TLH, in which there is no vaginal approach and the cuff is closed laparoscopically. Tubes and ovaries may also be removed via these techniques.

CLINICAL APPROACH

Hysterectomy rates in the United States are decreasing slightly, from 5.5 per 1000 women in 1990 to 5.1 per 1000 women in 2004. Abdominal hysterectomy is the most common approach, constituting 63% of all types in 1997. In April 2008, French gynecologists reported their experience comparing vaginal hysterectomy to LAVH in women who had not had prior vaginal delivery. They noted that there was less OR time, shorter hospital stay, and less cost to the patient when the vaginal approach was used. Further, as they progressed through the study and became increasingly comfortable with the vaginal approach, they relied less on the laparoscope for assistance.[3] Newer techniques such as supracervical or laparoscopic hysterectomies do not have any advantages over vaginal or abdominal hysterectomies, especially in terms of avoiding complications, including urinary and sexual function. Urinary incontinence is more frequent in women who have supracervical hysterectomy than in women randomized to vaginal hysterectomy, and there is no difference in sexual function in either group, regardless of hysterectomy technique or presence of a residual cervix.[4] **Leaving the cervix in situ as a result of a supracervical laparoscopic procedure has been associated with an increase in later trachelectomy procedures for cyclical monthly bleeding from the cervix, for cervical dysplasia, and for prolapse of the cervical**

stump, all of which can be eliminated by removing the cervix at VH. If these new technologies are being questioned, it is appropriate to reiterate the benefits of VH. This discussion will focus on the indications for vaginal hysterectomy and compare vaginal hysterectomy to other hysterectomy techniques in terms of uterine size, safety, length of hospital stay, cost, and patient satisfaction, including cosmetic results and sexual function.

Indications

Vaginal hysterectomy is performed only one-third as frequently as abdominal hysterectomy in the United States. The use of systematic guidelines and algorithm protocols makes it possible to transform many, if not most, abdominal hysterectomies into vaginal procedures. Many expert national bodies and professional organizations have published the indications for hysterectomy.[14] An abbreviated list of their indications includes **leiomyomata in uteri, abnormal uterine bleeding, endometriosis, pelvic relaxation, pelvic pain, endometrial hyperplasia with atypia, adenocarcinoma of the endocervix when invasive disease has been excluded, and as a prophylactic procedure to include bilateral oophorectomy when there is a positive family history of ovarian cancer.** There are traditional contraindications to VH that need to be reevaluated in the light of contemporary experience. **Many authors have demonstrated that the enlarged uterus may be removed vaginally.**[5,6,7,8] **Nulliparity is not a contraindication to vaginal hysterectomy, nor is a history of cesarean section. The absolute number of cesarean sections is not shown to increase the number of surgical complications.**[9] **Planned removal of adnexal pathology does not preclude the vaginal approach, nor does a history of prior abdominal surgery.**

There is concern in our specialty about the declining percentage of hysterectomies being done via the vaginal approach. Perhaps these numbers can stabilize if conditions that were traditionally viewed as being relative or absolute contraindication to vaginal hysterectomy can be perceived less dogmatically, and the decision regarding hysterectomy route can be made as objectively as possible, taking into account the pathology likely to be encountered, the desires of the patient, the experience of the surgeon, and the expense to be encountered.[10]

Uterine Size

Within reason, an enlarged uterus is not a contraindication to vaginal hysterectomy.[11] **Morcellation, bivalving, or coring facilitates removal of the large uterus**, and complication rates are generally lower with the vaginal approach. Blood loss seems to be related to the size of the uterus, as does operating time, which increases in a linear fashion according to uterine weight. Studies demonstrate comparable blood loss with either the VH or the TAH.[4] However, in comparison to TAH, the operating time for removing the enlarged uterus is not necessarily increased when using the vaginal approach. VH patients generally leave the hospital sooner than TAH patients. Comparisons of VH to LAVH for removal of the enlarged uterus indicate that the complication rate is higher for the LAVH, and that VH is preferable. Uteri weighing up to 280 g probably should be able to be removed vaginally by a skilled gynecologist—if vaginal removal is paramount, consider referral to an experienced vaginal surgeon when the uterine weight is expected to exceed this amount, or use an abdominal approach.

In removing the large uterus, once the uterine arteries have been secured, if leiomyomata are encountered that make removing the rest of the organ in situ difficult, then the cervix should be divided vertically with the scalpel until the body of the uterine corpus is encountered. Grasp each side of the amputated cervix with either Massachusetts clamps or single- or double-toothed tenacula, and then reduce the size of the corpus uteri by coring it centrally with the scalpel or Mayo scissors until the reduced size of the uterus allows its removal. A myoma screw is occasionally helpful at this juncture, allowing the surgeon to obtain a grasp of a myoma with one hand while the other hand uses an instrument to excise the tumor. Patience is rewarding during this process, and blood loss is rarely a problem if the uterine arteries were secured properly when the cervix was severed. The use of the operating headlight, a long-handled scalpel, and long Mayo scissors facilitates this portion of the operative procedure.

Safety

Published articles have also noted improved secondary outcomes with VH compared to TAH, specifically regarding febrile episodes and unspecified infections.[6] In those instances where VH could not be performed, they note that LH was preferable to AH, but at the greater risk of injury to the bladder or ureter. **Further studies indicate that there is a significant learning curve with both VH and LH, noting that the incidence of bleeding and bowel injuries associated with VH and the incidence of ureteral and bladder injuries with LH both tend to decrease with increasing experience of the gynecologic surgeon.** Several studies note that blood loss from VH is less than that from either TAH or LH.[12,13] Obese women suffer fewer complications if they have VH rather than TAH. They have less OR time, less ileus, less postoperative fever and wound infections, fewer urinary tract infections, and a shorter hospital stay.

Length of Stay

Several studies have evaluated length of stay relative to type of hysterectomy performed. They conclude that VH patients had a shorter hospital stay than TAH patients, usually staying at least a day less in the hospital postoperatively. VH procedures require less operating time than LH or TAH procedures, and VH patients usually convalesce more quickly than TAH patients and are able to resume normal activity more quickly.

Cost

VH typically costs less than TAH or LH or its variants because there is less utilization of OR time, the hospital stay is shorter, and the cost of OR equipment for reusable vaginal instruments is far less than that of disposable instruments for LH.[12,14] Like supracervical LH procedures, VH can also be performed in an outpatient fashion. Using carefully designed protocols based on good scientific evidence for proper patient selection, several authors report on the efficacy and reduced cost of performing VH on an outpatient basis, some discharge patients within 12 hours of admission, and note cost reductions of 20% to 25% compared to procedures requiring longer hospitalization. VH is consistently considered the most cost-effective approach. In this era of managed care, some insurance companies are still making the mistake of paying more for TAH and LH procedures than for VH approaches. It is estimated that the expense of hysterectomy is inflated by a factor of 200% to 300% because of the use of TAH and LH instead of VH. Adding the cost of the OR expense to the cost of anesthesia time yields an expense of about $50 per minute for gynecologic surgery. For the typical hospital being reimbursed a standard fee for similar procedures, the choice of VH over TAH and LH will make a huge difference in hospital costs when all of the cases are totaled at the end of a fiscal year.

Education

TAH is easier to teach and learn than VH. The view of the operative field is better for both the resident and the attending gynecologist with an open abdomen than that which can be obtained with both the surgeon and the assistants looking into the vagina. Nonetheless, responsible national organizations, hospital leadership groups, and residency training programs and education bodies recognize the benefits of VH. Implementation of the goal of making VH the standard approach requires change at the local level to implement the national efforts to increase the percentage of hysterectomies performed vaginally.[15] Published reports indicate that a change in approach is possible, and that with a concerted effort, in 3 to 7 years some hospitals have completely reversed the percentages of hysterectomies done abdominally and vaginally. Residency programs that wish to increase the percentage of VH procedures have reported being able to do so over the course of several years, without a concomitant increase in the complication rate. In most hospital settings, the senior gynecologists with many years of operating experience are the most proficient vaginal surgeons. Many articles have suggested that, in addition to increasing the number of VH procedures in residency, **the concept of using these senior physicians as mentors for newly minted gynecologists will increase the proficiency of the new staff members as vaginal surgeons.**[16]

Sexual Function and Cosmetic Results

Claims that leaving the cervix in place as an advantage of supracervical hysterectomy for better sexual function and orgasmic response have not been supported by any confirmatory studies in the medical literature. Extensive studies over the past several years have shown that improvements in sexual desire, activity, and coital frequency all increase after recovery from hysterectomy, whether VH or TAH. Scores for vaginismus, lack of orgasm, loss of sexual interest, and dyspareunia all decreased after recovery from hysterectomy.[17] Women who have had TAH have more of a negative body image because of the abdominal scar, and they have more postoperative pain and a slower recovery than did the patients in the VH groups.[17] **Women who were sexually active prior to hysterectomy tend to remain sexually active following hysterectomy, without encumbrance from the pathology necessitating hysterectomy in the first place.**

Technique

Gynecology is the only specialty in which the physician is uniquely trained to work inside the vagina. A successful vaginal surgeon appreciates the finesse of his/her skill, and learns that millimeters of exposure and meticulous dissection measure the difference between success and failure when working vaginally. He/she learns to regard the Heaney clamp as a functional extension of his/her hands, Russian forceps as transmitting a tactile sense which he/she can discern in his/her fingertips, and a needle driver in his/her grasp as secure and steady in an operative site where he/she is specifically trained to operate (Figures 22–1 through 22–5).

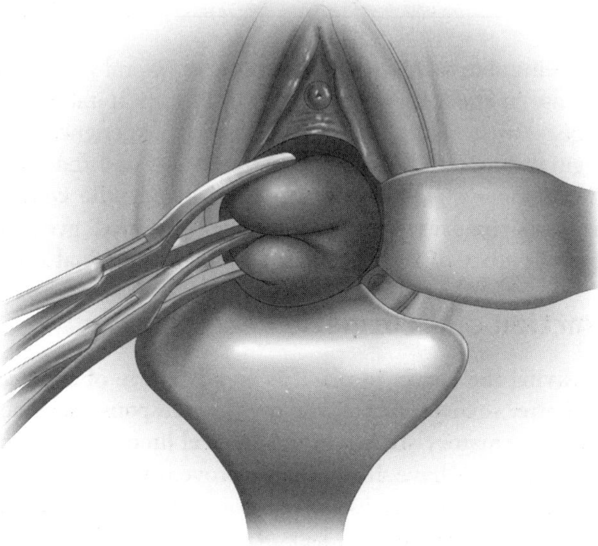

Figure 22–1. Vaginal mucosa incised circumferentially. *(Reproduced, with permission, from Brunicardi FC, Andersen DK, Billiar TR, et al.* Schwartz's Principles of Surgery, *9th ed. New York: McGraw-Hill, 2010:1505.)*

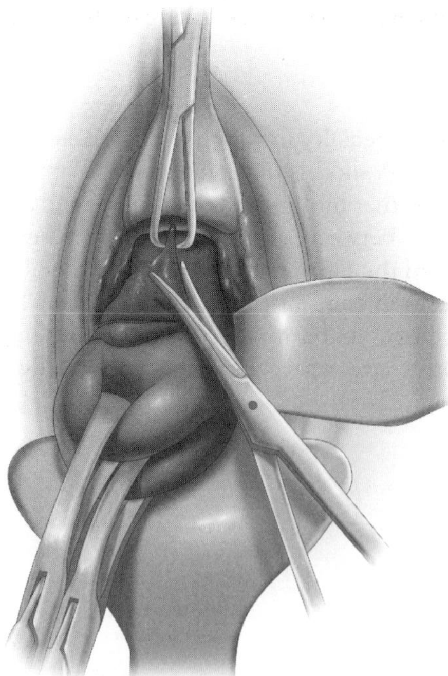

Figure 22–2. The anterior cul-de-sac is entered sharply. *(Reproduced, with permission, from Brunicardi FC, Andersen DK, Billiar TR, et al.* Schwartz's Principles of Surgery, *9th ed. New York: McGraw-Hill, 2010:1505.)*

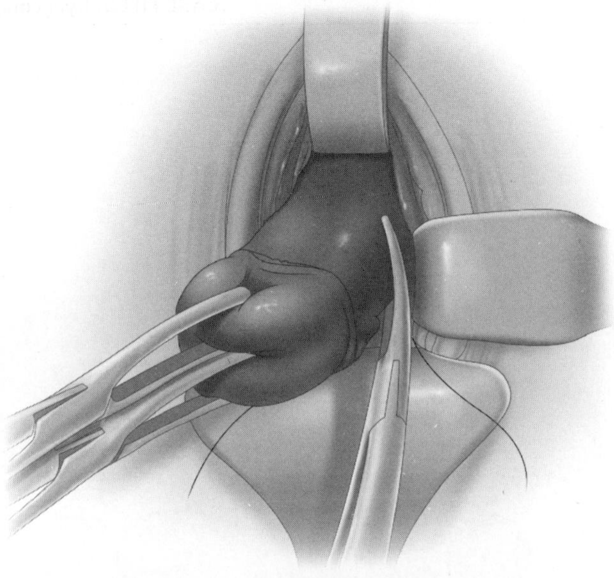

Figure 22–3. The pedicles are suture-ligated. *(Reproduced, with permission, from Brunicardi FC, Andersen DK, Billiar TR, et al.* Schwartz's Principles of Surgery, *9th ed. New York: McGraw-Hill, 2010:1505.)*

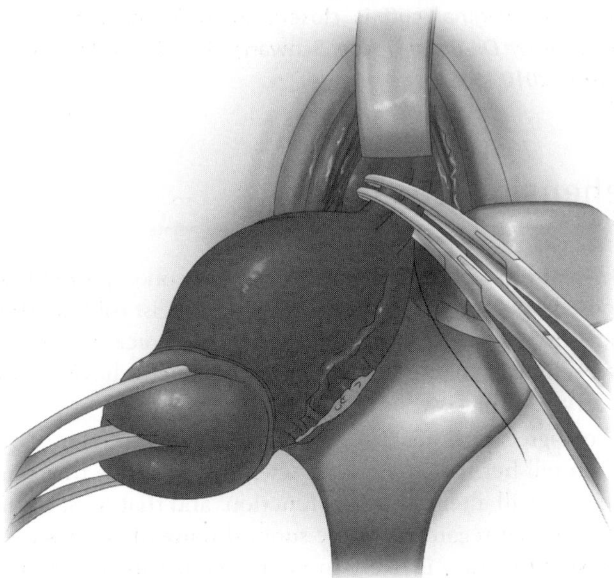

Figure 22–4. The uterus is completely excised. *(Reproduced, with permission, from Brunicardi FC, Andersen DK, Billiar TR, et al.* Schwartz's Principles of Surgery, *9th ed. New York: McGraw-Hill, 2010:1505.)*

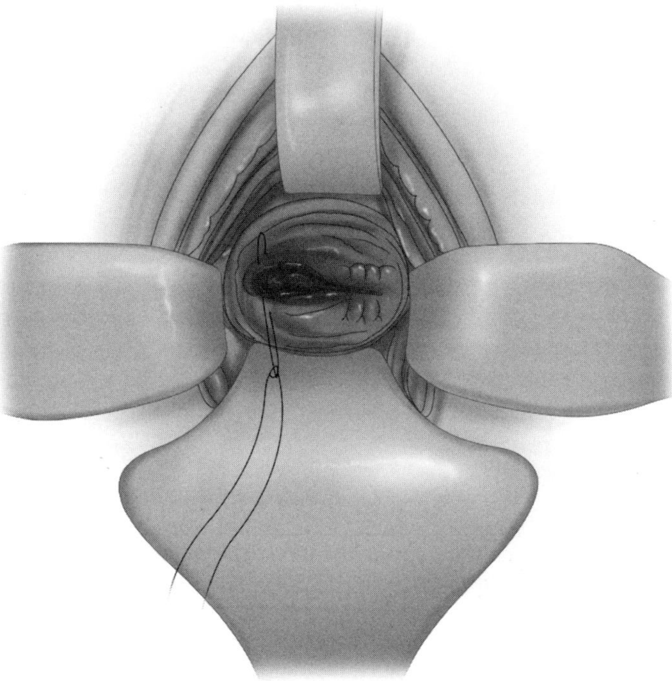

Figure 22–5. The vaginal cuff is closed. *(Reproduced, with permission, from Brunicardi FC, Andersen DK, Billiar TR, et al.* Schwartz's Principles of Surgery, *9th ed. New York: McGraw-Hill, 2010:1505.)*

Comprehension Questions

22.1 A 42-year-old woman consults you for a second opinion regarding her proposed hysterectomy. The initial gynecologist told her that a supracervical hysterectomy was the procedure of choice, rather than vaginal hysterectomy, because she would not be able to have orgasm without her cervix. What is your response?

A. You agree with her first gynecologist.

B. You tell her that there is no scientific evidence that removing her cervix will alter her sexual function, and that most studies demonstrate that regardless of the surgical route of her hysterectomy, her sexual function is likely to improve once she completely recovers from her surgery.

C. You tell her that you will refer her for sexual counseling postoperatively.

D. You plan to treat her with testosterone following surgery.

22.2 A 37-year-old patient has symptomatic uterine leiomyomas, and ultrasound confirms an enlarged uterus which you estimate weighs 250 g. Her friends tell her that she should have an abdominal hysterectomy because her uterus is too big to be removed safely via the vaginal route. What do you tell her?

A. You agree with her friends and schedule her for an abdominal hysterectomy.
B. You propose a laparoscopic hysterectomy as an alternative.
C. You tell her that you believe you can do the hysterectomy vaginally, and that you will begin using that approach, but that you are prepared to operate abdominally if necessary to complete the operation safely.
D. You propose myomectomy as an alternative.

22.3 A 35-year-old woman weighing 275 lb (124.74 kg) requires hysterectomy for menorrhagia not responsive to hormone therapy or endometrial ablation. She is afraid of vaginal hysterectomy because she believes that she will bleed excessively. What do you tell her?

A. You agree with her and schedule an abdominal hysterectomy.
B. You ask her to store blood in the blood bank for use at surgery.
C. You tell her that most scientific studies have indicated that her blood loss will be less vaginally than abdominally.
D. You schedule her for laparoscopic hysterectomy.

ANSWERS

22.1 **B.** The route of hysterectomy does not have any advantage in terms of sexual function. The cervix is not necessary for orgasm.

22.2 **C.** An enlarged uterus is not a contraindication to vaginal hysterectomy.

22.3 **C.** Several studies have shown that vaginal hysterectomy is associated with less blood loss than either abdominal or laparoscopic hysterectomy.

Clinical Pearls

See Table 1-2 for definition of level of evidence and strength of recommendation

- Infiltrate the vaginal mucosa at six equidistant sites around the cervix at the proposed incision site with a mixture of 1% with 1:100,000 epinephrine, or vasopressin, to reduce intraoperative blood loss (Level B).
- Use a headlight, or instruments such as retractors or suction instruments with a light source attached, when performing vaginal surgery. Standard OR lights are rarely bright enough, do not focus sharply, and never are at an optimum angle for seeing how to work in the vagina (Level C).
- If the vaginal hysterectomy is not accompanied by colporrhaphy, avoid the use of a Foley catheter. Tell the patient she will arrive in the recovery room with a full bladder, and that she will be encouraged to void in recovery. If unable to void, she may be straight-catheterized twice over the next 6 to 8 hours, and should have a Foley placed only after the third failed voiding attempt. Over 75% of patients will never need a Foley (Level B).
- Close the vaginal cuff vertically rather than horizontally if there is concern about maintaining adequate vaginal length. Horizontal closure shortens the vagina by about 1 cm; vertical closure does not significantly change vaginal length (Level B).

REFERENCES

1. Bump RC, Mattiasson A, Bø K, et al. The standardization of terminology of female pelvic organ prolapse and pelvic floor dysfunction. *Am J Obstet Gynecol.* 1996;175:10-17.
   The classic treatise describing the POPQ system for quantifying pelvic organ prolapse.
2. Johnson N, Barlow D, Lethaby A, Tavender E, Curr E, Garry R. Surgical approach to hysterectomy for benign gynaecological disease. *Cochrane Database Syst Rev.* 2006 Apr;19(2):CD003677.
3. Le Tohic A, Dhainaut C, Yazbeck C, Hallais C, Levin I, Madelenat P. Hysterectomy for benign uterine pathology among women without previous vaginal delivery. *Obstet Gynecol.*2008;111:829-837.
4. Gimbel H, Zobbe V, Anderson BM, Filtenborg T, Gluud C, Tabor A. Randomised controlled trial of total compared with subtotal hysterectomy with one-year follow up results. *BJOG.* 2003;110:1309-1318.
5. Paparella P, Sizzi O, Rosetti A, De Benedittis F, Papaarella R. Vaginal hysterectomy in generally considered contraindications to vaginal surgery. *Arch Gynecol Obstet.* 2004;270:104-109.
6. Makinen J, Johansson J, Tomas C, et al. Morbidity of hysterectomies by type of approach. *Hum Reprod.* 2001;16:1473-1478.

7. Jacobsen G, Shaber R, Armstrong M, Hung Y. Hysterectomy rates for benign indications. *Obstet Gynecol.* 2006;107:1278-1283.
8. Doucette R, Sharp H, Alder S. Challenging generally accepted contraindications to vaginal hysterectomy. *Am J Obstet Gynecol.* 2001;184:1386-1389.
9. Poindexter Y, Sangi-Haghpeykar H, Poindexter A, et al. Previous cesarean section. A contraindication to vaginal hysterectomy? *J Reprod Med.* 2001;46:840-844.
10. Julian TJ. Vaginal hysterectomy. An apparent exception to evidence-based decision making. *Obstet Gynecol.* 2008;111:812-813.
11. Unger J. Vaginal hysterectomy for the woman with a moderately enlarged uterus weighing 200 to 700 grams. *Am J Obstet Gynecol.* 1999;180:1337-1344.
12. Levy B, Luciano D, Emery L. Outpatient vaginal hysterectomy is safe for patients and reduces institutional cost. *J Minim Invasive Gynecol.* 2005;12:494-501.
13. Olah K, Khalil M. Changing the route of hysterectomy: the results of a policy of attempting the vaginal approach in all cases of dysfunctional uterine bleeding. *Eur J Obstet Gynecol Reprod Biol.* 2006;125:243-247.
14. Lefebvre G, Allaire C, Jeffrey J, et al. SOCG clinical guidelines. Hysterectomy. *J Obstet Gynaecol Can.* 2002;24:37-61.
15. Kovac S. Transvaginal hysterectomy: rationale and surgical approach. *Obstet Gynecol.* 2004;103:1321-1325.
    The definitive paper justifying vaginal hysterectomy, with an excellent algorithm to determine the correct surgical approach for a given patient.
16. Gutl P, Greimel E, Roth R, Winter R. Women's sexual behavior, body image and satisfaction with surgical outcomes after hysterectomy: a comparison of vaginal and abdominal surgery. *J Psychosom Obstet Gynaecol.* 2002;23:51-59.
17. Taylor S, Romereo A, Kammerer-Doak D, Rogers R. Abdominal hysterectomy for the enlarged myomatous uterus compared with vaginal hysterectomy with morcellation. *Am J Obstet Gynecol.* 2003;189:1579-1582.
18. Darai E, Soriano D, Kimata P, Laplace C, Leduru F. Vaginal hysterectomy for enlarged uteri, with or without laparoscopic assistance; randomized study. *Obstet Gynecol.* 2001;97:712-716.
19. Falcone T, Walters MD. Hysterectomy for benign disease. *Obstet Gynecol.* 2008;111:753-767.
    A definitive paper in the "clinical expert series" from the green journal.

Case 23

A 63-year-old woman, G4P4, presents to her gynecologist with a chief complaint of a large nontender mass protruding "several inches" out of her vaginal introitus. She relates a history of a vaginal hysterectomy 15 years earlier for vaginal prolapse. She denies any urinary or fecal incontinence, and relates that the mass exiting the vagina precludes satisfactory sexual intercourse. She is in good health otherwise, has an active lifestyle, and wants to be able to return to her golf and tennis activities as soon as possible.

- ➤ What is the most likely diagnosis?
- ➤ What is your next step?

ANSWERS TO CASE 23:

Vaginal Vault Prolapse, Sacrospinous Ligament Fixation, and Uterosacral Ligament Fixation

Summary: A 63-year-old woman, who is physically active, presents with a large bulge exiting the vaginal introitus. Examination reveals that she has Grade 4 vaginal vault prolapse, using the Baden-Walker staging system (see Table 23–1).

- **Most likely diagnosis:** Vaginal vault prolapse post-hysterectomy.
- **Next step:** Make a preoperative evaluation, discuss treatment options with the patient, and then proceed with sacrospinous ligament fixation or uterosacral ligament fixation.

ANALYSIS

Objectives

1. Be able to offer the patient appropriate options for therapy for pelvic organ prolapse based on evaluation of her symptoms, her physical findings, and her concerns regarding surgery.
2. Understand the potential surgical complications of sacrospinous ligament fixation (SSLF) and uterosacral ligament fixation (USLF).
3. Know how the SSLF and USLF procedures compare to each other regarding advantages and disadvantages, and to other solutions for pelvic organ prolapse.

Table 23–1 BADEN-WALKER SYSTEM FOR THE EVALUATION OF PELVIC ORGAN PROLAPSE ON PHYSICAL EXAMINATION

Grade posterior urethral descent, lowest part other sites
Grade 0: Normal position for each respective site
Grade 1: Descent halfway to the hymen
Grade 2: Descent to the hymen
Grade 3: Descent halfway past the hymen
Grade 4: Maximum possible descent for each site

Data from Baden WF, Walker T. Fundamentals, symptoms and classification. In: Baden WF, Walker T, *Surgical Repair of Vaginal Detects*. Philadelphia, PA: J.B. Lippincott; 1992, p. 14.

Considerations

This case is a 63 year-old woman in good health and physically active with vaginal vault prolapsed after hysterectomy. After a careful physical examination to ensure that there is no complicated reason for the prolapse, such as a pelvic tumor or ovarian cancer with ascites, the patient should be counseled on the options of therapy. In a patient who is a poor surgical candidate and not sexually active, a colpocleisis procedure is an option. In summary, this patient's problem is a common complaint. As the "Baby Boomers" enter their postmenopausal years, many of them are going to experience pelvic organ prolapse and require the attention of gynecologists. Some 200,000 operative procedures for prolapse are performed annually in the United States, and some 25% to 29% of these surgical procedures are going to fail to achieve and/or to maintain their intended result over the rest of the patient's lifetime. **Not every patient who presents with pelvic organ prolapse is a surgical candidate, and knowing which patient will best avoid surgery is an important lesson to discern.** Multiple surgical procedures have been described and performed for pelvic organ prolapse. The SSLF procedure has been a relatively popular vaginal approach to vaginal vault prolapse in the United States for about the past 25 years, and more recently the USLF has been widely used for vaginal vault prolapse. There are some unique benefits and risks for each procedure, and the gynecologic surgeon needs to know these to be able to discuss these operations knowledgeably with the patient and to be able to perform one of these operations on her if the patient and her surgeon decide that this is the preferred approach for her problem.

APPROACH TO Sacrospinous Ligament Fixation

David Nichols and Clyde Randall popularized SSLF in the early 1980s in the United States. In the years since, several other vaginal approaches to vaginal vault prolapse have been introduced, including uterosacral ligament suspension, endopelvic fascial suspension, and other abdominal and laparoscopic approaches described for prolapse. Sze and Karram indicate that 40 separate operations have been described for these vaginal hernias.[1] Of the 40 described, the two most frequently performed procedures in the Unites States today are the SSLF and the USLF.

CLINICAL PRESENTATION

Etiologic factors probably include menopause and advancing age, a history of vaginal delivery, especially of large babies requiring operative vaginal deliveries, disorders of connective tissue, and any condition that increases intra-abdominal pressure, such as obesity or chronic constipation. No studies demonstrate that weight loss will reverse extant prolapse, although weight loss and pelvic floor exercises may be beneficially combined with watchful waiting, and surgery may be avoided if symptoms do not worsen. While the use of estrogen creams will facilitate the surgical procedure itself, by making the vaginal mucosa thicker and more pliable, there is no data to support the use of estrogen either systemically or topically to reverse or treat pelvic organ prolapse.

Most parous women will have some degree of pelvic relaxation on physical examination, but the symptomatology she experiences does not necessarily have a direct relationship to her degree of prolapse. The presence of some prolapse without symptoms does not merit treatment, and no studies have been able to prove that there are effective measures that can prevent the condition from worsening. The patient's history, general medical condition, and severity of symptoms must be carefully weighed when considering a therapeutic choice. Nonsurgical approaches include the use of a pessary, biofeedback training, and pelvic-floor rehabilitation. For the medically fragile patient, these less vigorous solutions may be a prudent first choice, with surgery being entertained only for worsening symptoms not responsive to a nonsurgical approach. Regardless of which surgical procedure is being considered, most authorities agree that the prolapse patient should be given the option of pessary use before proceeding to a surgical alternative.[2] In general, most women may be successfully fitted with a pessary, even those with the more severe grades of prolapse (see Table 23–2 for grading stage of prolpase). However, the long-term success rate for pessary use is probably related to severity of prolapse, and many patients prefer surgery to long-term pessary use.

Recent prospective studies have shown that prolapse actually has the potential to wax and wane in individual women, being worse in some years than in others, with the pelvic structures presenting higher or lower in the pelvis when measured using the pelvic organ prolapse quantification (POP-Q) system.[2] Based on this prospective study, it is also reasonable to tell a patient that excepting unusual circumstances, her prolapse is not likely to worsen dramatically over short periods of time.

Many patients are especially embarrassed discussing the symptoms associated with pelvic organ prolapse and will be hesitant to volunteer specific symptoms of urinary or fecal incontinence, or of having to splint and/or brace the perineum or vaginal floor to evacuate stool. The gynecologist must ask these questions and know this information to plan the correct therapeutic approach.

Choice of Surgical Procedure

If surgery is indicated for vaginal vault prolapse, the considerations include the fact that there is less apical failure with the abdominal sacrocolpopexy, and less postoperative stress urinary incontinence and dyspareunia with the abdominal approach, but at the expense of more complications, including all of those that accompany an abdominal procedure, especially bowel obstruction. The age and overall general health of the patient may tip the scales in favor of either the SSLF or the USLF procedure. Surgical series of patients older than 80 years describe successful repairs with good results, but with some

Table 23–2 STAGES OF PELVIC ORGAN PROLAPSE

Stages are based on the maximal extent of prolapse relative to the hymen, in one or more compartments.

Stage 0: No prolapse; anterior and posterior points are all −3 cm, and C (cervix) or D (posterior fornix) is between TVL (total vaginal length) and (TVL − 2) cm.

Stage I: The criteria for stage 0 are not met, and the most distal prolapse is > 1 cm above the level of the hymen < −1 cm).

Stage II: The most distal prolapse is between 1 cm above and 1 cm below the hymen (at least one point is −1, 0, or +1).

Stage III: The most distal prolapse is > 1 cm below the hymen but no further than 2 cm less than TVL.

Stage IV: Represents complete procidentia or vault eversion; the most distal prolapse protrudes to at least (TVL − 2) cm.

Pelvic Organ Prolapse Quantification System

Six vaginal sites used in staging prolapse:

Points Aa and Ba anteriorly

Points Ap and Bp posteriorly

Point C for the cervix or vaginal apex

Point D for the posterior fornix (not measured after hysterectomy)

Three additional measurements:

GH—genital hiatus

PB—perineal body

TVL—total vaginal length

Data from Bump RC, Mattiasson A, Bo K, et al. The standardization of terminology of female pelvic organ prolapse and pelvic floor dysfunction. *Am J Obstet Gynecol.* 1996; 175:10–17.

increased risk of blood loss in this patient population.[3] For the patient who wishes to remain sexually active, a distinct advantage of the SSLF or the USLF is the fact that the vagina is not shortened by this procedure, and there is usually no painful coitus following SSLF or the USLF. For women who are potentially too medically compromised for a major surgical procedure and who do not plan to be sexually active, colpocleisis may be considered. The surgeon and the patient need to decide together what procedure to use, depending on the physical findings, the potential for complications based on the patient's history, and what if any surgical procedure has failed previously. The SSLF and USLF procedures have the advantage of a transvaginal approach and a lower complication rate, albeit with a slightly higher failure rate over an extended time frame. For the patient wanting to avoid a laparotomy, this may be a minor consideration.

Recent studies, especially those using MRI data, have confirmed the importance of apical support of the vagina when repairing prolapse, and have demonstrated that an adequately supported vaginal cuff, whether obtained via SSLF or abdominal sacrocolpopexy, is capable of obviating some minor anterior or posterior wall repairs, as some minimal degrees of both cystocele and rectocele will disappear when the vagina is firmly anchored at its apex. This is not to state that large defects in the anterior and posterior wall should not be repaired if they are present—the best long-term results occur when all visible vaginal hernias are fixed. Further, apical support frequently maintains or restores vaginal length.[4] The opposite result, undesirable vaginal foreshortening, is not uncommon following colporrhaphy. Finally, these same studies demonstrate that the long-term success rate of all types of surgery for prolapse is substantially enhanced when apical support is performed as a distinct part of the operative procedure.[1,4,5,6,7]

Details of the Sacrospinous Ligament Fixation Procedure

As initially popularized, the SSLF procedure was a unilateral operation, affixing the right side of the vaginal apex to the right sacrospinous ligament. The operation optimally required direct visualization of right sacrospinous ligament, penetration of the ligament with a Deschamps ligature carrier, and retrieval of the suture with a hook to pull the suture back out of the operative site. Then, using a free needle, the suture is passed through the vaginal mucosa, affixing the vaginal cuff to the ligament. The original operation is exacting in its requirements for expert knowledge of the anatomy, superb dissection technique, excellent assistance for visualization, and readily available support if there is injury to the abundant vasculature in the region of the sacrospinous ligament. Regardless, the operation has been quite successful in attaching the vaginal cuff to the posterior pelvis and eliminating vaginal vault prolapse. An evaluation comparing direct visualization with a needle driver, the Deschamps ligature carrier, or the Miya hook suggests that the direct visualization approach may cause the least number of complications, but this requires the greatest degree of surgical dissection to obtain this degree of visualization.[8]

Two refinements to the classic operative procedure merit consideration now. The first is to perform the operation using a Capio device (Boston Scientific Corporation, Natick, MA), a laparoscopic "throw-and-catch" suturing instrument that allows the surgeon to place sutures through the sacrospinous ligament without the degree of visualization required with the classic operation, and with less risk of vascular or neurologic complication, because of the smaller instrument and needle size. Second, one may consider doing the operation as a bilateral procedure if there is enough room at the vaginal cuff to facilitate this. A two-point suspension will lessen the risk of failure; also, if one side needs to be removed for postoperative pain, the contralateral side may remain in place and provide adequate long-term support. The bilateral approach requires that there should not be undue tension on the vaginal apex as the cuff is stretched between the sacrospinous ligaments. The theoretical concerns of bowel compromise arising from the bilateral procedure have not been demonstrated in the literature.

Initial descriptions of the operative procedure described the placement of absorbable suture into the ligament, and later reports detail the use of delayed absorbable or permanent suture. There are no randomized, prospective trials indicating a clear benefit for one over the other, but the longer the suture remains in place, the greater the potential for beneficial fibrosis to affix the cuff to the ligament. Some experts suggest that there is a better long-term success rate with permanent suture, but if postoperative pain due to suture placement is a problem, it is likely to persist for as long as the suture remains in place.

Sacrospinous Ligament Fixation Complications

Complications of the procedure include hemorrhage, nerve injury, and damage to adjacent pelvic structures, including the subsequent onset of stress urinary incontinence. Hemorrhage is most common and will respond to direct ligation or the placement of vascular clips if the injured vessel can be seen and repaired. The inferior gluteal artery is probably the artery most frequently injured in doing the SSLF procedure. Alternative methods for control include consulting an invasive radiologist for arterial embolization. Venous injury may respond to packing the operative site firmly with laparotomy packs for as long as necessary to obtain hemostasis.

Pain is a not infrequent complication of SSLF, occurring some 3% to 5% of the time, and is due to involvement of nerve tissue in or near the coccygeal-sacrospinous ligament complex. Attention to placing the suture at least two finger-breadths medial to the ischial spine will avoid most of these problems, **but there is significant aberrant nerve supply to this region, and postoperative pain is not uncommon.** Minor pain is usually self-limited, and will resolve within 6 weeks. **Severe pain involving the buttocks and posterior thigh requires removal of the sacrospinous ligament suture.** Removal of the nerve-entrapping suture will result in dramatic pain relief within a few hours in most cases. Case reports indicate that removal of suture as long as 2 years after initial suture placement will provide prompt pain relief for entrapped nerve tissue.[9] Injury to bowel and bladder are uncommon, but need to be recognized and repaired when they occur.

Sexual function following SSLF is usually improved or unchanged following the operation, if care is taken not to constrict the diameter of the vagina at its apex, especially if concurrent colporrhaphy is performed.[10]

The SSLF procedure will realign the long axis of the vagina into a more posterior orientation in the pelvis than had previously been the case, and this may result in new-onset stress urinary incontinence. The rate of cystocele formation following SSLF ranges from 18% to 92%.[1] Preoperative urologic evaluation may delineate those patients with prolapse-reduced urinary incontinence who are most likely to experience this problem, and the planned operative procedure may benefit from the inclusion of anterior colporrhaphy or the placement of a tension-free vaginal tape (TVT) midurethral sling to prevent the occurrence of postsurgical incontinence.

Details of the Uterosacral Ligament Fixation Procedure

The USLF procedure may be done in conjunction with vaginal hysterectomy and colporrhaphy procedures, or as a standalone procedure in the patient who presents with vault prolapse following prior hysterectomy. With the vaginal cuff open following vaginal hysterectomy, or after opening the vaginal apex in vaginal vault prolapse cases, any enterocele present is opened and the hernia sac is excised and closed with a purse-string suture. Cut a laparotomy pack in half and place the half with the tail into pelvis, elevating the bowel out of the way. Narrow Briesky-Navritol retractors facilitate visualization at this part of the operation. Grasping the vaginal cuff at the 5 and 7 o'clock positions respectively and tugging with an Oschner clamp with one hand while palpating over the region of the ischial spines with the other index finger will confirm identification of the uterosacral ligament in the region posterior and medial to the spines. The ligament may be grasped with a long Allis clamp, and sutures (3-4 in number) placed through the ligament. It is important to go from lateral to medial when placing the sutures, to avoid the potential for ureteral injury. These sutures may be delayed absorbable, or permanent, but permanent suture should not be tied leaving the knots in the vagina. The sutures placed through the ligaments are then directed through the anterior and posterior vaginal mucosal (or submucosal surfaces, in the case of permanent suture), and tied after any colporrhaphy procedures are completed, elevating the vaginal cuff to the level of the ischial spines.

Uterosacral Ligament Fixation Complications

At the conclusion of the USLF procedure, it is routine to perform cystoscopy to be sure that there is no ureteral injury. IV furosemide and indigo carmine dye injected 5 to 7 minutes prior to cystoscopy will quickly and easily demonstrate normal ureteral function. The rate of ureteral injury has been reported to be as high as 11%.[6] The failure rate for the USLF procedure is reported to be in the 13% to 15% range.[6,7] Significant postoperative pain is not usually a problem following the USLF, nor are hemorrhage at the time of the procedure and infection, especially if prophylactic antibiotics are used preoperatively.

SSLF versus USLF?

When experienced gynecologic surgeons who have extensive experience with these operative procedures are asked which of the two they prefer, they usually choose the USLF over the SSLF. The USLF results in a more anatomic alignment of the vagina and has less postoperative pain. While there is the potential for ureteral injury, this should be detected and corrected at the time of surgery, with minimal prospect for long-term sequela. The SSLF increases the risk of cystocele, and the pain which can occur following this operation from pudendal nerve fiber entrapment is dramatic.

Comprehension Questions

23.1 A 58-year-old patient had a seemingly uneventful bilateral SSLF procedure for vaginal vault prolapse. On the day following surgery, she complains of extreme pain in the left buttocks radiating down the posterior left thigh, not relieved with morphine. What is your next course of action?

A. Consult the pain management service.
B. Consult a neurologist.
C. Take the patient back to the OR and remove the suture from the left sacrospinous ligament.
D. Send the patient for physical therapy.

23.2 A 63-year-old patient had SSLF for vaginal vault prolapse. At her 6-week postoperative check, she has apparently healed completely, with good support of the vaginal apex, but she complains of stress urinary incontinence which was not previously present. What is your next step?

A. Prescribe an anticholinergic drug.
B. Ask her to do Kegel exercises.
C. Urodynamic testing.
D. Counsel the patient regarding the need for an artificial urethra.

23.3 Your 61-year-old patient sought another opinion after you told her she needed anterior and posterior vaginal repairs and an SSLF or a USLF. The gynecologist she saw told her that she did not need either the SSLF or the USLF, and that they were unnecessary, complicated, and dangerous procedures, and the problem could be solved without doing anything more than anterior and posterior repairs. How do you counsel the patient at this point?

A. At this point, it is probably best to agree with her consultant gynecologist and opt for the anterior and posterior colporrhaphy procedures.
B. Tell her that without vaginal apical support, all other vaginal repair work is likely to fail, and discuss with her the relative risks and benefits of SSLF and USLF.
C. Offer her a pessary instead of surgical management.
D. Suggest only an abdominal sacrocolpopexy initially and vaginal repairs later if her problems persist.

ANSWERS

23.1 **C.** Severe pain following SSLF is due to nerve entrapment. If conservative measures fail, then surgical removal of the involved suture is the therapy of choice. Pain relief is usually prompt and dramatic once the suture is removed.

23.2 **C.** Urodynamic testing is needed for this patient. A sling will likely be necessary to restore the urethrovesical (U-V) angle altered by the SSLF procedure. Patients who have a SSLF procedure should be counseled that they may develop urinary incontinence that did not exist before the procedure. Some gynecologists will perform a prophylactic urinary procedure in anticipation of this complication.

23.3 **B.** The key to long-term vaginal wall support, especially anteriorly, is adequate support of the vaginal apex. The "gold standard" is abdominal sacrocolpopexy, and patients may be offered an abdominal approach as part of your preoperative discussion of surgical options, but the long-term potential for success of vaginal hernias requires adequate apical support, regardless of how it is achieved.

Clinical Pearls

See Table 1-2 for definition of level of evidence and strength of recommendation

- The major complication of the SSLF procedure is pain (Level A).
- If the patient complains of severe pain in the buttocks, radiating down the posterior thigh, remove the suture from the sacrospinous ligament on the involved side (Level B).
- When placing sutures in the sacrospinous ligament, leave the suture long enough to facilitate suture removal if this later becomes necessary (Level C).
- When doing the USLF procedure, do not cut the sutures after tying the knots until you are sure that there is no ureteral compromise. Wait until cystoscopy confirms the ureters are clear (Level B).
- Suspend the apex first, and then decide whether anterior or posterior colporrhaphy is still necessary (Level C).
- Do not do either of these operations for the first time without a more experienced gynecologist who is skilled in this procedure as your first assistant (Level C).

REFERENCES

1. Sze EHM, Karram MM. Transvaginal repair of vault prolapse: a review. *Obstet Gynecol.* 1997;89:466-475.
2. The American College of Obstetricians and Gynecologists. Pelvic organ prolapse. ACOG Practice Bulletin No. 85. *Obstet Gynecol.* 2007;110:717-730.
3. Nieminen K, Heinonen PK. Sacrospinous ligament fixation for massive genital prolapse in women aged over 80 years. *BJOG.* 2001;108:817-821.
4. Lowder JL, Park AJ, Ellison R, et al. The role of apical vaginal support in the appearance of anterior and posterior vaginal prolapse. *Obstet Gynecol.* 2008;111:152-157.

5. David-Montefiore E, Barranger E, Dubernard G, Nizard V, Antoine JM, Darai E. Functional results and quality-of-life after bilateral sacrospinous ligament fixation for genital prolapse. *Eur J Obstet Gynecol Reprod Biol.* 2007;132:209-213.
6. Silva WA, Pauls RN, Segal JL Rooney CM, Kleeman SD, Karram MM. Uterosacral ligament vault suspension: five year outcomes. *Obstet Gynecol.* 2006;108:255-263.
7. Shull BL, Bachofen C, Coates KW, Kuehl TJ. A transvaginal approach to repair of apical and other associated sites of pelvic organ prolapse with uterosacral ligaments. *Am J Obstet Gynecol.* 2000;183:1365-1373.
8. Miyazaki FS. Miya hook ligature carrier for sacrospinous ligament suspension. *Obstet Gynecol.* 1987;70:286-288.
9. Pollak J, Takacs P, Medina C. Complications of three sacrospinous ligament fixation techniques. *Int J Gynaecol Obstet.* 2007;99:18-22.
10. Holley RL, Varner RE, Gleason BP, Apffel LA, Scott S. Sexual function after sacrospinous ligament fixation for vaginal vault prolapse. *J Reprod Med.* 1996;41:355-358.
11. Bradley CS, Zimmerman MB, Qi Y, Nygaard IE. Natural history of pelvic organ prolapse in postmenopausal women. *Obstet Gynecol.* 2007;109:848-854.
12. Pohl JF, Frattarelli JL. Bilateral transvaginal sacrospinous colpopexy: preliminary experience. *Am J Obstet Gynecol.* 1997;177:1356-1361.
13. Kettel LM, Hebertson RM. An anatomic evaluation of the sacrospinous ligament colpopexy. *Surg Gynecol Obstet.* 1989;168:318-322.

Case 24

A 59-year-old G4 P4004 woman presents with a complaint of a bulge that is exiting her vagina, which is bothersome and she desires surgery. The patient had a vaginal hysterectomy 15 years earlier for uterine prolapsed. Two years ago, she had a vaginal sacrospinous ligament fixation (SSLF) for vaginal vault prolapsed. She does not complain of any urinary incontinence, and states that her health is otherwise excellent. She is frustrated with the failure of the prior vaginal SSLF procedure and is skeptical of another vaginal procedure for this condition.

➤ What is the most likely diagnosis?

➤ What is your next step?

ANSWERS TO CASE 24: Abdominal Sacral Colpopexy

Summary: A 59-year-old G4P4004 woman, who has had a prior vaginal hysterectomy and later vaginal sacrospinous ligament fixation, presents with a recurrent vaginal defect.

- **Most likely diagnosis:** Vaginal vault prolapse following previous vaginal sacrospinous ligament fixation.
- **Next step:** Evaluate the patient for surgical repair, most likely to consist of abdominal sacral colpopexy (ASC).

ANALYSIS

Objectives

1. Learn the advantages and disadvantages of ASC.
2. Learn the types of materials to be used in the performance of this operation.
3. Learn the complications associated with this operation.

Considerations

This 59 year old woman presents with recurrent vaginal vault prolapse following a prior operation, which unfortunately is not an uncommon experience. Likewise, as in the case of this patient, many patients will not consent to another operation essentially identical to the one that failed in the first place. Unfortunately, operations for vaginal vault prolapse fail about 25% of the time. It is the wise surgeon who can offer his patient either the vaginal or abdominal approach for correction of a previous failed surgical procedure. The patient who presents with vaginal vault prolapse is not always a surgical candidate, however, and the surgeon must discuss nonsurgical options with his patient before deciding on the surgical approach (see Case 23). As the population in the United States ages, the number of patients presenting for potential surgical repair of vaginal vault prolapsed will inevitably increase significantly. ASC has been referred to as the "gold standard" operation for vaginal vault prolapse, because it has the lowest incidence of recurrence, ranging from 78% to 100%.[1] Proponents of the operation suggest that it is the procedure of choice for the younger, physically active woman who wants to have one operation last her for a lifetime, since it is statistically less likely to fail than a vaginal or laparoscopic approach. Those who prefer other operative procedures point to the laparotomy incision, the increased complication rate, and the higher costs. Comparing operative approaches is necessary for the surgeon discussing these with his/her patient, but the data is mixed, the advantages of one over another are not clearly delineated, and there is no clear answer to which operation is the "best." In the absence of contraindication, an abdominal sacral colpopexy is likely the best option for this patient.

APPROACH TO Abdominal Sacral Colpopexy

The basics of the ASC operation consist of a laparotomy approach to gain access to the pelvis, affixing a graft to the vaginal apex and possibly laying it under the posterior peritoneum, and then attaching it superiorly to the anterior surface of the first sacral vertebra. Multiple variants of this operation have been described, and some are discussed here.

CLINICAL APPROACH

ASC has been performed using a strip of fascia derived from the patient's own fascia lata, a portion of her own abdominal wall fascia, xenograft material, and synthetic materials (Figure 24–1). When sewing the graft to the vaginal apex, care should be taken to place the permanent suture into the vaginal muscularis, but not all the way through the vagina and into the vaginal mucosa. Some surgeons make a "Y" of the synthetic tissue they attach to the vaginal apex and secure it to both the dorsal and ventral vaginal surfaces. The graft should be placed under the posterior peritoneum, and attention paid to avoiding the course of the right ureter coursing along the right side of the graft. The graft should be sewn into the ventral surface of the S1 vertebrae with at least two permanent monofilament sutures, and **there should not be any tension on the graft** as it courses from the top of the vagina to the sacral promontory. Use of this location on the S1 level has been the standard location for some time, and has been shown to be optimal for being able to visualize and avoid the middle sacral artery and to maintain the vaginal angle least likely to result in stress urinary incontinence postoperatively. Placing several sutures into the portion of the mesh covering the vaginal segment of graft to distribute tension equally is a key surgical concept.

The issue of which graft material to use is still not clearly defined, but there has been enough experience to indicate that cadaveric fascia should no longer be used. Not enough literature exists to state whether synthetic or biological material is preferable, or which is more prone to cause erosion, or which will yield the overall best result. Other variables, such as patient age, vaginal health, estrogen use, concurrent antibiotic usage, and operative technique differences, will make this a difficult question to answer. The ideal graft does not yet exist. Autologous fascia is not going to be rejected and is not likely to erode through the vagina, but it is more prone to failure than synthetic materials.[4]

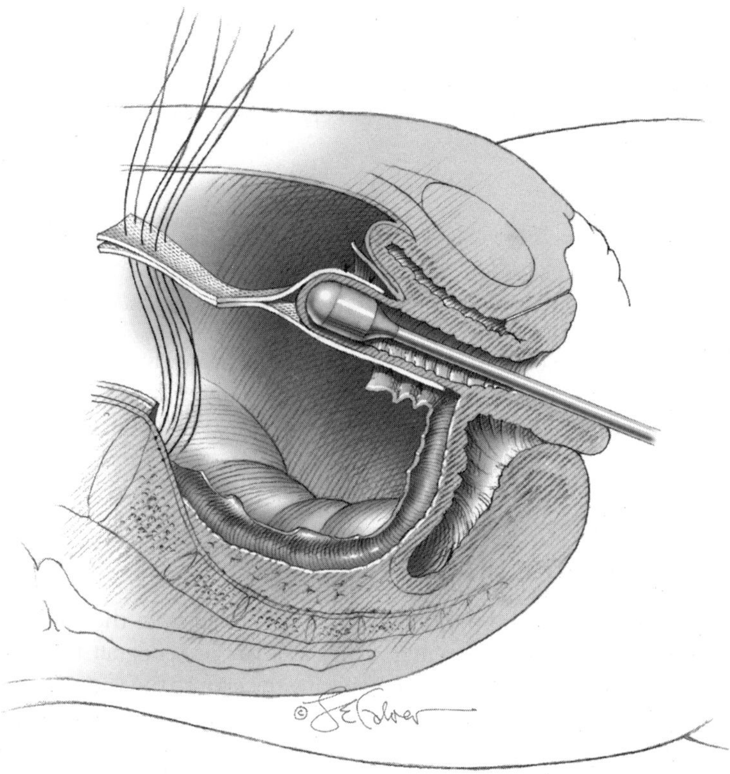

Figure 24–1. Abdominal sacrocolpopexy suing a polypropylene bridge from the sacral promontory to the vaginal apex. (*Reproduced, with permission, from Schorge JO, Schaffer JI, Halvorson LM, et al.* Williams Gynecology. *New York: McGraw-Hill, 2008.*)

Synthetic material pore size has been shown to be a factor in the development of infection and mesh erosion at all sites in the pelvis (Case 25).

Peritoneal closure over the mesh used for suspension to avoid the potential for mesh erosion and bowel obstruction is not clearly demonstrated to be effacacious in the literature. Bowel erosion is a relatively rare complication (~1.1%), and therefore this question is not going to be answered quickly with randomized studies. There is little harm in reperitonealization, however, and the benefit seemingly outweighs any risk involved, but studies have shown that this is no guarantee to avoid bowel erosion.

Whether concurrent hysterectomy increases the risk for infection and graft erosion is still controversial, with some studies suggesting that hysterectomy increases this risk, and others show no difference.[4] The theoretical risk is that hysterectomy accompanying ASC would allow bacteria to enter into the site.

Complications

Overall bowel function seems to improve for women who have ASC, but the data are limited. Causality is hard to discern in this regard, though, because for some patients bowel dysfunction may antedate prolapse, and the opposite may be true for others. This may be because straining to effect satisfactory bowel activity is reduced following successful ASC, and the procedure may create enough beneficial fibrosis to eliminate some defecatory dysfunction. In other patients, the surgery may result in scarring and pain with defecation that did not predate the surgery. Whitehead and colleagues found that[1] woman in 20 will have significant gastrointestinal morbidity, including problems such as ileus and small bowel obstruction, and that the older patient is at increased risk for these complications.[2]

Bladder function following the procedure is related to the degree of voiding dysfunction the patient had prior to the procedure, and whether any concomitant procedures were done at the time of the ASC. As with other procedures involving vaginal suspension, ASC can change the urethrovesical angle and create urinary incontinence for the woman who did not have this problem preoperatively. The gynecologist then has to decide whether to do a routine prophylactic operation for urinary incontinence if none is present when performing ASC, or wait until after the procedure to see if there is incontinence and then operate for urine loss.

Complications of ASC and their mean occurrence rate include urinary tract infection (10.9%), wound problems, including hematoma and infection (4.6%), hemorrhage and/or transfusion (4.4%), cystotomy (3.1%), enterotomy (1.6%), ureteral injury (1%), and deep vein thrombosis (3.3%). Mesh erosion occurred in 3% of patients reported in the largest review article. The Cochrane review of ASC concluded that the abdominal approach had less apical failure, but a greater propensity for complications, while encountering less stress incontinence and postoperative dyspareunia.

Successful surgeons list some key concepts for best surgical outcomes: (1) use graft tissue rather than trying to approximate either the vagina or the uterus to the sacrum; (2) place the graft at the S1-S2 level; (3) do not strip the abdominal vaginal apex down to the mucosal level before affixing the synthetic graft material to it; (4) place the graft between the anterior vagina and the sacrum without too much tension to reduce the risk of postoperative stress incontinence; (5) use many sutures in the vaginal end of the graft to equilibrate tension on the graft and the vagina.[4]

Whether the abdominal or vaginal approach is preferable for a given patient with vaginal vault prolapse is not clear from the extant literature. Prospective, randomized trials do not exist to answer this question, and therefore factors which will determine the answer to this question will, of necessity, involve the patient's age, the strength of her tissue, her lifestyle, the durability of the proposed operative procedure, and the opinion and experience of the surgeon taking care of the patient. All of the above are pertinent when discussing the best approach for a given patient with vaginal prolapse.

Comprehension Questions

24.1 A 55-year-old woman presents to the gynecologist's clinic with the complaint of "there's something falling out of my vagina." She had undergone an abdominal hysterectomy for uterine fibroids 15 years previously. She denies leakage of urine. On examination, she is noted to have a third-degree vaginal vault prolapse. The gynecologist counsels her about the options of abdominal sacrocolpopexy versus sacral ligament fixation to address the problem. As compared to ASC, which of the following complications is seen more often with SSLF?

A. Urinary tract infection
B. Wound infection
C. Hemorrhage and/or transfusion
D. Nerve injury

24.2 The gynecologist explains to the patient in question 24.1 that ASC has been referred to as the "gold standard" for repair of vaginal vault prolapse. Which of the following is the reason for this label?

A. ASC is more cost-effective than vaginal procedures.
B. ASC is less likely to fail and result in recurrent prolapse.
C. ASC is associated with less pain than vaginal procedures.
D. ASC is less likely to result in hemorrhage than vaginal SSLF and USLF.

24.3 A 69-year-old woman is noted to have a vaginal vault prolapse after a vaginal hysterectomy performed 25 years previously for pelvic pain. The patient is in fairly good health and is very active physically and sexually. She is 5 ft 4 in tall and weighs 180 lb (82 kg). After being counseled about the various options, she agrees to sacral spinous ligament fixation. Which of the following is the most important preoperative management in her case?

A. Lose 10 lb (4.5 kg) of weight prior to surgery.
B. Identify and treat any urinary tract infection.
C. Identify and treat bacterial vaginosis.
D. Apply topical estrogen to the vagina.

ANSWERS

24.1 **D.** Nerve injury is rare, occurring only in 1% to 2% of patients. With sacrospinous ligament procedures, the pudendal nerve can be entrapped.

24.2 **B.** ASC is considered the "gold standard" because there is less apical failure with this operation than with vaginal procedures for vault prolapse.

24.3 **D.** In a woman who is remote from menopause, the vaginal epithelium is typically thin and atrophic. Vaginal surgery is difficult in this circumstance and can lead to a greater incidence of wound breakdown and infection. The technical aspects of vaginal surgery are likewise difficult. Topical estrogen cream to the vaginal region can assist to allow the vaginal epithelium to be more pliable, thicker, and easier to manipulate in the OR.

Clinical Pearls

See Table 1-2 for definition of level of evidence and strength of recommendation

- ASC is occasionally complicated by bleeding from the site of attachment of the graft tissue to the anterior surface of the sacral vertebrae (Level B).
- Visualize and avoid small arterioles coursing over the bone surface. If bleeding occurs, have some sterile orthopedic thumbtacks available to push into the vertebra or bone wax to stop the bleeding (Level C).
- The "vaginal hand" instrument, consisting of a rigid vaginal dilator attached to a right-angle retractor, is placed into the vagina to delineate the apex of the vault from within the laparotomy incision. This instrument provides an easy method to manipulate the vagina while maintaining a sterile laparotomy field (Level C).
- A thorough bowel preparation prior to this operation facilitates packing the empty bowel out of the way to gain access to the pelvic floor for correct placement of the graft (Level B).

REFERENCES

1. Nygaard IE, McCreery R, Brubaker L, et al. Abdominal sacrocolpopexy: a comprehensive review. *Obstet Gynecol.* 2004:805-823.
   A definitive review of a challenging topic.
2. Whitehead WE, Bradley CS, Brown MB, et al. Pelvic floor network. Gastrointestinal complications following abdominal sacrocolpopexy for advanced pelvic organ prolapse. *Am J Obstet Gynecol.* 2007;197:78.e1-7.
3. The American College of Obstetricians and Gynecologists. Pelvic organ prolapse. ACOG Practice Bulletin No. 85. *Obstet Gynecol.* 2007;110:717-730.
4. Bensinger G, Lind L, Lesser M, Guess M, Winkler HA. Abdominal sacral suspensions: analysis of complications using permanent mesh. *Am J Obstet Gynecol.* 2005;193:2094-2098.
5. Wu JM, Wells EC, Hundley AF, Connolly A, Williams KS, Visco AG. Mesh erosion in abdominal sacral colpopexy with and without concomitant hysterectomy. *Am J Obstet Gynecol.* 2006;194:1418-1422.
6. Maher C, Baessler K. Surgical management of posterior vaginal wall prolapse: an evidence based literature review. *Int Urogynecol J.* 2005;17:84-88.

Case 25

A 64-year-old woman presents with a chief complaint of a mass protruding from her vagina. She denies stress urinary incontinence, but she has to splint her posterior vagina to have bowel movements. She had vaginal surgery for a similar problem 5 years ago, and she brought copies of the operative reports. Your review of her records reveals that she had a routine anterior and posterior colporrhaphy, but no other pelvic surgery was performed at that time. She had a vaginal hysterectomy 20 years earlier for vaginal prolapse. Her past medical history includes an appendectomy for a ruptured appendix and two subsequent laparotomies for intestinal obstruction following the appendectomy. Physical examination confirms that the vaginal cuff exits the vagina with a Valsalva maneuver, and she also has extremely thin, atrophic vaginal mucosa. Repositioning the vaginal cuff at the apex and asking the patient to repeat the Valsalva maneuver demonstrates a large second-degree cystocele and a large second-degree rectocele.

➤ What is the most likely diagnosis?

➤ What is the best therapy for this condition?

ANSWERS TO CASE 25: Vaginal Vault Prolapse Post-hysterectomy

Summary: A 64-year-old woman presents with vaginal vault prolapse following prior hysterectomy and anterior and posterior repairs. She is not a good candidate for abdominal surgery because of intestinal obstruction following appendectomy surgery. She has failed conventional vaginal repair surgery.

➤ **Most likely diagnosis:** Recurrent vaginal vault prolapse and failed conventional cystocele and rectocele repair.

➤ **Best therapy:** Vaginal paravaginal defect repair using biological graft tissue, and posterior colporrhaphy using biological graft tissue. Support of the vaginal apex, whether by sacrospinous ligament fixation or uterosacral ligament suspension is critical to the long-term success of the operative procedures to repair the cystocele and the rectocele.

ANALYSIS

Objectives

1. Become familiar with the concepts for using graft tissue in vaginal reconstructive surgery.
2. Know the indications for using graft tissue in vaginal reconstructive surgery.
3. Learn the contraindications and complications associated with the use of graft tissue in the vagina.

Considerations

This case report details a 64-year-old patient who had undergone previous surgery for pelvic organ prolapse without long-term success. Her vaginal tissue is thin, atrophic, and weak, and she is not likely to benefit from an operative procedure which duplicates prior failed attempts. Additionally, she is not likely to consent to an abdominal operation which will place her at risk for another episode of intestinal obstruction. Facing such a surgical challenge, some gynecologists would consider the use of graft tissue to reinforce the vaginal repairs which this patient requires.

The initial approach to this patient should include urologic evaluation to see if her urinary continence is due to the fact that the urethra is kinked because of the degree of prolapse she is experiencing. Whether she will need a mid-urethral sling as part of the combined operative procedures for repair of pelvic floor relaxation, or later, if urinary incontinence develops following surgery, needs to be discussed preoperatively. Randomized trials have shown that the patient who is stress continent prior to surgery for prolapse may become incontinent following surgery, and that placement of tension-free vaginal tape (TVT) as an adjunct to the prolapse surgery will statistically reduce the likelihood of postoperative stress incontinence.

Grafts have been employed in vaginal vault prolapse surgery for over 50 years, but their use is still controversial. The decision to proceed with the use of graft tissue should be considered only when the patient's endogenous tissue is inadequate for a nongrafted repair. Additionally, the prolapse should have a significant negative impact on the patient's quality of life, and the degree of prolapse should be to the vaginal introitus or beyond.[1]

Any discussion of graft tissue is incomplete without some consideration of the significant cost of using these materials. Several square inches of synthetic or biological materials usually cost about $1000. The cost equation also must include the increased cost of OR time to position these products correctly.[2,3]

APPROACH TO Using Graft Tissue in Vaginal Hernia Repairs

DEFINITIONS

XENOGRAFT: A surgical graft of tissue from one species to an unlike species (or genus or family).

MESH GRAFT: Prosthetic nonabsorbable porous material used to give strength or bulk for surgical repairs of pelvic organ prolapsed.

BIOLOGICAL GRAFT: A portion of living tissue that is used to join to another living tissue. It can be from the same organism (autologous) or same species, or different species (xenograft).

CLINICAL APPROACH

There are two broad categories of graft material available for use in vaginal hernia repairs, those being either synthetic or biological products. Within these two categories, there are many of material available. Any listing of the choices available is somewhat futile, as the field is being inundated on a regular basis with new products and materials too rapidly for the individual surgeon to remain current with the choices available. **Additionally, there is a dearth of randomized, prospective, controlled trials clearly demonstrating the superiority of one product over another.**[3] No matter which type of graft tissue is chosen, surgeons should not believe that graft tissue use will compensate for mediocre performance in the OR, or for choosing a patient who is not a good candidate for graft surgery. Many authorities in this field are of the opinion that the use of any type of graft tissue should be reserved for those select patients in whom a conventional operative procedure has already resulted in failure.[4]

This is a controversial arena with a dearth of prospective randomized clinical trials to substantiate claims of effectiveness and safety. ACOG published a practice bulletin in February 2007 in reaction to the FDA warning of numerous vaginal mesh erosions and complications and the plethora of graft products and "kits" for the correction of pelvic organ prolapse. The initial ACOG publication described these products as "experimental." Enough protest ensued over the use of the word "experimental" that the Practice Bulletin was withdrawn and republished in August 2007 without the use of that descriptive language.[3] However, surgeons should not, based on the current state of the art, be using graft tissue indiscriminately just because it is possible to do so, and the discerning surgeon should be able to determine those situations that appropriate and inappropriate for the use of graft tissue.

Synthetic Graft Tissue

A comparison of synthetic to biological material demonstrates that the synthetic product may have, at least initially, greater success rates, but the biological product is probably better tolerated for a longer duration of time. **Synthetic grafts are indeed permanent, and erosion of the graft through a vaginal or intestinal wall into the vagina or the bowel lumen is a lifetime risk after graft placement.** Surgical case series that report several months to a few years of successful symptom relief do not predict the future safe compartmentalization of synthetic mesh in anterior or posterior hernia repairs. Vaginal tissue ages, atrophies, and loses its innate tensile strength, which predisposes the graft tissue to erode through a previously intact vaginal wall.

Permanent graft products are most likely to be successfully incorporated into the hernia spaces they are designed to reinforce if their pore size is large enough to allow ingrowth of new endogenous fibrous tissue and blood supply. Synthetic graft products with small, tight interstices are less prone to be well integrated into the surrounding tissue, which may result in graft erosion or infection. When using synthetic graft tissue for repairing cystoceles and rectoceles, the vaginal mucosal thickness covering the graft should be as thick as possible, to reduce the risk of erosion and to ensure a good blood supply to the endogenous tissue overlying the graft.

If graft erosion of synthetic mesh occurs into the vagina, it may respond to several weeks of topical application of an estrogen cream to encourage overgrowth of vaginal epithelium. If this is not successful, trimming the protuberant mesh until it is flush with or slightly beneath the mucosal surface may stimulate successful overgrowth of vaginal mucosa. Infected mesh must be removed.

The consequence of graft tissue eroding through the vaginal mucosa has created a new descriptive term, "hispareunia," describing the phenomenon experienced by the male partner of a patient who encounters sharp, stubby synthetic graft material eroding through the vagina with the potential to lacerate his penis.[5]

Biological Graft Tissue

The ideal biological graft is sterile, noncarcinogenic, inert, durable, inexpensive, easy to use, and maintains its shape. Biological grafts are contraindicated in patients with the following conditions: heavy smoking, morbid obesity, poorly controlled diabetes, on systemic corticosteroids, immunocompromised, active pelvic or vaginal infection, or prior pelvic irradiation. Biological graft tissue may be autologous graft tissue from rectus fascia of fascia lata, or allograft tissue from fascia lata or dura mater, or xenograft tissue from porcine or bovine sources. Xenograft tissue has been treated to remove the cellular component, leaving only a collagen matrix, which has minimal potential to trigger a rejection phenomenon. Recent evidence indicates that cadaveric fascial tissue in abdominal sacrocolpopexy should no longer be used. The variable thickness and strength of cadaveric dermis, compared to the consistency of bovine and porcine source tissue, make the latter preferable to the former. Clear superiority of bovine versus porcine tissue has not been demonstrated in any long-term prospective trials. Xenograft tissue does have the advantage of providing a scaffold-type matrix for endogenous tissue to use in fabricating the ingrowth of new fibrous tissue with its own neovascularization, but it degenerates over time and does not provide the long-term strength of synthetic material.

In summary, grafts are probably more useful in repairing the anterior rather than the posterior vaginal wall. Patient selection is critical, and patients should be counseled, in a carefully described and documented consent process, that although grafts are being used more commonly, this technology is still relatively new and expensive, with unique potential complications. Gynecologic surgeons need to gain knowledge and experience with graft materials if they plan to use them to correct pelvic floor defects, and be able to handle the complications which may ensue following graft placement. Given the rapid introduction of new graft products, surgeons should demand data demonstrating that new materials are safe and effective.[6]

Comprehension Questions

25.1 A healthy 55-year-old woman presents with a symptomatic cystocele, rectocele, and enterocele. She had a vaginal hysterectomy for uterine prolapse performed 10 years previously. Which operative procedure should be *avoided* in this patient?

A. Anterior and posterior colporrhaphy using synthetic graft material, sacrospinous ligament fixation
B. Conventional anterior and posterior colporrhaphy, enterocele repair via sacrospinous ligament fixation or uterosacral ligament suspension
C. Laparoscopic sacrospinous ligament fixation with conventional anterior and posterior colporrhaphy
D. Abdominal sacrocolpopexy, Burch procedure, conventional posterior colporrhaphy

25.2 A 58-year-old patient returns 6 weeks following vaginal repair surgery for recurrent cystocele. She is afebrile, but complains of persistent vaginal discharge. She has not been using any medication vaginally. Bovine graft tissue was used to repair the cystocele, and a 1.5×1.0 cm portion of graft material is visible 3 cm inside the introitus in the anterior repair suture line. What is the therapy of choice?

A. Return the patient to the operating room and remove the graft.
B. Start the patient on oral antibiotic therapy.
C. Trim the exposed graft in the clinic.
D. Instruct the patient to begin using estrogen vaginal cream.

25.3 A 48-year-old woman weighing 265 lb (120.20 kg), with a 10-year history of systemic lupus erythematosus presents with cystocele and rectocele. She states that multiple types of pessaries have not controlled her prolapse symptoms. She is taking oral steroids and methotrexate to control her lupus. What vaginal graft tissue is indicated for repairing this patient's prolapse?

A. Polypropylene mesh
B. Fetal bovine fascia
C. Porcine mesh
D. None of the above

ANSWERS

25.1 **A.** The use of graft tissue is not usually needed the first time when a patient has vaginal repair surgery if her endogenous tissue is satisfactory. Graft tissue can lead to erosion, infection, or pain.

25.2 **D.** Vaginal estrogen cream use for several weeks will stimulate the vaginal mucosa to cover the visible graft tissue. This has very little systemic absorption and works well in strengthening the tissue locally.

25.3 **D.** The use of any type of graft tissue is contraindicated in morbidly obese patients, and in patients who are using systemic steroids.

Clinical Pearls

See Table 1-2 for definition of level of evidence and strength of recommendation

- Soak the graft in an antibiotic solution before using it to reduce the risk of postoperative infection (Level B).
- Sew the graft into place—do not simply lay it into a cystocele or rectocele space and expect it to stay in the intended position. These materials have a propensity to migrate and bunch if not anchored with suture (Level B).
- Cover the defect with the graft such that it lays flat and smooth, but not under tension (Level C).
- Use the carpenter's adage of "Measure twice, cut once" when working with graft tissue. This material is too expensive to waste. Be sure you do not create "a square peg to go into a round hole." Make a pattern using some sterile paper, and then cut the graft using the pattern as a guide. Err on the side of making it too big and then trim excess graft on the edges after suturing it into place (Level C).

REFERENCES

1. Davila GW, Drutz H, Deprest J. International Urogynecological Association: the usage of grafts in pelvic reconstructive surgery symposium 2005. *Int Urogynecol J.* 2006;17:S51-S55.
2. Norton P. New technology in gynecologic surgery: is new necessarily better? *Obstet Gynecol.* 2006;108:707-708.
3. American College of Obstetricians and Gynecologists. Pelvic organ prolapse. ACOG Practice Bulletin No. 85. *Obstet Gynecol.* 2007;110:717-730.
4. Botros SM, Sand PK. Cystocele and rectocele repair: more success with mesh? *OBG Mgmt.* 2006;18:30-43.
5. Brubaker L. Partner dyspareunia (hispareunia). *Int Urogynecol J.* 2006;17:311.
6. Karram M. Pelvic organ prolapse: which operation for which patient? *OBG Mgmt.* 2006;18:72-84.

Case 26

A 46-year-old G2P2002 woman complains of leakage of urine with coughing and sneezing that has worsened over the last several years requiring her to use two to three pads per day despite pelvic floor exercises. She complains that this has adversely affected her social life and is seeking treatment for her condition. She also has occasional urgency and frequency but denies leakage of urine associated with the urge to void. She denies any difficulty emptying her bladder. The rest of her medical history is unremarkable with the patient having had two vaginal deliveries without complications and no prior surgeries. A gynecologic examination is performed and the patient is found to have a normal vagina, a small mobile uterus without significant prolapse, and no palpable adnexal masses.

- ➤ What is the most likely diagnosis?
- ➤ What further physical examination should be performed?
- ➤ What further testing should the patient undergo?
- ➤ What minimally invasive surgical options are available for the treatment of stress urinary incontinence (SUI) with a hypermobile urethra?

ANSWERS TO CASE 26: Stress Urinary Incontinence

Summary: This is a 46-year-old G2P2002 woman who complains of urinary leakage with activities associated with increased abdominal pressure. She also has urgency and frequency, but this has not been associated with leakage. She has no prior surgeries and an unremarkable history other than two vaginal deliveries.

- **Most likely diagnosis:** Stress urinary incontinence.
- **Additional physical examination:** The urethra should be examined for urethral hypermobility by direct visualization and/or a Q-tip test (placement of a cotton swab into the urethra to judge urethral mobility). Additionally, a supine empty stress test (SEST) may be performed if the patient has voided recently and a post void residual (PVR) should be determined by in-and-out catheterization or bladder ultrasound.
- **Additional testing:** The patient should have a urinalysis to rule out a urinary tract infection that may be worsening her condition. Additionally, the patient should undergo urodynamic testing to further evaluate her lower urinary tract to determine if her leakage is caused by SUI, detrusor overactivity, or both (mixed incontinence).
- **Treatment for SUI with urethral hypermobility:** Mid-urethral slings are an excellent treatment for women who suffer from SUI with urethral hypermobility.

ANALYSIS

Objectives

1. Know the workup for urinary incontinence.
2. Know the indications for different incontinence surgeries.
3. Be familiar with the intra- and postoperative complications of incontinence surgeries.

Considerations

This is a 46-year-old parous woman who has a history of urinary incontinence associated with coughing and sneezing. She has had two prior vaginal deliveries, which are risk factors for this condition. The history is very important to determine if the patient has any "red flags" to indicate a more complicated condition other than pure genuine stress incontinence. These red flags include nocturia, urgency, frequency, dysuria, delay from cough to leakage, or prior urinary incontinence surgery. This patient complains also of urgency and frequency, but these symptoms don't seem to be related to urinary incontinence; nevertheless, these complaints may indicate a mixed incontinence. Cytometric evaluation would be important to evaluate for the degree of stress versus urge incontinence, since these findings would guide therapy.

APPROACH TO
Stress Urinary Incontinence

DEFINITIONS

DETRUSOR OVERACTIVITY: A urodynamic observation characterized by involuntary detrusor contractions during the filling phase which may be spontaneous or provoked.

MIXED URINARY INCONTINENCE: The complaint of involuntary leakage associated with urgency and also with exertion, effort, sneezing, or coughing.

STRESS URINARY INCONTINENCE: The complaint of involuntary leakage on effort or exertion, or on sneezing or coughing.

URGE URINARY INCONTINENCE: The complaint of involuntary leakage accompanied by or immediately preceded by urgency.[1]

CLINICAL APPROACH

Multiparous patients who complain of SUI without a history of prior incontinence procedures usually tend to have hypermobile urethras from what is thought to be injury to supportive structures during the birthing process. Women with SUI and hypermobile urethras are excellent candidates for mid-urethral slings whereas those with nonhypermobile urethras may be better suited for treatment by way of intraurethral bulking agents or bladder neck slings. Currently, there are numerous products on the market, and more being introduced every day, with some devices having been studied in more depth than others. The best procedure for the patient is the one that the surgeon is comfortable performing and best suits the patient's specific problem. When using mid-urethral slings, it has become increasingly clear that the sling material should be made of monofilament polypropylene with interstices sufficiently wide to allow tissue incorporation and penetration of neutrophils to combat infection. Prior to surgery, the patient should be examined by some method of objective testing to further evaluate the patient's complaint.

DIAGNOSTICS

Typically before an incontinence procedure is performed, the patient undergoes urodynamic testing. This may be as simple as placing a 16-Fr red rubber catheter through the urethral meatus into the bladder and filling the bladder with sterile saline through a 60-mL syringe attached to the catheter with the plunger removed. By filling with gravity, the saline enters more slowly than pushing the fluid with the syringe's plunger. It also allows the meniscus of the syringe to be observed. A rise in the meniscus indicates a bladder contraction. In this situation, the patient may be better served by multichannel urodynamics to further evaluate the lower urinary tract. As the bladder is filled, the patient's first sensation and first urge to void may be recorded. Once capacity or 250 to 300 mL is reached, whichever is achieved first, the catheter is removed. The patient is asked to perform Valsalva maneuver and cough several times, and the practitioner should look for leakage that would imply SUI. If leakage is not seen with the patient supine, the patient should be asked to stand upright with stress testing repeated.

The advantage of simple cystometrics is that it is inexpensive and can be performed in a clinic setting without complicated and expensive equipment. However, this technique does not allow the recording of bladder pressures during stress maneuvers to determine the leak point pressure (LPP), which is the abdominal pressure sufficient to overcome the continence mechanism to result in leakage of urine. It is also unable to determine if the leakage seen is caused by a detrusor contraction during the stress maneuvers.

Complex or multichannel urodynamics involves placing one catheter through the urethra into the bladder to measure vesical pressure and another into the rectum or vagina to measure abdominal pressure. These catheters are then connected to a computer that then displays the pressures generated on a computer screen. The detrusor pressure is then calculated by subtracting the abdominal pressure from the vesical pressure. The fill rate can be controlled and usually varies from 50 to 80 mL/min. Needle electrodes can also be placed into the striated urethral sphincter or patch electrodes applied to the perineum to assess the muscle activity of the striated sphincter. LPP testing is performed at different intervals usually starting at 150 mL to evaluate for SUI. Detrusor overactivity is diagnosed by a rise in detrusor pressure signifying an increase in bladder pressure without an increase in abdominal pressure. Leakage during cough or Valsalva without a rise in detrusor pressure indicates SUI. Other tests that may be performed include a urethral pressure profile or maximum urethral closure pressure (MUCP). The MUCP is performed by placing a urethral catheter into the bladder and then slowly removing the catheter. A peak is then generated as the pressure increases as the catheter passes through the continence mechanism with the MUCP being the maximal pressure recorded. This test as well as a low LPP may help identify patients with intrinsic sphincter deficiency (ISD).

TREATMENT

History

In the early 1900s, slings were first placed at the bladder neck to treat SUI.[2] In 1942, Aldridge was the first to describe using autologous rectus fascia at the bladder neck.[3] This procedure which has been modified by different surgeons is the basis for the modern day bladder neck sling. Placed at the level of the bladder neck and proximal urethra, these slings are tunneled by a variety of techniques behind the pubis through the retropubic space and can be secured to itself, the rectus fascia, the periosteum of the pubis, or by way of bone anchors. Tensioned correctly, the sling gives support and an adequate amount of compression to prevent incontinence while not causing obstruction sufficient to result in voiding dysfunction. After Aldridge in 1949, Marshall described the first retropubic colposuspension for the treatment of SUI. Called the Marshall-Marchetti-Krantz (MMK), this procedure entailed placing sutures into the endopelvic fascia along the bladder neck and into the periosteum.[4] By suspending the endopelvic sutures to Cooper ligament instead of the periosteum, the MMK was modified and renamed the Burch colposuspension. Its first results were published in 1968.[5] The Burch colposuspension has been one of the most widely used and studied incontinence procedures. Although the bladder neck sling and Burch colposuspension have comprised the majority of incontinence procedures performed since the 1950s, today they have been largely replaced by the mid-urethral slings developed in the 1990s that continue to evolve into less invasive procedures.

Types of Slings

Bladder Neck Slings As the name implies, bladder neck slings are placed at the level of the bladder neck which is located by using the balloon of a Foley catheter. These slings are placed by passing suture down through the retropubic space into an incision at the level of the bladder neck/proximal urethra, anchored into each end of the sling material and passed through the retropubic space in reverse fashion where the suture is then tied anchoring the sling into place. Materials used in bladder neck sling construction can be autologous (ie, rectus facia, fascia lata), allograft (ie, cadaveric fascia, cadaveric dermis), xenograft (ie, porcine dermis, bovine pericardium, submucosal intestine), or synthetic (ie, polypropylene). Some studies have demonstrated autologous slings to be superior to those constructed from allograft material.[6] Bladder neck slings are commonly used to treat patients with severe ISD and/or a nonhypermobile urethra, previously failed mid-urethral sling procedures, and patients with high risk for synthetic mesh extrusion or erosion. In a comparison study between an intraurethral bulking agent and autologous pubovaginal sling in patients with ISD and largely nonhypermobile urethras, the pubovaginal sling had a much greater objective success rate (81% vs 9%, $P < .001$), thus demonstrating its good efficacy in this cohort of patients that has been historically difficult to treat.[7]

Complications of bladder neck slings include incidental cystotomy and new-onset urgency. Incomplete emptying and detrusor overactivity may also result from bladder outlet obstruction from a sling tensioned too tightly. This surgical technique has been well studied with proven durability. The downside of this technique is the required suprapubic incision, increased vaginal dissection, and tissue harvesting with autologous slings that increase operative time and risk of morbidity.

Mid-urethral Slings In 1990 Petros and Ulsten published a theory paper where they described both stress and urge symptoms being derived from a common anatomical site, a lax vagina. They proposed that this laxity may derive from the vaginal wall itself or the supporting structures of the vaginal wall which include ligaments, muscles, and connective tissue insertions.[8] Based on this theory, the tension-free vaginal tape (TVT) procedure was created to restore urethral support by a tunneled strip of monofilament polypropylene mesh placed at the mid-urethra. The mesh is passed by a trocar that is tunneled from a suburethral incision at the mid-urethral level through the endopelvic fascia and into the retropubic space. It then passes through the layers of the anterior abdominal wall and out through the skin just above the pubis. This was first performed under local anesthesia with a mean operative time of 22 minutes and a cure rate of 84% at 2 years in patients with SUI and urethral hypermobility.[9] Some data suggest that in patients with a low MUCP, a nonhypermobile urethra, or both the cure rate may be 60% or significantly lower.[10] Other studies have shown better success in patients with ISD.[11] Complications of this procedure include voiding dysfunction from 4% to 20% and mesh extrusion reported by some at 3%.[12,13] Though rare, bowel injury and vascular injury have been reported.[14,15] Cystoscopy is required intraoperatively to rule out an incidental cystotomy during passage of the trocars. Modifications have been made where this type of retropubic mid-urethral sling may be passed through the abdominal wall and downward through the sub-urethral incision. It appears that this surgery is well suited for patients with SUI or mixed urinary incontinence with a hypermobile urethra.

In 2004, DeLorme published results of a modified mid-urethral sling to decrease the risk of cystotomy as well as bowel injury called the transobturator tape (TOT).[16] Skin incisions are made at the level of the clitoris where the adductor longus tendon insertion is located at the labial fold. A trocar is then passed through the obturator fossa and out through the suburethral incision at the level of the mid-urethra. A polypropylene mesh is then attached and the trocar is reversed bringing the mesh out through the skin (Figure 26–1). Although cystoscopy is not required by the manufacturers of these products, it is suggested as urethral injury may occur and bladder injury, though rare, has been reported.[17] Modifications to this procedure have been made

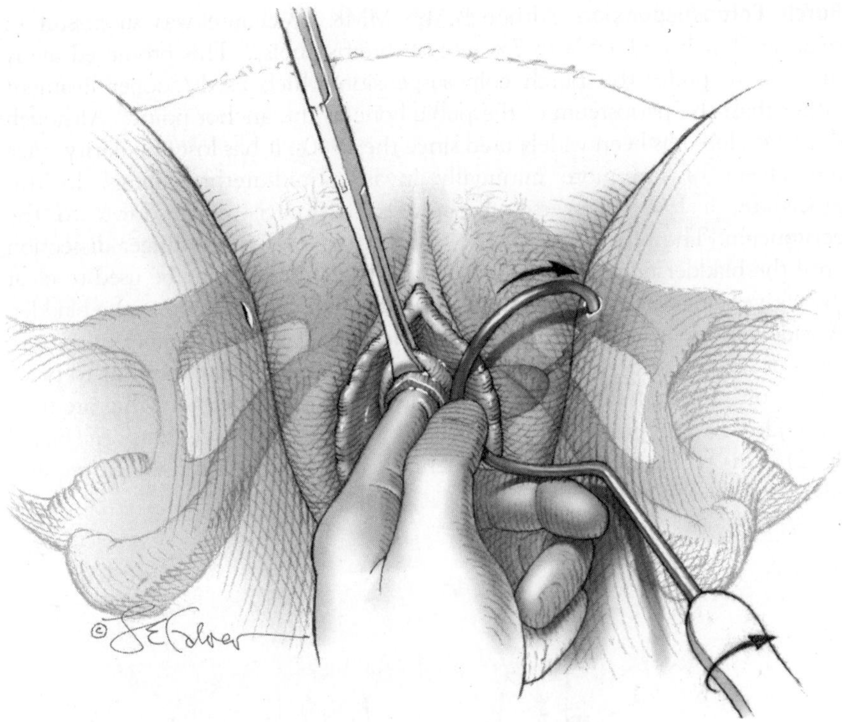

Figure 26–1. TOT being tensioned with mesh at the level of the mid-urethra and one arm of the sling visible at the level of the clitoris. (*Reproduced, with permission, from Schorge JO, Schaffer JI, Halvorson LM, et al.* Williams Gynecology. *New York: McGraw-Hill, 2008:983.)*

allowing the trocar to be passed in the opposite direction from the sub-urethral incision out through the obturator foramen. In a review comparing the retropubic approach to the transobturator approach, it appeared that the both methods had similar cure rates. The transobturator approach had less risk of voiding difficulties but higher risk of groin/thigh pain, vaginal injuries, and erosion of mesh.[18] Some data suggest that the TOT may not be as successful in patients with ISD defined as an LPP less than 60 cm H_2O.[19] Based on these data, the transobturator sling is safe and effective in treating patients with the diagnosis of SUI or mixed incontinence with urethral hypermobility. From limited reports, a retropubic mid-urethral sling may have better efficacy in patients with a low LPP or MUCP.

Newer slings that pass through the prepubic space and "mini" slings, which pass under the urethra through a single incision and have no point of exit, are now available on the market. However, at this time, data are too limited to comment on their role in the treatment of SUI.

Burch Colposuspension Although the MMK procedure was successful in treating SUI, it had a 5% to 7% rate of osteitis pubis.[20] This prompted many surgeons to prefer the Burch colposuspension which used Cooper ligament rather than the periosteum of the pubic bone as the anchor point.[5] Although this procedure has been widely used since the 1960s, it has lost popularity since the advent of the more minimally invasive mid-urethral slings. In this procedure, a low transverse abdominal incision is made down to the peritoneum. The retropubic space is then entered by gentle finger dissection until the bladder neck is visualized. Different techniques may be used to clear the perivesical fat to better visualize the endopelvic fascia lateral to the bladder. A wide variety of techniques have been described as far as number of sutures, types of sutures, and suture placement are concerned. It is important to place sutures into the endopelvic fascia at the level of the bladder neck that are then suspended to Cooper ligament and tied without excessive tension (Figure 26–2). This technique may also be performed laparoscopically which requires advanced laparoscopic skills.

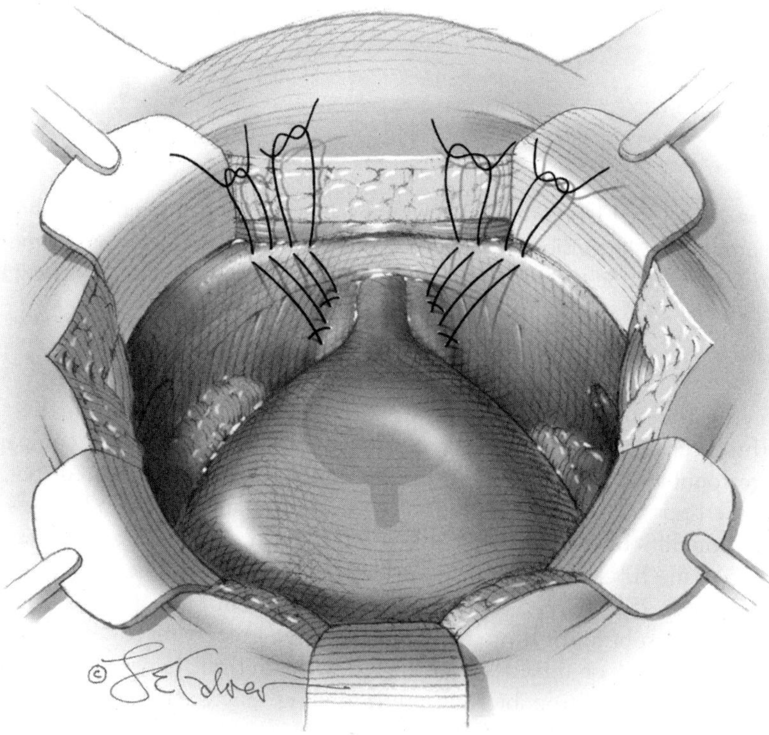

Figure 26–2. Burch colposuspension with two sutures placed into the endopelvic fascia at the level of the bladder neck and two sutures just distal along the urethra. All four sutures are suspended to Cooper ligament loosely. *(Reproduced, with permission, from Schorge JO, Schaffer JI, Halvorson LM, et al.* Williams Gynecology. *New York: McGraw-Hill, 2008:979.)*

Currently, this procedure is indicated in the treatment of SUI with urethral hypermobility and may best benefit those patients undergoing an open abdominal procedure such as abdominal hysterectomy or sacral colpopexy. The continence rate at 1 year is approximately 85% to 90% and about 70% at 5 years.[21] Common complications include bleeding from the venous plexus of the retropubic space or inadvertent placement of suture into the bladder which can be avoided by intraoperative cystoscopy. Postoperative voiding difficulties may last up to 6 months though often resolve. Changes in anatomy may predispose patients to posterior wall defects, and between 12% and 18.5% of patients may have detrusor overactivity. Those who have had prior unsuccessful surgery, particularly with a low MUCP, the elderly, and those with poor tissue from weaker collagen may be at risk for increased failure.[20] A National Institutes of Health (NIH)-sponsored trial also has shown the Burch colposuspension to be protective against new-onset SUI in patients undergoing abdominal sacral colpopexy.[22]

Comparisons

Although data are limited in comparing these different surgical treatments, a few large studies deserve mention. The autologous pubovaginal sling was recently compared to the Burch colposuspension in a prospective, randomized, multicenter NIH-sponsored trial. In this study at 24 months, success for treating SUI was significantly higher in the fascial sling group (66% vs 49%, $P < .001$) though the procedure was associated with more urinary tract infections, difficulty voiding, and postoperative urge incontinence.[23] When comparing the TVT to older procedures with good success such as the Burch colposuspension, one randomized, controlled trial with 5-year follow-up found no statistically significant difference between the groups in terms of a 1-hour pad test. The Burch group had an increase in enterocele and rectocele while the TVT had tape-related complications in 8% of patients.[24] Currently, multicenter studies are underway comparing the TOT to the TVT to better understand the differences between these procedures.

Comprehension Questions

26.1 A 34-year-old woman complains of urinary incontinence that is worsening. Which of the following statements regarding treatment of the incontinence is most accurate?

A. Cystometric evaluation is necessary before performing a surgical procedure.
B. The presence of nocturia is consistent with SUI.
C. Mid-urethral sling procedures have been noted to be equivalent to Burch urethropexy procedures in terms of efficacy.
D. Urge incontinence is best treated by urethropexy.

26.2 A cystometric evaluation that is consistent with genuine SUI demonstrates which of the following?

A. Small bladder capacity
B. Detrusor contractions
C. Normal sphincter pressure
D. Residual volume of 200 mL

26.3 In comparing the advantages of a TVT versus a TOT, which of the following statements is most accurate?

A. TOT seems to have more voiding dysfunction than TVT.
B. TOT seems to have a lower rate of cystotomy.
C. TOT is better suited for patients with a hypermobile urethra.
D. TOT is better suited for patients with a lower urethral closure pressure.

ANSWERS

26.1 **C.** Patients with pure SUI do not usually have nocturia, urge, or urinary frequency. If the history and physical examination are consistent with genuine stress incontinence, a formal cystometric evaluation does not need to be performed prior to surgery. Urge incontinence is treated medically rather than surgically.

26.2 **C.** Patients with genuine stress incontinence may have normal or somewhat lower urethral sphincter pressures. They usually have normal bladder capacity and no component of urge or dysuria and absence of detrusor contractions.

26.3 **B.** TOT procedures seem to have a lower rate of voiding dysfunction and lower rate of cystotomy. TVT procedures seem to be better suited for patients with a hypermobile urethra or lower urethral closing pressures.

Clinical Pearls

See Table 1-2 for definition of level of evidence and strength of recommendation

- Patients with ISD, especially those as defined by a nonhypermobile urethra, may be best treated by a bladder neck sling (Level B).
- Though data are limited, autologous rectus fascial slings may be more efficacious than slings constructed from allograft or xenograft material (Level C).
- Mid-urethral slings composed of wide-spaced monofilament polypropylene have lower complications than those composed of multifilament weave (Level B).
- The TVT may be more efficacious than the TOT in treating patients with a hypermobile urethra and low LPP or MUCP (Level B).
- The TOT appears to have less voiding dysfunction than the TVT and a lower rate of cystotomy (Level B).
- The Burch colposuspension is an effective procedure that may be considered in patients already undergoing an abdominal incision who require incontinence surgery for SUI (Level B).

REFERENCES

1. Abrams P, Cardozo L, Fall M, et al. The standardisation of terminology of lower urinary tract function: report from the Standardisation Sub-committee of the International Continence Society. *Neurourol Urodyn.* 2002;21:167-178.
2. Kobashi KC, Leach GE. Stress urinary incontinence. *Curr Opin Urol.* 1999;9:285-290.
3. Aldridge AH. Transplantation of fascia for relief of urinary stress incontinence. *Am J Obstet Gynecol.* 1942;44:398-411.
4. Marshall VF, Marchetti AA, Krantz KE. The correction of stress incontinence by simple vesicourethral suspension. *Surg Gynecol Obstet.* 1949;88:509-518.
5. Burch JC. Urethrovesical fixation to Cooper's ligament for correction of stress incontinence, cystocele, and prolapse. *Am J Obstet Gynecol.* 1961;81:281-290.
6. Howden NS, Zyczynski HM, Moalli PA, Sagan ER, Meyn LA, Weber AM. Comparison of autologous rectus fascia and cadaveric fascia in pubovaginal sling outcomes. *Am J Obstet Gyecol.* 2006;194:1444-1449.
7. Maher CF, O'Reilly BA, Dwyer PL, Carey MP, Cornish A, Schlutter P. Pubovaginal sling versus transurethral Macroplastique for stress urinary incontinence and intrinsic sphincter deficiency: a prospective randomised controlled trial. *BJOG.* 2005;112(6):797-801.
8. Petros PE, Ulsten UI. An integral theory of female urinary incontinence. Experimental and clinical considerations. *Acta Obstet Gynecol Scand Suppl.* 1990;153:7-31.
9. Ulsten U, Henriksson L, Johnson P, Varhos G. An ambulatory surgical procedure under local anesthesia for treatment of female urinary incontinence. *Int Urogynecol J Pelvic Floor Dysfunct.* 1996;7(2):81-85.

10. Clemons JL, LaSala CA. The tension-free vaginal tape in women with a non-hypermobile urethra and low maximum urethral closure pressure. *Int Urogynecol J.* 2007;18:727-732.
11. Segal JL, Vassallo BJ, Kleeman SD, Hungler M, Karram MM. The efficacy of the tension-free vaginal tape in the treatment of five subtypes of stress urinary incontinence. *Int Urogynecol J.* 2006;17:120-124.
12. Salin A, Conquy S, Elie C, et al. Identification of risk factors for voiding dysfunction following TVT placement. *Eur Urol.* 2007;52(3):782-787.
13. Giri SK, Sil D, Narasimhulu G, Flood HD, Skehan M, Drumm J. Management of vaginal extrusion after tension-free vaginal tape procedure for urodynamic stress incontinence. *Urology.* 2007;69:1077-1080.
14. Kobashi KC, Govier FE. Perioperative complications: the first 140 polypropylene pubovaginal slings. *J Urol.* 2003;170(5):1918-1921.
15. Sivanesan K, Abdel-fattah M, Ghani R. External iliac artery injury during insertion of tension-free vaginal tape: a case report and literature review. *Int Urogynecol J.* 2007;18:1105-1108.
16. Delorme E, Droupy S, de Tayrac R, Delmas V. Transobturator tape(Uratape): a new minimally-invasive procedure to treat female urinary incontinence. *Eur Urol.* 2004;45:203-207.
17. Smith PP, Appell RA. Transobturator tape, bladder perforation, and paravaginal defect: a case report. *Int Urogynecol J.* 2007;18(1):99-101.
18. Latthe PM, Foon R, Toozs-Hobson P. Transobturator and retropubic tape procedures in stress urinary incontinence: a systemic review and meta-analysis of effectiveness and complications. *BJOG.* 2007;114(5):522-531.
19. O'Conner RC, Nanigian DK, Lyon MB, Ellison LM, Bales GT, Stone AR. Early outcomes of mid-urethral slings for female stress urinary incontinence stratified by Valsalva leak point pressure. *Neurourol Urodyn.* 2006;25(7):685-688.
20. Bidmead J, Cardozo L. Retropubic urethropexy (Burch colposuspension). *Int Urogynecol J.* 2001;12:262-265.
21. Lapitan MC, Cody DJ, Grant AM. Open retropubic colposuspension for urinary incontinence in women. *Cochrane Database Syst Rev.* 2003;1:CD002912.
22. Brubaker L, Cundiff GW, Fine P, et al. Abdominal sacrocolpopexy with Burch colposuspension to reduce urinary stress incontinence. *N Engl J Med.* 2006;354(15): 1557-1566.
23. Albo ME, Richter HE, Brubaker L, et al. Burch colposuspension versus fascial sling to reduce stress urinary incontinence. *N Engl J Med.* 2007;355(21):2143-2155.
24. Ward KL, Hilton P, on behalf of the UK and Ireland TVT Trial Group. Tension-free vaginal tape versus colposuspension for primary urodynamic stress incontinence: 5-year follow up. *BJOG.* 2008;115:226-233.

Case 27

A 42-year-old G3P3003 woman is in lithotomy position to undergo a total laparoscopic hysterectomy for a symptomatic 14-week leiomyomatous uterus. Her medical, surgical, and gynecologic histories are unremarkable except for a history of three cesarean sections. An umbilical incision is made with easy entry through the fascia for placement of a Hassan trocar. Several thin filmy adhesions are noted and taken down. The hysterectomy is then started by identifying and ligating the uterine-ovarian ligaments and round ligaments with a tissue sealing device using thermal energy. Upon creation of the bladder flap, the bladder is noted to be adherent to the lower uterine segment. This is taken down sharply with some difficulty.

Once the uterine arteries are skeletonized bilaterally, they are ligated using the tissue sealing device. When the pedicle is divided, it appears that the device has moved and brisk bleeding is noted from what appears to be the right uterine artery pedicle. The pedicle is quickly grasped and an absorbable suture is used to ligate the area of bleeding. The rest of the hysterectomy is then performed up to amputation of the cervix from the vagina without difficulty. During closure of the vaginal cuff, the bladder is noted to be in close proximity to the suture line of the cuff closure.

- ➤ Where are potential points of injury to the urinary tract during this hysterectomy?
- ➤ What are possible complications of unrecognized injury?
- ➤ What is the next step in management of this patient?

ANSWERS TO CASE 27: Urinary Tract Injury During Gynecologic Surgery

Summary: This is a 42-year-old G3P3003 woman with three prior cesarean section deliveries and a 14-week leiomyomatous uterus who is undergoing a total laparoscopic hysterectomy. During surgery, further ligation by suture was required at the right uterine artery pedicle to obtain hemostasis. The bladder was also adherent to the lower uterine segment and cervix. During closure of the vaginal cuff, the suture line was noted to be in close proximity to the bladder.

- **Points of injury:** The bladder is at risk during creation of the bladder flap as well as closure of the vaginal cuff. The ureter is at greatest risk during ligation of the ovarian and uterine vessels. In this case, the ovarian vessels were not at risk as the uterine-ovarian ligament was divided. However, when dividing the uterine artery, further ligation was required to achieve hemostasis.
- **Unrecognized injury:** Unrecognized injuries to the bladder could result in urinoma formation, urinary peritonitis, or vesicovaginal fistulas. With foreign bodies present, the bladder is at risk for bladder calculi and recurrent infections. Unrecognized injury to the ureter could also result in urinoma formation as well as hydronephrosis and loss of renal function caused by ureteral stricture or ligation.
- **Next step:** Cystourethroscopy with intravenous indigo carmine is a minimally invasive diagnostic method to ensure ureteral patency and absence of bladder wall injury from cystotomy or foreign body (suture, mesh, etc). When thermal energy is used, injury to the urinary tract may present in a delayed fashion. Careful dissection of the ureter would also need to be performed to evaluate the distance of the suspected site of injury from the point of application of thermal energy.

ANALYSIS

Objectives

1. Know the possible complications to the urinary tract during gynecologic surgery.
2. Know the indications for cystourethroscopy in gynecologic surgery.
3. Know the parts that comprise a cystourethroscope and appropriate uses of these parts for intraoperative use during gynecologic procedures.

Considerations

This is a 42-year-old woman with three prior cesarean sections who is undergoing a total laparoscopic hysterectomy for a symptomatic 14-week leiomyomatous uterus. There was significant difficulty developing the bladder flap and vesicovaginal space. Additionally, incomplete ligation of the right uterine artery pedicle required further lateral suture ligation deeper into the surrounding tissue. Finally, the bladder was noted to be in close proximity to the suture line during vaginal cuff closure. These events have led the right ureter and bladder to be placed at significant risk for injury. The retroperitoneal space may be opened at the time of surgery to allow identification of the ureter and its course to assure the surgeon of ureteral patency. Near the area where the uterosacral ligament inserts into the uterus, the ureter may be as close as 0.9 ± 0.4 cm from the cervical portion of the uterosacral ligament.[1] Cystoscopy provides an easy, less invasive method to check the patency of the ureter at the ureteral orifice in the bladder. It is especially helpful in cases where there is no abdominal access during surgery or in those patients with multiple adhesions or poor exposure that lead to a difficult retroperitoneal dissection. The bladder is also at risk for cystotomy during a difficult sharp dissection from the lower uterine segment and vagina which may not have been readily identifiable. If bladder fibers are immediately adjacent to the cuff closure, visual inspection alone may not be sufficient to recognize if the suture line incorporates bladder tissue. Cystourethroscopy allows for close inspection of integrity of the bladder lumen, presence of foreign bodies, and ureteral patency.

APPROACH TO Ureteral Injury

DEFINITIONS

BRIDGE: The portion of the cystourethroscope that connects the sheath to the telescope and often contains one or more operative ports.

INDIGO CARMINE: A substance that is injected, usually intravenously, which colors the urine blue to aid in identification of the ureteral orifices and diagnosis of ureteral obstruction.

SHEATH: The portion of the cystourethroscope which is introduced into the urethral meatus and contains ports for distending media.

TELESCOPE: The portion of the cystourethroscope that contains the lens and eyepiece.

CLINICAL APPROACH

Cystourethroscopy

History

In 1805, Bozzini was the first to describe cystoscopy of the female bladder.[2] Several modifications were made over the nineteenth century. In 1894, Kelly described a different technique that is well known. The cystoscope used was a hollow tube that used gas to distend the bladder. The patient was placed in a knee-chest position while cystoscopy was performed using a head mirror to channel light for visualization.[3] Since the advent of fiber optics, many changes have been made to the original models.

The Instrument

The cystourethroscope may either be a flexible scope or rigid scope. The flexible cystoscope is a single unit scope with the tip ranging from 15- to 18-Fr in diameter. A lever near the viewing lens allows the tip to be deflected up to 290 degrees in a single plane. The optics and light source are made of fiberoptic bundles that allow the device to function when bent.[4]

In contrast, the rigid cystoscope is composed of a lens, bridge, and sheath (Figure 27–1) which allow different parts to be interchanged, depending on the need of the operator. The sheath usually contains two ports for inflow and outflow of distending media. Normal saline is commonly used for diagnostic cystourethroscopy whereas glycine or sorbitol is often used when electrocautery is used. Typical sizes range from 17 to 23 Fr. Often 17 Fr is preferred for diagnostic cystourethroscopy since the smaller size facilitates passage of the scope through the urethral meatus.

The bridge functions to connect the sheath to the telescope. Bridges also contain one or more ports allowing for the passage of distending media, ureteral catheters, or other working instruments for operative cystoscopy. Often during ureteral catheterization, difficulty may be encountered in finding the right angle to easily access the ureteral orifice. Use of an Albarrán bridge may facilitate catheterization by adjusting an external knob that deflects the tip of the catheter downward at the end of the sheath. This bridge also helps to stabilize the ureteral catheter in the working channel.

Similar to the other parts of the cystourethroscope, telescopes also are available in different models with each having a different viewing angle. The most common angles are 0, 15, 30, and 70 degrees. Often a 30-degree telescope will suffice for examination of the bladder and urethra as well as such operative procedures as ureteral catheterization and intraurethral bulking. If difficulty is encountered when trying to visualize the entire bladder, a 70-degree telescope will improve visualization. Similarly, a 0- or 15-degree

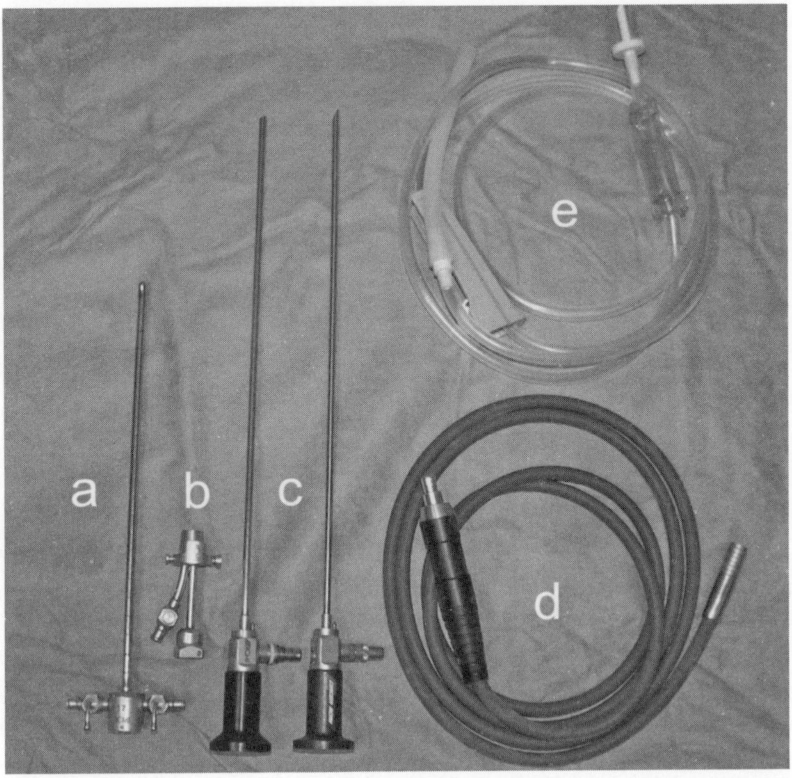

Figure 27–1. **A.** Sheath; **B.** bridge; **C.** telescopes; **D.** light source; **E.** tubing for distending media.

telescope will improve visualization of the urethra during diagnostic or operative procedures. The telescope also has a coupling for the light source, and a camera may be attached to the eyepiece to display the picture on a monitor.

Indications

The role of cystourethroscopy has become so important that an ACOG committee opinion has been issued, describing its role in the use of general obstetrician-gynecology practice. In the committee opinion, it is suggested that general obstetrician-gynecologists can perform cystourethroscopy for diagnostic and a few operative procedures.[5] Specifically, the most important indications listed are to rule out cystotomy and intravesical and intraurethral foreign bodies such as mesh and suture (Figure 27–2) as well as ensure ureteral patency. Other indications would include any symptoms or diseases related to the lower urinary tract. Surgical procedures such as the tension-free vaginal tape (TVT) procedure, Burch colposuspension, and high uterosacral

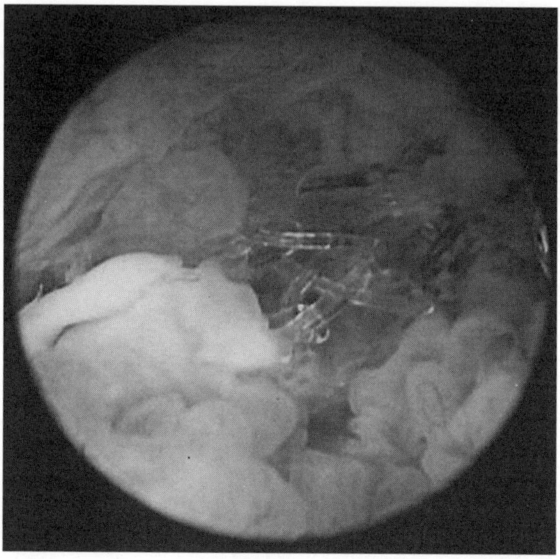

Figure 27–2. Cystoscopy was performed and reveals TVT mesh in the lumen of the urethra.

ligament suspension require intraoperative cystourethroscopy whereas McCall culdoplasty, colpocleisis, and advanced or difficult laparoscopic and vaginal procedures may be other indications.[5] Although not listed in the above procedures, cystourethroscopy is also helpful in ruling out intraoperative injury to the bladder and urethra with other mid-urethral slings, bladder neck slings, and mesh placed into the vesicovaginal space.

When performing cystoscopy, it is important to visualize the entire bladder mucosa and urethra. It is helpful in holding the camera in the proper orientation while the telescope is rotated by the light source to change the angle as the entire scope is moved. Performing a bladder survey helps to rule out other conditions such as cystitis, polyps, and suspected carcinoma. When surveying the urethra, there should be inflow of distending media to obtain a complete circumferential view.

Indigo Carmine Dye

This text focuses on the use of indigo carmine, as other more advanced techniques of detecting ureteral obstructions such as ureteral stenting and retrograde pyelography are beyond the scope of this chapter. Indigo carmine is available in one ampule of 5 mL containing 40 mg of indigotindisulfonate sodium which becomes a deep blue solution when mixed in water. It is largely excreted by the kidneys usually within 10 minutes of injection intravenously and can be seen jetting from the ureteral orifice (Figure 27–3). Intramuscular injection can be performed but requires larger quantities and additional time for excretion.

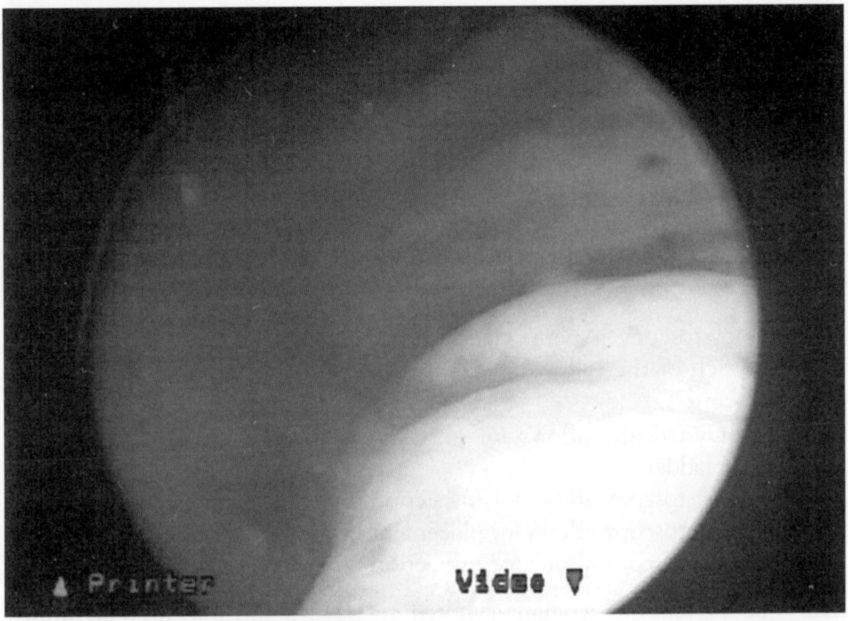

Figure 27–3. Indigo carmine spilling from the ureteral orifice.

Indigo carmine is contraindicated in patients with a prior adverse reaction to its use. Weak ejection of blue dye from the ureteral orifice does not necessarily rule out a partial obstruction that may need further evaluation.[6]

Rates of Injuries

Since hysterectomy is one of the most common surgical procedures performed on women, Vakili et al. performed a prospective study examining the rate of urinary tract injury at the time of hysterectomy by using universal cystoscopy.[7] With 471 patients enrolled, they had a 1.7% rate of ureteral injury and 3.6% rate of bladder injury. Ureteral injury was found to be significantly higher at the time of prolapse surgery whereas bladder injury was significantly higher when concurrent anti-incontinence procedures were performed. The most important aspect of this study is that only 12.5% of ureteral injuries and 35.3% of bladder injuries were diagnosed prior to cystoscopy. The authors concluded that the overall rate of injury to the urinary tract during hysterectomy was 4.8%, and prolapse and anti-incontinence procedures increased this risk. In the authors' opinion, the use of cystoscopy should be considered with hysterectomy.[7]

In a retrospective review by Gustilo-Ashby et al., 700 consecutive patients were reviewed to determine the incidence of ureteral obstruction during vaginal surgery for pelvic organ prolapse specifically. Their surgeries consisted of uterosacral ligament suspension, proximal and distal McCall culdoplasty, anterior colporrhaphy, and colpocleisis. In their study, 5.3% of patients had no spillage from one or both ureters with a false-positive and false-negative cystoscopy rate of 0.4% and 0.3%, respectively. Intraoperative cystoscopy had a sensitivity of 94.4% and specificity of 99.5% for ureteral injury, making it a valuable diagnostic test in this review.[8]

Comprehension Questions

27.1 A cystoscopy is performed after a routine abdominal hysterectomy. Which of the following statements is the best rationale for the cystoscopy?

A. Cystoscopy allows for ensuring that no sutures perforated the bladder.
B. Cystoscopy allows for inspection of bladder endometriosis.
C. Cystoscopy allows for placement of stents after hysterectomy.
D. Cystoscopy allows for inspection of ureteral injury.

27.2 A 44-year-old woman is noted to have a possible ureteral injury. Cystoscopy is contemplated. Which of the following is the best adjuvant to assist in the interpretation of the cystoscopic findings?

A. IV radio opaque dye
B. IV indigo carmine
C. Methylene blue in the bladder
D. Saline in the cul-de-sac

27.3 A 30-degree rigid cystoscope is placed into the bladder, but the entire bladder is difficult to visualize. Which of the following is the best method to address this problem?

A. Change to a 0-degree cystoscope.
B. Change to a 70-degree cystoscope.
C. Change to a flexible cystoscope.
D. Document what is visualized and stop the procedure.

ANSWERS

27.1 **D.** In studies, only 12.5% of ureteral injuries were discovered prior to cystoscopy after hysterectomy. Thus, routine cystoscopy can allow for discovery of unsuspected ureteral injury Although it is valid to use cystoscopy to examine the bladder for sutures, this complication is less common during a routine uncomplicated hysterectomy.

27.2 **B.** Indigo carmine is concentrated in the kidneys and excreted into the bladder. Cystoscopy allows inspection of the ureteral orifices to see if there is efflux of urine through both ureteral openings.

27.3 **B.** The 70-degree cystoscope allows for inspection of the entire bladder when the 30-degree cystoscope may be insufficient to visualize the entire bladder.

Clinical Pearls

See Table 1-2 for definition of level of evidence and strength of recommendation

- The cystourethroscope is composed of a sheath, bridge, and telescope.
- Lenses with different angles may assist in evaluating the bladder and urethra. Lenses of 0, 15, and 30 degrees are commonly used to evaluate the urethra whereas 30- and 70-degree lenses are commonly used to evaluate the bladder (Level B).
- Cystourethroscopy aids in the detection of urinary tract injuries, especially when concomitant prolapse and anti-incontinence procedures are performed (Level B).
- Use of indigo carmine intravenously given 10 minutes prior to cystourethroscopy may aid in locating the ureteral orifices and detect ureteral obstruction (Level B).
- The ureteral orifices are most easily found by locating the intertrigonal ridge which is an elevation of the bladder mucosa just proximal to the urethral-vesical junction (Level B).
- In patients with significant prolapse, placement of a sponge stick into the vagina may restore anatomy sufficiently to aid in identification of the ureteral orifices (Level C).
- Overdistending the bladder may make it more difficult to locate the ureteral orifices (Level B).
- When passing ureteral catheters, an Albarrán bridge may facilitate passage of the ureteral catheter into the orifice (Level C).

REFERENCES

1. Buller JA, Thompson JR, Cundiff GW, et al. Uterosacral ligament: description of anatomic relationships to optimize surgical safety. *Obstet Gynecol.* 2001;97: 873-879.
2. Bozzini P. Lichtleiter, eine erfindung zur anschung inerer theile, und krukheiten nebst abbildung. *J Pract Arzeykunde.* 1805;24:107.
3. Kelly HA. The direct examination of the female bladder with elevated pelvis: the catheterization of the ureters under direct inspection, with and without elevation of the pelvis. *Am J Obstet Dis Wom Child.* 1894;25:1-9.
4. Cundiff GW, Bent AE. Cystourethroscopy. In: Bent AE, Cuniff GW, Swift SE, et al., eds. Ostergard's *Urogynecology and Pelvic Floor Dysfunction.* 5th ed. Philadelphia, PA: Lippincott Williams & Wilkins; 2003.
5. American College of Obstetricians and Gynecologists. The role of cystourethroscopy in the generalist obstetrician-gynecologist practice. ACOG Committee Opinion No. 372. *Obstet Gynecol.* 2007;110:221-224.

6. American Regent, Inc. Indigo Carmine. http://www.americanregent.com/documents/Product27PrescribingInformation.pdf. Accessed August 12, 2010.
7. Vakili B, Chesson RR, Kyle BL, et al. The incidence of urinary tract injury during hysterectomy: a prospective analysis based on universal cystoscopy. *Am J Obstet Gynecol.* 2005;192:1599-1604.
8. Gustilo-Ashby AM, Jelovsek JE, Barber MD, et al. The incidence of ureteral obstruction and the value of intraoperative cystoscopy during vaginal surgery for pelvic organ prolapse. *Am J Obstet Gynecol.* 2006;194:1478-1485.

Case 28

A 40-year-old G3 P3003 Caucasian woman with a body mass index (BMI) of 24 kg/m^2 has dysfunctional uterine bleeding unresponsive to hormonal therapy. The patient is desirous of permanent sterilization, and opts for a total abdominal hysterectomy. She denies any symptoms of urinary or fecal incontinence. Her general physical examination is unremarkable, except that her uterus is at the upper limits of normal size and slightly tender to bimanual examination. She has adequate vaginal support of both the anterior and posterior vaginal walls. On the day of her surgery, an emergency in the adjoining OR just preceding the patient's general anesthesia induction required a quick substitution of one anesthesiologist for another, and during the physician transfer procedure, the patient did not receive her scheduled dose of cefazolin, 1 g intravenously just prior to having general anesthesia. Her vaginal hysterectomy (VH) is complicated by an 850-cc blood loss, though no intra- or postoperative transfusion is required. On postoperative day 1, her 4:00 AM oral temperature is 101.5°F, and her 8:00 AM temperature is 101.8°F.

- ➤ What is the most likely diagnosis?
- ➤ What is your next step?
- ➤ What potential complications may ensue?
- ➤ When should the prophylactic antibiotics be administered?

ANSWERS TO CASE 28: Febrile Morbidity/Pelvic Infection Complicating Vaginal Hysterectomy

Summary: A 40-year-old woman underwent a VH without receiving her scheduled dose of preoperative antibiotic. She has an 850-cc blood loss, and has two elevated temperatures 4 hours apart on the morning of postoperative day 1.

- **Most likely diagnosis:** Febrile morbidity/probable pelvic infection following vaginal hysterectomy.
- **Next step:** Treat the pelvic infection. Perform an examination to rule out other causes of fever, and likely start antibiotic therapy.
- **Potential complications:** Development of pelvic abscess, allergic reaction to antibiotic therapy, development of septic pelvic thrombophlebitis.
- **Prophylactic antibiotics:** Administration of antimicrobial agents usually prior to surgery or a procedure used to decrease febrile morbidity such as wound infection.

ANALYSIS

Objectives

1. Know why, how, and when to use prophylactic antibiotic therapy when performing vaginal surgery.
2. Be able to construct the differential diagnosis for the febrile patient following vaginal hysterectomy.
3. Learn how to treat postoperative pelvic infection following vaginal surgery.
4. Be able to recognize and treat pelvic abscess and septic pelvic thrombophlebitis following vaginal surgery.

Considerations

This 40-year-old Caucasian woman had a VH without receiving preoperative antibiotics, and she sustained an 850-cc blood loss at the time of surgery.[1] She has febrile morbidity on postoperative day 1, with two elevated temperatures 4 hours apart. The differential diagnosis of fever following vaginal surgery depends to some extent on which postoperative day the elevated temperature occurs. On postoperative day 1, the differential should include infection at the surgical site, such as cuff cellulitis, or atelectasis, or infection at a nonsurgical site, such as the urinary tract, the respiratory tract, or at the IV site.[1] A directed physical examination and appropriate laboratory and imaging studies will help to delineate the source of the fever if the patient appears significantly ill, but these workups are usually not likely to yield much useful clinical information.[2,3] Febrile responses occurring later in the postoperative course suggest the possibility of a pelvic abscess or pelvic vein thrombosis.

APPROACH TO Evaluation and Management of Fever after Vaginal Hysterectomy

DEFINITIONS

FEBRILE MORBIDITY: Temperature of 100.4°F or greater on two separate occasions at least 4 hours apart, after the first 24 hours after surgery.

VAGINAL CUFF CELLULITIS: Infection of the vaginal mucosal and submucosal tissue involving vaginal bacteria.

CLINICAL APPROACH

Prophylactic Antibiotic Usage

Febrile morbidity is the most common complication of VH, although this is less likely to occur with vaginal than with abdominal hysterectomy. A major review has shown that some of the difference in rates of febrile morbidity may relate to the increased use of prophylactic antibiotics in VH versus TAH, specifically 7.2% versus 16.8%.[4] Both routes of hysterectomy experience decreased febrile morbidity if prophylaxis is used. Overall, the literature suggests that the incidence of febrile morbidity varies from 10% to 30% for all types of hysterectomy.[4] This case illustrates the two major risk factors for febrile morbidity following VH: those being failure to use prophylactic antibiotics and experiencing excessive blood loss.

There is a unique circumstance that merits therapy before the day of surgery. Studies have shown that the patient with bacterial vaginosis is at increased risk for postoperative pelvic cuff cellulitis. This should be searched for and treated at a preoperative visit prior to the scheduled surgical procedure, with therapy consisting of 4 days of therapy with metronidazole.

The rationale for using a prophylactic antibiotic prior to vaginal hysterectomy rests on the premise that the vagina is a "clean contaminated" space, and that no amount of sterile preoperative preparation is going to make this a sterile operative field. Upon transcervical surgical entry into the peritoneal cavity via the vagina, the operative site is exposed to a plethora of aerobic and anaerobic bacterial organisms with the potential to cause infection. Using antibiotics preoperatively enhances the patient's own immune response and lowers the number of bacteria at the surgical site. The efficacy of single-dose antibiotic prophylaxis does not require that the drug used be bactericidal against all of the organisms in the vagina.

Conceptually, prophylactic antibiotic usage requires that the drug used be relatively inexpensive, safe, and effective. A detailed analysis of the drugs available for use for this purpose is available elsewhere in American College of Obstetricians and Gynecologists publications,[5] and different hospitals may have unique pathogens, which require modification of any blanket recommendations. Also, efficacy and sensitivity patterns are subject to change, so hospital infection control committees should monitor the patterns of prophylaxis usage and benefit for their particular environment and make specific drug recommendations accordingly. **Given the overwhelming evidence regarding the effectiveness of prophylactic antibiotic usage, hospital quality committees should enforce their usage as a routine preoperative protocol for indicated surgical procedures, unless there is some compelling reason for the surgeon to cancel this order.**

Within that context, current studies suggest that a single dose of a cephalosporin, usually cefazolin, 1 or 2 g IV is the drug of choice for prophylaxis, especially for vaginal and abdominal hysterectomy. The drug is low cost, has a long (1.8 hours) half-life, a low incidence of allergic reactions, and is relatively free of side effects. Antibiotics significantly more expensive than cefazolin will decrease the theoretical cost-benefit ratio implicit in supporting the prophylaxis concept. Cefazolin is also similar in its profile of effectiveness against anaerobes to other cephalosporins. Anaphylaxis with cephalosporins occurs less than 0.02% of the time, and this is only slightly increased in patients with known penicillin allergy. Of the four types of immunopathologic responses to β-lactam antibiotics, only the immediate hypersensitivity-type reaction to penicillin should preclude the use of a cephalosporin for prophylaxis. For those patient that have significant allergy to beta lactam agents, other choices include:

- Clindamycin 600 mg IV and Gentamicin 1.5 mg/kg IV
- Metronidazole 500 mg IV and Gentamicin 1.5 mg/kg IV

Timing of administration of antibiotic therapy preoperatively is important. Most studies demonstrate that the antibiotic should reach therapeutic tissue levels prior to the initial incision, and this is best accomplished by administering antibiotic 30 to 60 minutes prior to the initial incision, which effectively means that the antibiotic should be given just prior to the induction of general anesthesia. While the strongest evidence is for the use of a single dose of antibiotic prior to the onset of VH, there are other recommendations in the literature for the use of more than one dose. Some experts suggest that the object of the preventative therapy is to have therapeutic drug levels on board for the duration of the operative procedure and, therefore, if the case is exceptionally long, that is, greater than 2 hours, a subsequent dose of prophylactic antibiotic can be considered at sequences of one to two times the drug's half-life.[5] Given that excess blood loss is also a major risk factor for infection, another antibiotic dose at the conclusion of the case is a consideration. Different studies have suggested that blood loss amounts of 750 to 1500 cc may prompt additional antibiotic dosing. Bacterial resistance is a risk factor for more than routine prophylactic antibiotic usage, so the use of more than a single dose should be approached with caution.

Treatment of Infection/Pelvic Cellulitis

As the ptient case demonstrates, febrile morbidity may occur following VH. When used appropriately, antibiotic prophylaxis has reduced postoperative infection rates from 5% to 10% to about 4% for most gynecologic procedures, infection may result. Pelvic cellulitis is the most likely diagnosis in the illustrative case report. The patient may complain of pelvic pain and a slight increase in vaginal discharge, but neither pelvic examination nor imaging procedures are likely to demonstrate a mass within 24 hours of surgery. Laboratory results may likely demonstrate an elevated white blood (cell) count (WBC) of greater than 13,000/mm^3, with a left shift to greater than 90% bands and polymorphonuclear leucocytes. The value of an extensive fever workup for febrile morbidity following gynecologic procedures has been questioned.[3] Comparing groups of patients with postoperative infection did not demonstrate the value of multiple laboratory or imaging studies, and the approach to the patient with fever following VH should be specific to the individual situation. The therapy of choice is a single agent IV antibiotic, usually not the drug used for prophylaxis.

Again, knowledge of hospital antibiotic resistance patterns is important, but in general, single agent cephalosporin therapy is indicated, such as cefotetan, cefotaxime, cefoxitin, or ceftriaxone. Other choices include ampicillin/sulbactam, piperacillin, mezlocillin, or ticarcillin/clavulanic acid.

Treatment of Infection/Infected Hematoma and Pelvic Abscess

Febrile responses persisting beyond 48 to 72 hours of antibiotic suggest the presence of an abscess or an infected hematoma, and imaging studies such as ultrasound or CT may show a mass.[6] These abscesses usually require surgical drainage, usually in the OR with sedation or anesthesia to allow for transvaginal access to the mass, bluntly opening the cuff enough to facilitate drainage. If imaging studies suggest that the hematoma or abscess is not accessible via the vaginal route, ultrasound- or CT-guided needle or catheter drainage is a consideration. IV antibiotic therapy must continue until the patient becomes afebrile for 24 to 48 hours. The concept of continuing prolonged oral antibiotic therapy for several days after the patient is afebrile is no longer viable and only serves to increase antibiotic resistance.

In general, cultures for anaerobic organisms are costly and not done routinely. Additionally, the antibiotic choices must be made long before the culture results are available. If the fever persists despite therapy for 48 to 72 hours, reevaluation of the cultures and antibiotic choices is in order, and consultation with the infectious disease service is a consideration. Another study of febrile morbidity in patients following VH or TAH has shown that blood cultures were not cost-effective, and that none demonstrated bacteremia in febrile patients.

"Drug fever," as indicated by persistent temperature elevation in the patient with no sign of infection after an exhaustive evaluation, and eosinophilia on the complete blood (cell) count (CBC) should be entertained as a diagnosis.

Treatment of Infection/Septic Thrombophlebitis

If the febrile response continues in spite of 72 hours of antibiotic therapy, the diagnosis of septic pelvic thrombophlebitis should be considered. Physical examination signs are variable and may include pelvic tenderness and pain over the upper thigh along with edema, suggesting ileofemoral vein involvement. Imaging studies such as CT or MRI may show the involved region, with the radiographic criteria for diagnosis, including (1) venous enlargement, (2) the vessel wall having a low-density lumen, and (3) contrast media enhancing a sharply defined vessel wall.[6] Medical therapy is indicated for this problem, not another surgical procedure. Some practitioners will add heparin therapy to the antibiotic regimen. Prolonged therapy is often required for adequate response. Oral anticoagulants are not required following defervescence.

Comprehension Questions

28.1 Which of the following classes of antibiotics is usually the first choice for use as a prophylactic antibiotic in vaginal surgery?

A. Cephalosporins
B. Penicillins
C. Quinolones
D. Tetracyclines

28.2 When pelvic cellulitis is suspected following vaginal hysterectomy, which of the following therapeutic measures should constitute your initial approach?

A. Consult the infectious disease service.
B. Begin therapy with heparin.
C. Begin triple antibiotic therapy with ampicillin, gentamycin, and metronidazole.
D. Begin single-drug therapy with a drug not used for prophylaxis.

28.3 Once the patient described in question 28.2 has responded to IV antibiotic therapy with a normal temperature and no longer appears ill, which of the following is the best next step?

A. Oral antibiotic therapy should commence and continue for another 5 to 7 days.
B. Blood cultures should be obtained to be sure that the patient is well.
C. Antifungal agents should be begun.
D. Antibiotic therapy may end 24 hours following the last elevated temperature.

ANSWERS

28.1 **A.** The cephalosporins, as a class, are generally preferred for antibiotic prophylaxis in vaginal surgery. They are effective, relatively inexpensive, and safe, rarely causing anaphylaxis.

28.2 **D.** Therapy for straightforward pelvic cellulitis should begin with single agent antibiotic therapy. The other treatment options listed should be reserved for infectious problems that do not resolve easily.

28.3 **D.** Continuing antibiotic therapy either IV or orally, after the patient is well, only serves to increase the potential for bacterial resistance and to cause drug fever.

Clinical Pearls

See Table 1-2 for definition of level of evidence and strength of recommendation

- Timing is critical in using prophylactic antibiotics—have the anesthesia service administer your antibiotic of choice before the initiation of general anesthesia, usually within the hour prior to your incision (Level A).
- Keep blood loss to a minimum—the greater the blood loss, the greater the chance for infection (Level B).
- Work quickly and efficiently. The longer the case, the greater the potential for infection. If the case is obviously going to last significantly longer than 2 hours, consider a second dose of prophylactic antibiotic at the 2-hour mark (Level B).
- Consider doing VH without electrocautery. Cauterized tissue provides a nidus for infection, and meticulous surgical technique combined with a lidocaine/epinephrine mixture injected at the vaginal cuff prior to the initial incision significantly reduces blood loss (Level B).

REFERENCES

1. Culligan P, Heit M, Blackwell L, Murphy M, Graham C, Snyder J. Bacterial colony counts curing vaginal surgery. *Inf Dis Obstet Gynecol.* 2003;11:161-165.
2. Swisher E, Kahleifeh B, Pohl J. Blood cultures in febrile patients after hysterectomy. *J Reprod Med.* 1997;42:547-550.
3. Schey D, Salom E, Papadia A, Penalver M. Extensive fever workup produces low yield in determining infectious etiology. *Am J Obstet Gynecol.* 2005;192:1729-1734.
4. Peipert J, Weitzen S, Cruickshank C, Story E, Ethridge D, Lapane K. Risk factors for febrile morbidity after hysterectomy. *Obstet Gynecol.* 2004;103:86-91.
5. American College of Obstetricians and Gynecologists. Antibiotic prophylaxis for gynecologic procedures. ACOG Practice Bulletin No. 74. *Obstet Gynecol.* 2006;108:225-234.
6. Brown C, Lowe T, Cunningham F, Weinreb J. Puerperal pelvic thrombophlebitis: impact on diagnosis and treatment using x-ray computed tomography and magnetic resonance imaging. *Obstet Gynecol.* 1986;68:789-794.

Case 29

A 45-year-old Caucasian G4 P4004 woman with uterovaginal prolapse is scheduled for a planned procedure of vaginal hysterectomy, anterior and posterior colporrhaphy, and sacrospinous ligament fixation. Except for her uterovaginal prolapse, the patient is in good health and has no chronic diseases. On the day of surgery, the patient is positioned in "candy cane" hanging stirrups, and the initial parts of the operation are accomplished without any noticeable complication. A Capio device (Boston Scientific, Boston, MA) is employed to place the permanent suture used for securing the vaginal apex to the right sacrospinous ligament. Following the patient's recovery from general anesthesia, she complains of difficulty walking and getting her right foot to function normally.

➤ What is the most likely diagnosis?

➤ What is your next step?

ANSWERS TO CASE 29: Complications from Vaginal Surgery

Summary: A 45-year-old woman has a vaginal hysterectomy, anterior and posterior colporrhaphy, and right sacrospinous ligament fixation. She awakens with difficulty walking and altered ability to make her right foot function normally.

- **Most likely diagnosis:** Right foot drop from compression of the common perineal nerve by pressure on the nerve by the stirrup at the site of the lateral epicondyle.
- **Next step:** Reassure the patient that this is likely a transient problem. Consult physical therapy for assistance in rehabilitation to restore normal foot function.

ANALYSIS

Objectives

1. Recognize the types of neuropathy related to vaginal surgery.
2. Describe the various mechanisms and preventative strategies of nerve injury associated with vaginal surgery: positioning of the patient, intraoperative injury, and nerve entrapment/injury.
3. Describe the classic presentations of nerve injury and the therapy for these conditions.

Considerations

This patient's immediate postoperative complaint of right foot drop is a known complication of vaginal surgery, especially if the patient was positioned in hanging stirrups which did not have adequate lateral padding to prevent compression of the common peroneal nerve at the lateral epicondyle. This is but one of the types of neuropathy that may occur in association with vaginal surgery. Knowing how to avoid these types of neurologic injury and how to recognize and treat them promptly when they occur is an essential tool for the accomplished vaginal surgeon.

APPROACH TO
Neurologic Injury in Vaginal Surgery

DEFINITIONS

FOOT DROP: Weakness of the ability to dorsiflex the foot, usually due to peroneal nerve or sciatic nerve injury.

SCIATICA: Pain originating from the buttocks and radiating down the posterior aspect of the leg, usually due to irritation of the sciatic nerve.

CLINICAL APPROACH

Neurologic injury in vaginal surgery may arise from two distinct causes—injury due to incorrect preoperative positioning of the patient resulting in nerve stretching, and direct injury to nerve tissue during the actual surgical procedure. Prevention must therefore be twofold; the patient must be correctly positioned prior to the onset of the surgical procedure, and nothing should be done during the surgical procedure itself that will result in stretching or compression or vascular compromise of nerve tissue. Knowledge of the nerve supply to the pelvis is critical to avoid neurologic injury, especially in some of the vaginal operative procedures for reestablishing apical vaginal support where nerve tissue is intimately close to structures utilized for achieving restored vaginal vault integrity (Table 29–1).

How Nerve Injuries Occur in Vaginal Surgery

Most vaginal surgical procedures are accomplished with the patient in the dorso-lithotomy position. It has been demonstrated that vaginal retractors do not have the capability to compress the femoral nerve during vaginal surgery, but that injury to the **femoral nerve** may result from incorrect patient positioning. If the patient's hips are in excessive rotation, excessively flexed, and abducted, then the femoral nerve is placed at an 80- to 90-degree angle as it comes under the inguinal ligament, which is relatively nonpliable and fixed. This results in pressure, which may progress to ischemia to the femoral nerve, and neuropathy distal to the site of compression. The preferred lithotomy position for the patient having vaginal surgery is to have the thighs flexed and abducted, the knees should be flexed, and there should be minimal external rotation of the hips.[1,2]

Sciatic or peroneal nerve injury is relatively rare, occurring only 0.2% to 0.3% of the time. Sciatic nerve injury likewise is a positioning problem, resulting in excessive stretching of nerve tissue. This occurs if there is excessive hip flexion, excessive extension of the knees, or extreme external hip

Table 29–1 NERVES SUBJECT TO INJURY IN VAGINAL SURGERY

NERVE	ORIGIN	MOTOR FUNCTION	SENSORY FUNCTION
Genitofemoral	L1-L2	None	Upper labia, anterior superior thigh
Lateral femoral	L2-L3	None	Anterior and posterior lateral thigh
Cutaneous femoral	L2-L4	Hip flexion, adduction, knee extension	Anterior and medial thigh, medial calf
Sciatic	L4-S3	Hip extension, knee flexion	None
Common peroneal		Foot dorsiflexion Foot eversion	Lateral calf Dorsum of foot
Tibial		Foot plantar flexion Foot inversion	Toes Plantar surface of foot
Pudendal	S2-S4	None	Perineum

rotation.[3] The sciatic nerve is also vulnerable to injury if a surgical assistant leans on the inner thigh during the operation and places excessive tension on the nerve, stretching it during the operative procedure.[2] The **common peroneal nerve** is subject to compression injury most likely due to compression at its most vulnerable location, that being at the lateral fibular head, where it is most superficial. Injury to the peroneal nerve can be successfully avoided with adequate cushioning on the lateral aspect of the calf during vaginal surgery.

Many of the classic papers describing neurologic injury resulting from vaginal surgery were written when "candy cane" stirrups were in common use. Supporting the patient's legs with fully cushioned, multiadjustable (Allen) stirrups will eliminate many, if not most, of the cases of neurologic injury which result from improper positioning.

Injury to the **pudendal nerve** is not uncommon in association with sacrospinous ligament fixation. The pudendal nerve exits from the pelvis through the greater sciatic foramen, and then it lies directly behind the sacrospinous ligament along the lateral one-third of the ligament that attaches to the ischial spine. Nerve fibers are entrapped when the surgeon places the suture securing the vaginal cuff to the sacrospinous ligament too near to its origin at the ischial spine. Most experts describe the optimal suture placement as being 1.5 to 2 finger breaths medial to the ischial spine to avoid nerve entrapment.[4] Anatomic studies have indicated that suture placement should be through the medial one-third of the ligament to completely avoid the pudendal nerve complex.[5] Injury can occur with any of the devices used to place a suture through the sacrospinous ligament, including the Deschamps ligature carrier (Surgipro, Shawnee, KS), the Miya hook, Carrier device (Thomas Medical, Indianapolis, IN), or the Capio device. None seems uniquely designed to allow the surgeon to avoid the possibility of nerve entrapment, **though the likelihood of pudendal nerve injury is reduced to the extent that the suture can be placed through the front of the ligament, and avoid going around or toward the posterior aspect of the ligament where the nerve courses.** Injury to the pudendal nerve will result in the patient having persistent pain long after normal postoperative pain has resolved. Patients complain of perineal pain, pain in the buttocks on the affected side, and of being unable to sit comfortably. Patients need to be taken back to the OR as soon as this diagnosis is made, and the problematic suture needs to be removed. If this is recognized in the immediate postoperative period, then the suture may be placed more medially, or if the procedure has been done as a unilateral procedure, then the fixation may be done to the contralateral ligament. It is important to keep this particular neuropathy in mind, because this complication can occur even in the experience of the best of gynecologic surgeons, possibly because there is a demonstrable anatomic variability in the path of pudendal nerve fibers along the course of the sacrospinous ligament. This complication has been reported as being amenable to surgical correction by reexploration and removal of the offending suture up to 2 years following the initial surgical procedure. In that instance, pain relief was described as being "immediate." This nerve injury has also been reported following uterosacral ligament suspension of the vagina, occurring seven times in 182 procedures.[6]

Treatment Considerations

Fortunately, the incidence of neuropathy from vaginal surgery is relatively low, and recovery is generally complete in most instances, though this may take months rather than weeks if the problem is due to a stretch injury. Neurologic consultation and rehabilitation consisting of physiotherapy, a foot drop brace if indicated, and electrical stimulation of the involved musculature is frequently required. Physical therapy will be necessary if motor deficits are identified, as this will prevent atrophy and wasting of involved muscle groups innervated by the involved nerve. Some authors have also used medical therapy in the form of gabapentin as an adjunct to rehabilitation procedures.

Comprehension Questions

29.1 A 33-year-old woman underwent a vaginal hysterectomy due to dysfunctional uterine bleeding unresponsive to medical therapy. On postoperative day 1, the patient was noted to have difficulty walking. On examination, she has difficulty lifting her right leg off the bed. Her right patellar reflex is absent. Which of the following is the most likely mechanism for the nerve injury?

A. Intraoperative injury with suture
B. Intraoperative pressure with retractor
C. Hyperflexion of the hip
D. Lack of padding to the lateral leg

29.2 Which nerve is most subject to injury as a result of a sacrospinous ligament fixation procedure?

A. Femoral
B. Common peroneal
C. Pudendal
D. Sciatic

29.3 A 55-year-old woman is noted to have foot drop following a vaginal surgery. Which of the following findings would more likely indicate a sciatic nerve problem rather than peroneal nerve issue?

A. Lack of ankle reflex
B. Posterior leg pain
C. Lack of padding to the lateral fibular area
D. Sacrospinous ligament fixation as part of the procedure

ANSWERS

29.1 **C.** This patient likely has a right femoral nerve injury. The femoral nerve innervates the quadriceps muscles leading to difficulty walking and a diminished or absent patella reflex. The most common mechanism of femoral nerve palsy in vaginal surgeries involves hyperflexion of the hips leading to pressure and ischemia of the femoral nerve under the inguinal ligament.

29.2 **C.** The course of the pudendal nerve just behind the lateral aspect of the sacrospinous ligament, near the ischial spine, makes it vulnerable to injury while performing SSLF.

29.3 **B.** Injury to either the sciatic nerve and peroneal nerve will result in foot drop and diminished ankle reflex. Lack of padding to the fibular head leads to common peroneal nerve palsy. Buttocks or posterior leg pain is consistent with sciatic nerve damage.

Clinical Pearls

See Table 1-2 for definition of level of evidence and strength of recommendation

- When tying the sutures affixing the vaginal apex to the sacrospinous ligament, leave the cut ends of the suture long enough so that they can be readily identified to facilitate removal of the suture if pudendal nerve entrapment is diagnosed (Level C).
- Caution your surgical assistants not to put any pressure on the medial aspect of the patient's thigh while she is in lithotomy position (Level C).
- Make sure the patient is correctly positioned in the stirrups before the operation starts. Nerve injury prevention is much simpler, easier, and cheaper than treatment for postoperative neuropathy (Level B).

REFERENCES

1. Irvin W, Andersen W, Taylor P, Rice L. Minimizing the risk of neurologic injury in gynecologic surgery. *Obstet Gynecol.* 2004;103:374-382.
2. Burkhart FL, Daly JW. Sciatic and peroneal nerve injury: a complication of vaginal operations. *Obstet Gynecol.* 1966;28:99-102.
3. Alevizon SJ, Finan MA. Sacrospinous colpopexy: management of postoperative pudendal nerve entrapment. *Obstet Gynecol.* 1996;88:713-715.
4. Verdeja AM, Elkins TE, Odol A, Gasser R, Lamoutte E. Transvaginal sacrospinous colpopexy: anatomic landmarks to be aware of to minimize complications. *Am J Obstet Gynecol.* 1995;173:1468-1469.
5. Batres F, Barclay DL. Sciatic nerve injury during gynecologic procedures using the lithotomy position. *Obstet Gynecol.* 1983;62(suppl):92S-94S.
6. Flynn MK, Weidner AC, Amundsen CL. Sensory nerve injury after uterosacral ligament suspension. *Am J Obstet Gynecol.* 2006;195:1869-1872.

Case 30

A 23-year-old Caucasian woman presents to her gynecologist with a chief complaint of dyspareunia. She relates that she had recently had the onset of severe coital pain on several occasions, which had not previously been present. Specific questioning reveals that the patient localizes the pain to the vaginal vestibule, and that this is exacerbated by touching the region, or by her partner attempting vaginal entry. Physical examination is negative for any evidence of vaginal inflammation, and wet mount examination of the vaginal secretions is negative for the presence of any vaginal pathogens. The vaginal vestibule is exquisitely sensitive when the vaginal speculum is inserted into the vagina, and applying pressure on the perineum exacerbates the patient's pain sensation.

- ➤ What is the most likely diagnosis?
- ➤ What is the next step?

ANSWERS TO CASE 30: Vulvar Vestibulitis

Summary: A 23-year-old woman has dyspareunia localized to the vaginal vestibule. Physical examination reveals tenderness to pressure and touch in this region, with no evidence of any inflammatory process in the vagina.

➤ **Most likely diagnosis:** Vulvar vestibulitis.

➤ **Next step:** Rule out other causes of labial pathology, and then discuss treatment options with the patient for treatment of this diagnosis.

ANALYSIS

Objectives

1. Be able to recognize and treat the benign conditions that are commonly seen on the labia.
2. Know how to perform diagnostic biopsy procedures to confirm these diagnoses.
3. Understand those benign conditions which the generalist gynecologist should be able to treat surgically with confidence, how to do those procedures, and to discern those which should be referred to the gynecologic oncologist.

Considerations

This 23-year-old woman has a recent history of dyspareunia which on examination is localized to the vaginal vestibule. There is no evidence of inflammation or other lesions. There is no evidence of infection by wet mount. On examination, the vaginal vestibule is very sensitive to touch. A careful inspection of the vagina and vulva is important especially to try to identify herpes simplex virus or other neurologic processes. Pain can be assessed and mapped by touching a cotton-tipped applicator to the vulva. In the evaluation process, a herpes assay for polymerase chain reaction (PCR) or culture should be performed. A careful psychosocial history should be taken to assess for sexual abuse or physical abuse. Once infection is ruled out, biopsy may be considered. Vulvar vestibulitis is a diagnosis of exclusion, and usually there is some erythema. Different treatments may be considered, with surgical excision being most successful.

APPROACH TO Nonmalignant Vulvar Disease

DEFINITIONS

VULVAR VESTIBULITIS: A syndrome of severe pain of the vulvar introitus without inflammation.

VULVAR INTRAEPITHELIAL NEOPLASIA: Premalignant condition with dysplastic cells confined within the epithelium of the vulva.

BARTHOLIN GLAND CYST: Fluid within the greater vestibular gland causing swelling.

CLINICAL APPROACH

This chapter on vulvar surgery does not intend to describe surgical therapy for malignant vulvar disease. Rather, it is intended to define practical steps for the generalist gynecologist to use in making the diagnosis of labial disease, to delineate commonly encountered labial conditions amenable to surgical therapy, and to describe surgical approaches for those benign entities that will benefit from surgical therapy.

Vulvar lesions constitute a significant component of the gynecologist's clinical practice. Authors stress the necessity of the labial biopsy to confirm the pathology before embarking on a course of treatment.[1,2] The consultant gynecologist who makes the correct diagnosis and establishes the proper therapeutic plan is often the first physician to make a tissue diagnosis after multiple other physicians have tried a myriad number of ointments and creams without success. The gynecologist should have a close working relationship with the pathologist who is going to evaluate the tissue, and remember that communication with the pathologist regarding the patient's history and gross appearance of the lesion may improve his/her diagnostic acumen under the microscope.

VULVAR VESTIBULITIS

Vulvar vestibulitis as an entity has been initially described by Friedrich as consisting of (1) severe pain on vestibular touch; (2) tenderness when pressure is applied in the vaginal vestibule; (3) erythema of the vestibule.[3] Strenuous evaluation of the validity of these criteria has been established, and it has generally been upheld, except that the erythema of the vestibule has been questioned, and the pain and pressure components have been more accurately described, such that the pain in the vestibule has been described as having a "thermal" component, and the degree of severity is worse than that of severe dysmenorrhea. The etiology of this entity is still unclear, though studies have excluded the human papillomavirus (HPV) as causative, and no other infectious process has been implicated as being likely. Multiple therapeutic approaches have been utilized, though none have been demonstrated to be as effective as surgery for effective treatment of this problem. Success rates range from 36% to 100%, with the overall average being in the 60% range. Women younger than 30 years seem to benefit more from this procedure than those in older age ranges.[4]

The surgical procedure should include complete vestibulectomy, including excision of tissue up to the periurethral region if it is deemed to be involved on the basis of the preoperative evaluation. Undermining and advancement of the vaginal wall completes the operation. Complications of the surgical procedure include the lack of satisfactory lubrication in 24% and the development of Bartholin gland cysts in 6%, which occurs when the Bartholin gland duct is obstructed as part of the excision of the vaginal vestibule.[4]

Labial Biopsy

Office labial biopsy should be simple, fast, routine, and as painless as possible. Premedication of the area to be sampled with topical application of 2.5% lidocaine and 2.5% prilocaine prior to the sterile preparation and the injection of the local anesthetic will significantly reduce patient discomfort; many patients volunteer that they do not feel the injection itself if the cream has been on the labial surface for 5 minutes prior to the injection. Labial tissue has an abundant blood supply, so a mixture of lidocaine and 1:100,000 epinephrine is a good choice to provide good topical anesthesia and minimal bleeding at the biopsy site. Biopsy may be accomplished with tissue forceps and scissors or a punch biopsy instrument. Obtaining a full thickness of tissue down to the subcutaneous tissue is important; rarely is it necessary to remove so much tissue that suture closure for hemostasis is required. Most labial biopsy sites respond to simple application of silver nitrate and there is no need for antibiotic coverage. Homogenous appearing lesions should be sampled from the most representative site; the potential for labial squamous cell carcinoma to be surrounded by lichen sclerosus may require removal of a larger specimen or sampling of multiple biopsy sites.

Vulvar Intraepithelial Neoplasia

Vulvar intraepithelial neoplasia (VIN) should be considered as a diagnosis in the patient whose labial pruritus and chronic labial pain does not have a readily apparent explanation. This is a likely diagnosis in the patient who already has confirmed cervical dysplasia. The colposcope may also be used to evaluate the labia, and acetic acid applied to the labia will create the colposcopic appearance typically associated with dysplastic disease, which can then be confirmed with labial biopsy. Therapy depends on extent and severity of the disease process. Most VIN II and all VIN III lesions merit therapy; asymptomatic VIN I lesions may be followed expectantly in a reliable patient if she is willing to return for follow-up visits. Therapy may consist of topical imiquimod, fulguration, laser vaporization, or wide local excision. Before performing any procedure that eradicates tissue, such as fulguration or laser vaporization, it is critical to ascertain that there is no invasive disease present. Many of the procedures for treating VIN can be performed in the clinic with local anesthesia, or if the hospital OR is indicated, the surgery may frequently be done on an outpatient basis. **It is important to stress to the patient that no matter which modality of therapy is chosen, and no matter how thorough and complete the therapy is to remove the affected tissue, there is always the chance for recurrent disease.** Patients should be informed about the potentially premalignant nature of this disease process and the necessity for long-term follow-up.

Studies that have looked at cases series separated by several decades have noticed a distinct change in the nature of this disease process. Series from the 1960s to the 1980s describe women who average 50+ years of age, with many of these VIN lesions arising in area of lichen sclerosus and other skin abnormalities and not having an HPV infection association. Series from the 1990s report average patient ages dropping into the 30s, and showing a strong clinical correlation with positivity for HPV infection. Dysplasia elsewhere in the genital tract is strongly associated with VIN. Authors stress delay in diagnosis because VIN is confused with infection, and treatment for infection proceeds without a positive biopsy diagnosis. Smoking seems to be a cofactor in disease progression in many cases, and some cases can proceed from VIN to invasive disease in as little as 4 years.[1]

Surgical therapy needs to weigh the cosmetic and functional effects of excising excessive amounts of labia in the OR with a scalpel against using a laser too superficially to eradicate the disease process, which will likely allow for recurrent disease. Laser therapy of the labia minora should not go deeper than 1 mm, and therapy to the majora, the perineum, the fourchette, and skin around the anus should not exceed 2.5 mm. Any laser use should include consideration of the adjacent and deep thermal injury margins, which will increase the effective treatment area.

Bartholin Gland Surgery

Benign conditions of the Bartholin gland, such as cysts or abscesses, affect about 2% of women. Antibiotic therapy is usually prescribed for these lesions, but it is only marginally effective as definitive treatment, especially for cysts. Surgical therapy consists of hospitalization for marsupialization, or outpatient therapy using the Word catheter (WC), an attractive, inexpensive alternative therapy for these lesions.[5] The WC allows for a relatively painless, rapid return to normal activity, including intercourse, and treatment results are comparable to marsupialization surgery. If marsupialization is used, suturing the edges of the abscess cavity to facilitate an adequate drainage window and long-term drainage is preferable to simple incision and drainage of the abscess.[6] The CO_2 laser has been used effectively on an outpatient basis for Bartholin gland abscesses and cysts. The Bartholin gland lesion which does not quickly and completely respond to one of the surgical modalities discussed earlier merits further evaluation, as Bartholin gland malignancies are frequently treated as infectious processes before a cancer diagnosis is established. Recurrent abscesses or cysts require a tissue diagnosis before the assumption is made that the recurrent process is in fact due to infection and not neoplasia.[7] In contrast to initial outpatient therapy for cysts or abscesses, the decision to proceed with total excision of a Bartholin gland should not be made lightly. This is a challenging surgical procedure that should be done only after adequate informed consent and thorough familiarization with the operative procedure.

Labial Hypertrophy

Patient concerns regarding the size of their labia minora are not uncommon. Excessive size of the minora may be congenital, due to chronic stretching, irritation, or androgenic hormone therapy. Symptoms may include disparate appearance of one side versus the other, inability to wear tight fitting clothing, pain with exercise, or entrapment and resultant discomfort of the enlarged labia during coitus. Several reports describe patient satisfaction with operative procedures to reduce the size of the minora. Complications are infrequent, and the vast majority of surveyed patients would have the operation done again.[8] The laser has been used to accomplish this procedure in some instances, and a wedge resection technique has also been described to remove a central portion of the labia while leaving the lateral border intact.[9,10] Surgical techniques in this region need to be fastidious with appropriate attention to detail and hemostasis, including the use of small suture and delicate instruments.

Importantly, legitimate vulvar surgery does not include "vaginal rejuvenation," "designer vaginoplasty," "revirgination," or "G-spot amplification." Some practitioners are marketing these procedures heavily for the sole purpose of changing labial appearance or for enhancing sexual pleasure. No studies exist to demonstrate their efficacy, safety, or patient satisfaction, and they have the risk of significant complications, including infection, scarring, altered and/or diminished sexual response, and adhesion formation. Patients seeking these sorts of surgical procedures should be counseled about the normal variability of the appearance of their external genitalia and about normal sexual function not being dependent on labial appearance.[11]

Comprehension Questions

30.1 A 32-year-old woman is diagnosed with vulvar vestibulitis. She has searched the Internet and learned that surgery is an option for therapy. Under what circumstances should she consider surgical management?

A. If she has been unresponsive to other therapy
B. Only if she is older than 50 years of age
C. Only if a minimal amount of tissue can be removed
D. As a possible first line treatment

30.2 A 45-year-old woman is diagnosed on vulvar biopsy to have VIN II. The patient asks about risk factors. You explain that the VIN:

A. Has a relationship to HPV infection rates
B. Does not seem to be related to smoking
C. Is related to topical corticosteroid use
D. Is related to topical estrogen

30.3 Labioplasty

A. Is legitimate surgery for the proper indication
B. Has recently been noted to have scientific basis for therapy
C. Is relatively straightforward and is associated with few complications
D. Is an antiquated procedure and does not have a place in modern gynecology

ANSWERS

30.1 **A.** Surgery for vulvar vestibulitis provides better results than any other therapy for this disabling condition and is most effective in younger patients. Complete excision of all involved tissue provides the best functional result.

30.2 **A.** Vulvar dysplasia in recent years is associated primarily with HPV infection, and it is exacerbated by smoking. Alcohol intake is not known to be a contributing factor.

30.3 **A.** Valid indications for labial plastic surgery are well known and reasonable, but the combination of labioplasty with questionable and ill-defined therapeutic goals associated with some practitioners' heavy marketing efforts place these efforts in a non-professional category.

Clinical Pearls

See Table 1-2 for definition of level of evidence and strength of recommendation

- Pretreat the area on the labia to be biopsied with a topical anesthetic cream to reduce the pain of injection and the biopsy itself (Level B).
- At the preoperative visit for the patient who is to have labioplasty, especially for reduction in the labia minora, use a marking pen and a mirror and be sure that the patient is in agreement with the amount of tissue to be removed (Level C).

REFERENCES

1. Jones RW, Rowan DM. Vulvar intraepithelial neoplasia III: a clinical study of the outcome in 113 cases with relation to the later development of invasive vulvar carcinoma. *Obstet Gynecol.* 1994;84:741-745.
2. Baggish MS, Sze EHM, Adelson MD, Cohn G, Oates RP. Quantitative evaluation of the skin and accessory appendages in vulvar carcinoma in situ. *Obstet Gynecol.* 1989;74:169-174.
3. Bergeron S, Binik YM, Khalife S, Pagidas K, Glazer HI. Vulvar vestibulitis syndrome: reliability of diagnosis and evaluation of current diagnostic criteria. *Obstet Gynecol.*2001;98:45-51.
4. Traas MAF, Bekkers RLM, Dony JMJ, et al. Surgical treatment for the vulvar vestibulitis syndrome. *Obstet Gynecol.* 2006;107:256-262.
   A definitive treatise justifying surgery for this perplexing entity.
5. Andersen PG, Christensen S, Detlefsen GU, Kern-Hansen P. Treatment of Bartholin's abscess. Marsupialization versus incision, curettage and suture under antibiotic cover. A randomized study with 6 months' follow-up. *Acta Obstet Gynecol Scand.* 1992;71:59-62.
6. Haider Z, Condous G, Kirk E, Mukri F, Bourne T. The simple outpatient management of Bartholin's abscesses using the Word catheter: a preliminary study. *Aust N Z J Obstet Gynecol.* 2007;47:137-140.
7. Cardosi RJ, Speights A, Fiorica JV, Grendys EC Jr, Hakam A, Hoffman MS. Bartholin's gland carcinoma: a 15-year experience. *Gynecol Oncol.* 2001;82:247-251.
8. Pardo J, Sola V, Ricci P, Guilloff E. Laser labioplasty of labia minora. *Int J Gynaecol Obstet.* 2006;93:38-43.
9. Rouzier R, Louis-Sylvestre C, Paniel BJ, Haddad B. Hypertrophy of labia minora: experience with 163 reductions. *Am J Obstet Gynecol.* 2000;182:35-40.
10. Choi HY, Kim KT. A new method for aesthetic reduction of labia minora (the deepithelialized reduction of labioplasty). *Plast Reconstr Surg.* 2000;105:419-422.
11. American College of Obstetricians and Gynecologists. Vaginal "rejuvenation" and cosmetic vaginal procedures. ACOG Committee Opinion No. 378. *Obstet Gynecol.* 2007;110:737-738.

Case 31

A 43-year-old African American woman presents with a history of anemia from heavy menstrual bleeding not responsive to hormone therapy. She had a bilateral tubal ligation (BTL) at the time of her second cesarean section. She is not interested in any therapeutic procedure that cannot guarantee her that she will not bleed again in the future. She is otherwise in good health. On physical examination, she has a uterus that is at the upper limits of normal size, and some leiomyomata are palpable on examination. The estimated weight of the uterus is 250 g. Ultrasound of the uterus shows slight enlargement, and some leiomyomata, the largest of which is 2 to 3 cm in size. The patient opts for vaginal hysterectomy, and the chief resident is assigned to the case. After making a 180-degree incision around the anterior portion of the cervix, the resident encounters a fibroid and has some difficulty gaining access to the peritoneal cavity anteriorly, and clear, slightly yellow liquid exits the operative site. The fluid is slightly blood tinged. The resident quickly extends the incision around the posterior aspect of the cervix, and tries to force the duckbill retractor into the posterior cul-de-sac. A watery, foul-smelling, brown substance coming from the region of the posterior cul-de-sac is encountered.

- ➤ What are the most likely diagnoses?
- ➤ How would you confirm the diagnoses?
- ➤ What is the best therapy?

ANSWERS TO CASE 31: Incidental Cystotomy and Proctotomy

Summary: A 43-year-old woman with two prior cesareans and small fibroids presents for vaginal hysterectomy. While making the incision around the cervix, the surgeon encounters a yellow liquid anteriorly and a watery, brown substance coming from the posterior cul-de-sac.

- **Most likely diagnoses:** Incidental cystotomy and incidental proctotomy.
- **Confirmation of diagnoses:** Instill sterile milk into the bladder and see if it exits the wound anteriorly; place a gloved finger in the rectum and see if the finger is visible through the proctotomy site.
- **Best therapy:** Immediate operative repair of both the injury to the bladder and to the rectum.

ANALYSIS

Objectives

1. Know the approximate potential rates of bladder and bowel injury.
2. Consider what can be done at the time of vaginal hysterectomy to diminish the potential for injury to the bowel and bladder.
3. Become familiar with the most common type of injuries to occur when performing a vaginal hysterectomy.
4. Learn how to repair injuries to the bladder and rectum that may occur during the course of vaginal hysterectomy.

Considerations

This 43-year-old woman had both incidental cystotomy and proctotomy. Prompt identification of the injuries is important with repair. The bladder injury should be delineated and it should be assured that the laceration is sufficiently far from the ureteral orifices. An injury too close to the ureters can lead to stricture and obstruction. Laceration to the rectum likewise must be recognized. Typically, the rectum will be injured below the peritoneal reflection and can be repaired with a double layer closure. The exception is for a significant amount of devitalized tissue, cancer, or prior irradiated tissue.

Fortunately, injury to the bladder and to the bowel is relatively uncommon in vaginal hysterectomy. Injury to the ureter is distinctly rare in vaginal hysterectomy and will not be discussed further. While some studies fail to distinguish a significant difference in complication rates attributable to the route of hysterectomy, most studies indicate that the incidence of any injury with vaginal hysterectomy (VH) is less than that with either total abdominal hysterectomy (TAH) or with laparoscopically assisted vaginal hysterectomy (LAVH). Difficulty in performing a VH is more likely to result in injury to either the bladder or the bowel. Careful case selection is helpful in avoiding the vaginal route if the risk of potential complication is felt to be unacceptably high. **The experience of the operating gynecologist is a major determinant in deciding whether to attempt a challenging vaginal case.** While the percentages of hysterectomy done worldwide via the vaginal route are felt by most authorities to be too low, it is better to err on the side of caution and avoid the vaginal route if the risk of injury is deemed to be unacceptably high, or refer the patient to a more experienced gynecologic surgeon if the reasons for taking the vaginal route are compelling.

In the case cited above, the history of cesarean sections increases the risk for bladder injury, and, if the uterine fibroids are occluding the posterior cul-de-sac, rectal injury is a distinct possibility.

The potential for rectal injury is also increased by adhesions resultant of endometriosis, history of pelvic inflammatory disease, prior pelvic surgery, or any other process, which may compromise or obliterate the posterior cul-de-sac.

APPROACH TO Bladder and Bowel Injuries

DEFINITIONS

CYSTOTOMY: Surgical entry into the bladder.
PROCTOTOMY: Surgical entry into the rectum.

CLINICAL APPROACH TO BLADDER INJURY

The best solution regarding injuries to the bowel and bladder is to avoid them in the first place. Hemostasis and some hydrodissection are extremely beneficial in gaining access to both the anterior and posterior cul-de-sacs. The scalpel incision on the anterior cervix should be about 2.0 to 2.5 cm above the plane of the exocervix, and perpendicular to the long axis of the cervix. The incision is extended into a level of cervical tissue that permits easy index finger dissection of the outer layers of the uterine tissue upward in a cephalic direction. Dissection laterally on both sides of the anterior aspect of the cervix facilitates placement of a small Deaver type of retractor in the midline, which retracts the cut tissue cephalad. Placing the tip of the Metzenbaum scissors firmly into the tissue and opening both blades of the scissors laterally will usually expose the anterior peritoneal fold. The index finger of the non-scissor operating hand feels the distinctly "slippery" consistency of the anterior peritoneal fold as it slides back and forth between the surgeon's index finger and the underlying firm tissue of the anterior cervico-uterine junction. This peritoneal fold is distinctly visible at this point and should be grasped with tissue forceps, lifted slightly ventrally, and then incised sharply with Metzenbaum scissors in a line directly parallel to the long axis of the cervix. This should gain direct access into the anterior cul-de-sac, and a Heaney retractor should be placed into this opening. Clearly visible contents of the abdominal cavity and the lack of visible urine confirm entry into the correct plane.

A review of the literature reveals multiple rates of bladder injury in the performance of VH. The bladder is most likely injured when the surgeon is attempting to gain entry into the anterior cul-de-sac. The other potential for bladder injury happens as part of anterior vaginal wall repair with placement of a suture into the bladder as part of a plication stitch. This is best avoided by keeping the stitch lateral enough to avoid the bladder and by being alert for blood in the urine immediately following placement of these stitches. Bladder injury rates range from 0.2 to 10 per 1000 surgeries.[1] A history of prior cesarean increases the odds ratio for bladder injury to 2.04 (95% CI: 1.01-4.1, P = 0.46) for all types of hysterectomies.[2] Other historical events which have been shown to increase the risk for bladder injury include prior pelvic surgery, and obesity is shown to be problematic in some series but not in others. Nulliparity and nondescent of the uterus increase the potential for bladder injury, but neither of these are absolute contraindications to the vaginal route. Concurrent surgery for incontinence increases the risk for bladder injury, increasing from 3.1% in VH cases without repair to 12.5% where repair was performed. Cystoscopy can also occur during cesarean (Figures 31–1 and 31–2).

Women who sustain injuries to the bladder experience longer operating times, greater blood loss, longer hospital stays, greater postoperative morbidity, more febrile morbidity, and longer use of catheter drainage of the bladder. **The vast majority of bladder injuries sustained at VH can be managed vaginally without resorting to laparotomy.**

The technique of repair of the bladder injury involves placing two or three layers of absorbable suture, size 3-0, initially using the mucosal layer for approximation and hemostasis, and then a horizontal mattress layer to provide strength and to imbricate the mucosal layer closure. A third layer of interrupted mattress sutures may be indicated in especially large injuries, burying the initial submucosal muscular layer. The integrity of the closure should be tested by filling the bladder with milk via a catheter at the conclusion of the repair, and the catheter needs to remain in place for 5 to 7 days postoperatively, with appropriate antibiotic coverage to avoid urinary tract infection from the indwelling catheter.

Vesicovaginal fistula is a potential complication following cystotomy, but the likelihood of that happening is only in the range of 10%. **The risk is significantly higher in those cases in which the bladder injury is not recognized**

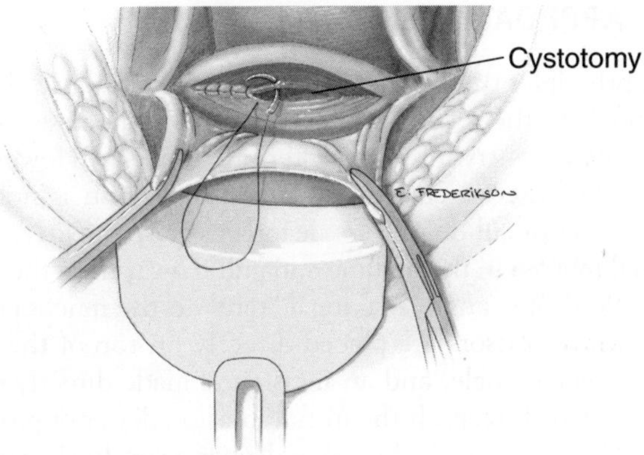

Figure 31–1. Bladder is repaired in two layers. First layer is mucosa. *(Reproduced, with permission, from Cunningham FG, Leveno KJ, Bloom SL, et al.* Williams Obstetrics, *23rd ed. New York: McGraw-Hill, 2010.)*

at the time of the initial surgical procedure. A recent study using diagnostic cystourethroscopy after all TAH, VH, and LAVH cases in the series determined that only 35.3% of bladder injuries were detected prior to cystoscopy, and the authors suggest that the routine use of cystoscopy should be considered at the conclusion of all types of hysterectomy.[3] "Cystoscopy should be performed intraoperatively to assess for bladder or ureteral damage after all prolapse or incontinence procedures during which the bladder or ureters may be at risk of injury."[4]

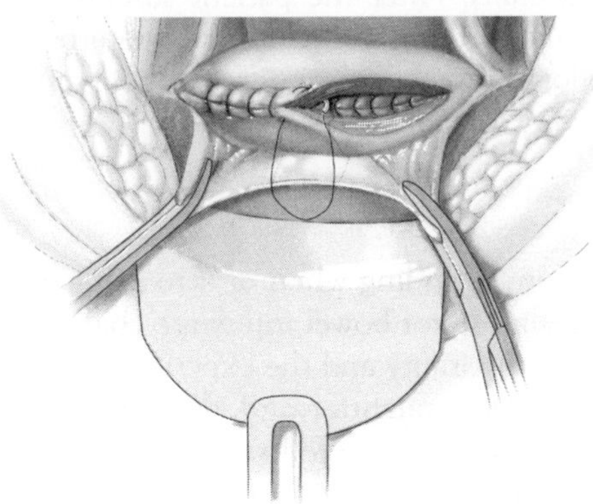

Figure 31–2. Bladder is repaired with second layer. *(Reproduced, with permission, from Cunningham FG, Leveno KJ, Bloom SL, et al.* Williams Obstetrics, *23rd ed. New York: McGraw-Hill, 2010.)*

CLINICAL APPROACH TO BOWEL INJURY

Many of the principles that apply to avoiding bladder injury also apply to prevention of injury to the rectum. Hemostasis and hydrodissection beneficially provide visibility for entry into the posterior cul-de-sac. However, in contrast to entry into the anterior cul-de-sac, lateral dissection is not helpful when entering the posterior cul-de-sac. Tissue forceps grasp the uterine border of the incised vaginal mucosa in the midline and pull it away from the cervico-uterine junction at a 90-degree angle, making a "tent" in the mucosa and underlying peritoneum. Mayo scissors are placed directly on top of the tissue forceps, at about a 45-degree angle, and an incision is made directly into the "tent" created by the tissue forceps. If the initial incision does not provide entry into the peritoneal cavity, pick up the tissue deeper again in the site of the initial incision and repeat the incision in the same tissue plane. Using the scissor tips to "open and spread" the tissue is not helpful in gaining entry posteriorly. If unable to gain entry at this point, stay close to the uterus and continue dissection posteriorly toward the top of the uterine fundus until entry can be gained into the cul-de-sac. **It is better to make incisions into the posterior uterus than into the bowel.**

If bowel injury is suspected, place a gloved finger into the rectum and see if rectal injury can be confirmed. If there is bowel injury, obtain visualization with enough dissection to see the extent of the injury and then approximate the mucosa with a running stitch of 3-0 absorbable suture. The muscularis is closed with interrupted inverting mattress sutures of 3-0 absorbable suture.

Bowel injuries are less common than bladder injuries. Large series reported an incidence of bowel injury with vaginal hysterectomy of 0.5%, with almost all occurring at the point of entry into the posterior cul-de-sac.[1] Rectovaginal fistula is a rare complication of this injury, as most are detected and repaired immediately and successfully. After the patient sustains a bowel injury, she should be kept on a liquid diet until bowel function returns and then on a low-residue diet for the following week. Judicious use of stool softeners and laxatives is indicated until recovery is complete.

CONCLUSION

Blanket recommendations regarding when or if to call a consultant urologist for bladder injury or a surgeon for bowel injury are challenging and obviously depend on the extent of the injury and the experience of the operating gynecologist. If the injury appears straightforward, the repair goes smoothly, and if the bladder or the bowel appears intact following repair, then consultation may not be required. If the limits of the injury are not easily delineated, the integrity of the repair cannot be confirmed, or if the degree of confidence in the result is less than satisfactory, then ask for help. Patients with chronic diseases of the urinary tract or of the intestinal tract which would predispose such a patient to a complicated recovery even without unintentional injury should definitely be evaluated intraoperatively by urology or surgery as needed. Community practice and standards of course also play an important role.

Comprehension Questions

31.1 Which of the following surgical approaches for hysterectomy is associated with the overall lowest incidence of bladder injury?

A. Abdominal hysterectomy
B. Laparoscopic hysterectomy
C. Vaginal hysterectomy

31.2 If incidental cystotomy is noted at the time of vaginal hysterectomy, which of the following should be the approach?

A. The location of the injury should be ascertained regarding the distance from the ureteral orifices.
B. The vaginal approach should be abandoned, and the case converted to an abdominal procedure.
C. The patient should undergo an intravenous pyelogram to assess the renal function.
D. A suprapubic catheter should be placed in the bladder.

ANSWERS

31.1 **C.** Vaginal hysterectomy results in the lowest incidence of bladder injury compared to all other surgical approaches.

31.2 **A.** Upon recognition of a bladder injury, its extent and location, especially with respect to the ureteral orifices, should be established. This assessment will indicate whether the bladder can be closed with a simple two layer closure or will require possible ureteral surgery and/or stents.

Clinical Pearls

See Table 1-2 for definition of level of evidence and strength of recommendation

- Early detection, preferably intraoperatively, of injury to the bowel or bladder will allow for immediate repair and greatly reduce the risk of significant harm to the patient, and to the reputation of the surgeon (Level B).
- Infiltration of the cervix with a mixture of 1% lidocaine and 1:100,000 epinephrine or 0.5% lidocaine and 1:200,000 epinephrine prior to the circumferential incision around the cervix will provide excellent hemostasis and allow for better visualization of anatomic landmarks and the potential to avoid injury (Level B).
- Using the more dilute solution will allow for instillation of a greater volume of fluid, and the principle of hydrodissection may create easier planes for entry into the anterior and posterior cul-de-sacs (Level C).
- The use of sterile milk to see the injury to the bladder may be preferable to the use of indigo carmine or methylene blue dyes, as both dyes tend to stain the tissue and may make visualization of the tissue to be repaired more difficult (Level B).
- When repairing injuries to the bladder, sutures should be tied such that the knot is outside of the bladder mucosa to avoid the potential for the knotted suture to cause bladder stones (Level C).
- When repairing rectal injuries, tie the suture such that the knot is inside of the rectal lumen, allowing the suture to slough into the bowel when healing is complete and the suture dissolves (Level B).
- If your surgical procedure results in an injury to the bowel or bladder, do not describe this as "inadvertent" in your written or dictated operative report. Synonyms for "inadvertent" include "careless" and "inattentive." Do not put yourself in the position of having to explain this wording in a deposition or trial for medical malpractice (Level C).

REFERENCES

1. Mathevet P, Valencia P, Cousin C, Meiller G, Dargent D. Operative injuries during vaginal hysterectomy. *Eur J Obstet Gynecol Reprod Biol.* 2001;97:71-75.
2. David-Montefiore E, Rouzier R, Chapron C. Surgical routes and complications of hysterectomy for benign disorders: a prospective observational study in French university hospitals. *Hum Reprod.* 2007;22:260-265.
3. Vakili B, Chesson R, Kyle B, et al. The incidence of urinary tract injury during hysterectomy: a prospective analysis based on universal cystoscopy. *Am J Obstet Gynecol.* 2005;192:1599-1604.
4. American College of Obstetricians and Gynecologists. Pelvic organ prolapse. ACOG Practice Bulletin No. 85. *Obstet Gynecol.* 2007;110:717-730.

5. Harkki-Siren P, Sjoberg J, Tiitinen A. Urinary tract injuries after hysterectomy. *Obstet Gynecol.* 1998;92:113-118.
6. Rooney C, Crawford A, Vassallo B, Kleeman S, Karram M. Is previous cesarean section a risk for incidental cystotomy at the time of hysterectomy? *Am J Obstet Gynecol.* 2005;193:2041-2044.
7. Carley M, McIntire D, Carley J, Schaffer J. Incidence, risk factors, and morbidity of unintended bladder or ureter injury during hysterectomy. *Int Urogynecol J Pelvic Floor Dysfunct.* 2002;13:18-21.
8. Dorairajan G, Rani P, Habeebullah S, Dorairajan L. Urological injuries during hysterectomies: a 6-year review. *J Obstet Gynaecol Res.* 2004;30:430-435.

Case 32

A 44-year-old African American, G3P2012, woman complains of increasing abdominal girth and urinary frequency for the past 6 months. She has noted that she has had difficulty buttoning her pants and has had to buy clothes several sizes larger. She denies dysuria, hematuria, or nocturia. She denies any change in bowel habits. She reports menstrual cycles every 30 days with a flow lasting for 7 days. She has no chronic medical conditions and no family history of gynecologic malignancies. Past surgical history includes a tubal ligation.

The pelvic examination reveals normal external female genitalia. The vaginal and cervix are without lesions. The uterus is 16-week size on palpation, irregular and mobile. Six months ago, the uterus measured 10-week size on examination. The patient's adnexa are not well palpated due to the midline mass. The rectal examination reveals a 3-cm firm mass that is continuous with the uterus. A pelvic ultrasound reveals multiple hypoechoic densities suggestive of fibroids, the largest measuring 8 cm in the fundal region.

- What is the most likely diagnosis?
- What are the indications for surgery in the presence of myomas?
- What is the best treatment for this patient?

ANSWERS TO CASE 32: Indications for Surgical Therapy for Fibroids

Summary: This is a 44-year-old multiparous woman has a rapidly enlarging pelvic mass which is most likely due to uterine fibroids. She has symptoms of increasing abdominal girth and urinary frequency. She does not desire more children.

- **Most likely diagnosis:** Uterine leiomyoma.
- **Indications for surgery:** The list of indications is lengthy, here are the common indications:
  1. Abnormal uterine bleeding not responsive to conservative therapy
  2. High level of suspicion for pelvic malignancy
  3. Myoma growth after menopause
  4. Infertility with distortion of endometrial cavity or tubal obstruction
  5. Recurrent pregnancy loss due to distortion of endometrial cavity
  6. Pain or pressure symptoms interfering with quality of life
  7. Urinary tract symptoms like frequency and/or obstruction
  8. Iron deficiency anemia secondary to chronic blood loss
  9. Adnexa cannot be palpated due to uterine enlargement
- **Best treatment:** Hysterectomy, possibly also bilateral salpingoophrorectomy. The route of hysterectomy should be tailored to the situation.

ANALYSIS

Objectives

1. Develop a differential diagnosis of a pelvic mass.
2. List symptoms caused by leiomyoma.
3. List indications for fibroid surgery.
4. List surgical treatment options for symptomatic uterine fibroids.

Considerations

This 44-year-old woman has worsening symptoms from her uterine fibroids, specifically the increasing pelvic pressure and menorrhagia. She does not desire more children. Medical therapy does not seem to be effective. Thus, surgical therapy should be considered. Myomas are the most common solid pelvic tumors in women. The benign monoclonal tumors develop from a chromosomal mutation in a single smooth muscle cell of the uterus. Leiomyomas contain fibrous tissue as well as smooth muscle cells and are bounded by a fibrous capsule. Approximately 20% to 40% of women will be diagnosed with a leiomyoma during their reproductive years, and it is the most common indication for hysterectomy.

APPROACH TO Uterine Fibroids

DEFINITIONS

MEIGS SYNDROME: Benign fibromas of the ovary associated with ascites and pleural effusion.

CARNEOUS DEGENERATION (aka Red degeneration): Necrosis of the leiomyoma that occurs because the myoma has outgrown its blood supply, especially in pregnancy. Clinically, it causes severe pain and local peritoneal inflammation. Carneous degeneration is associated with marked softening and red color of the fibroid. This type of degeneration occurs in 5% to 10% of pregnant women with leiomyomas.

TENESMUS: Ineffectual and painful straining with bowel movement or upon urination.

MONOCLONAL: Originating from a single cell. Monoclonal smooth muscle cells in the uterus that form leiomyoma often have aberrant chromosomes.

CLINICAL APPROACH

Symptoms

Most women with leiomyoma are asymptomatic. However, the size, number, location, and degeneration status of the myomas can determine the symptoms that the patient will experience. Myomas can range in size from subcentimeter to occupying the whole pelvic cavity. They can be subserosal, submucosal, or intramural in location. They can be pedunculated or prolapsed through the cervix. The myoma may become parasitic and derive its blood supply from an organ other than the uterus.

Aside from leiomyoma, other etiology for pelvic masses should be considered in order to plan for surgery. Differential diagnoses for pelvic and lower abdominal masses include follicular cyst, hemorrhagic corpora lutea, serous cystadenoma, benign cystic teratoma, mucinous cystadenoma, malignant ovarian tumors, Meigs syndrome, endometrioma, malignant uterine tumors, metastatic disease, benign or malignant masses of the fallopian tubes, diverticulitis, pregnancy, gestational trophoblastic disease, and adenomyosis.

Women with uterine fibroids may complain of abnormal uterine bleeding, pelvic pressure, and increasing abdominal girth. Although other bleeding patterns can be present, menorrhagia is the most common type of bleeding associated with myomas. Explanation for the cause of menorrhagia includes the obstructive effect of myomas, leading to ectasia of the endometrial venules, which causes congestion in the endometrium and myometrium, contributing to an increase in bleeding during menstrual cycle. The increased surface area from the enlarged uterine cavity can cause menorrhagia. Endometritis is often histologically seen in the endometrial tissue overlying the submucous myoma and can contribute to excessive menstrual flow. Aberrant angiogenesis and dysregulation of local growth factors have been linked to abnormal uterine bleeding in patients with leiomyoma. Persistent abnormal uterine bleeding can lead to iron deficiency anemia due to chronic blood loss.

Pelvic pain is rarely caused by leiomyoma. Myomas can cause acute pain if there is torsion of a pediculated myoma, cervical dilation from a prolapsing pediculated submucosal myoma, or carneous degeneration with pregnancy. More frequently, the pelvic discomfort is described as pelvic pressure. Pelvic pressure and increasing abdominal girth are a result of the enlarging leiomyoma. Urinary symptoms include urinary frequency, outflow obstruction, and compression of the ureters which can result from the myoma pressing on the bladder and pelvic side wall. Gastrointestinal symptoms include constipation and tenesmus which are due to pressure on the rectosigmoid by a myoma on the posterior wall of the uterus. An incarcerated uterus in the posterior cul-de-sac or a single large posterior wall myoma may cause rectal pressure, but this symptom is rare.

Rarely, myomas have been associated with infertility. When all the other causes of infertility are excluded, 2% to 3% of the infertility cases can be attributed to the presence of myomas. Mechanisms by which myomas can cause infertility include the following:

1. Alteration of the endometrial cavity may inhibit implantation.
2. Enlarged and deformed endometrial cavity can inhibit sperm transport.
3. Displacement of the cervix can block access by ejaculated sperm.
4. Alteration in uterine contractility may alter sperm movement.
5. Persistent blood or clots in endometrial cavity may inhibit implantation.
6. Tubal ostia may be obstructed or distorted.

In patients undergoing in vitro fertilization, decreased rates of implantation and pregnancy were noted in patients who had a endometrial cavity distorted by leiomyomas up to 50% of the time. Recurrent pregnancy losses have also been linked to myomas. Although no prospective studies comparing expectant management to myomectomy in asymptomatic women have been done, most clinicians conclude that surgery does improve pregnancy rates.

Malignancy associated with uterine fibroids is rare. A study done by Parker evaluated 1332 women who underwent hysterectomy or myomectomy for symptomatic leiomyoma; uterine sarcoma (leiomyosarcoma, endometrial stromal sarcoma, and mixed mesodermal tumor) was found in 0.23%. The incidence of leiomyosarcoma usually increases with age. Women in the reproductive years have a 0.1% risk and women undergoing uterine surgery for myomas have a risk of approximately 1.7%. The possibility of sarcoma in a uterine myoma is 10 times greater in a woman in her 60s than a woman in her 40s. Although malignancy is usually suspected if the leiomyoma displays rapid growth, the incidence of leiomyosarcoma is not related to the rate of growth or the uterine size. Considering the high prevalence of uterine fibroids, most researchers agree that sarcomas arise spontaneously in fibroid uterus. Of note, myomas tend to exhibit an accelerated rate of growth in the fifth decade of life, likely due to unopposed estrogen stimulation from anovulatory cycles in the perimenopausal period.

Some clinicians advocate treatment for asymptomatic uterine myomas if the uterine size is larger than 12 weeks' size due to inability to palpate the adnexa which may interfere with the detection of an ovarian tumor or cancer.

Summary of clinical settings that may require surgical therapy for myomas includes

1. Abnormal uterine bleeding not responsive to conservative therapy.
2. High level of suspicion for pelvic malignancy.
3. Myoma growth after menopause.
4. Infertility with distortion of endometrial cavity or tubal obstruction.
5. Recurrent pregnancy loss due to distortion of endometrial cavity.
6. Pain or pressure symptoms interfering with quality of life.
7. Urinary tract symptoms like frequency and/or obstruction.
8. Iron deficiency anemia secondary to chronic blood loss.
9. Adnexa cannot be palpated due to uterine enlargement.

Treatment

The choice and approach for therapy should take into account medical and social factors.

Considerations for treatment:

1. Age
2. Parity
3. Desire for childbearing
4. Extent and severity of symptoms
5. Size and number of myomas
6. Locations of myoma
7. Medical conditions
8. Possibility of malignancy
9. Proximity to menopause
10. Desire for uterine preservation

There are various options for management of leiomyomas. These include expectant management, medical management, surgical management, uterine artery embolization, high-frequency ultrasonography, laser treatment, cryotherapy, and thermablation. Surgical management includes hysterectomy and myomectomy. Hysterectomy is the most common treatment for leiomyomas because it is the only therapeutic option that provides a cure and eliminates the chance of recurrence. It is second to cesarean delivery as the most common major surgical procedure performed in women in the United States. Of note, all surgical alternatives to hysterectomy allow for the chance that new myomas may form or leiomyomas that were already present and were too small to be seen or intentionally not removed may grow significantly and may require another procedure. Also, complications from surgical procedures other than a hysterectomy may lead to a hysterectomy. Before proceeding with treatment, it is important to rule out adnexal or endometrial pathology. Pathology in either of these locations will determine which therapeutic option is chosen.

Comprehension Questions

32.1 A 43-year-old G3P3 woman has a 10-week irregular uterus on palpation. No adnexal masses are palpated. She reports normal menstrual cycles and no other symptoms. What is the best treatment for this patient?

A. Expectant management
B. Medical management
C. Myomectomy
D. Hysterectomy

32.2 A 43-year-old G1P1 woman complains of heavy menstrual bleeding lasting for 10 days for 3 months. She feels chronic fatigue. She has been on iron supplements. She has had a BTL and no other medical or surgical conditions. She does not smoke. Her pelvic examination reveals a 16-week size irregularly shaped uterus. Adnexa are not well palpated due to the midline mass. What is the next step in the management of this patient?

A. Expectant management
B. Oral contraceptives
C. Pelvic ultrasound
D. Hysterectomy

32.3 A 35-year-old woman is noted to have an irregular uterus with menorrhagia. The excessive bleeding with fibroids is caused by dysregulation of growth factors, the obstructive effect of leiomyoma, and which of the following?

A. Associated endometritis
B. Coagulopathy
C. Endometrial hyperplasia
D. Carneous degeneration

ANSWERS

32.1 **A.** Since this patient is asymptomatic, the small uterine myomas do not require treatment. Initially she should be examined every 6 months for uterine growth and the development of symptoms. Annual visits can resume when the clinician is confident that the leiomyomas are not enlarging.

33.2 **C.** Although this patient's history and physical are highly suggestive of uterine leiomyoma, other gynecologic conditions should be considered in the differential diagnosis prior to instituting therapy. Since the adnexa were not well evaluated with the pelvic examination, ovarian or adnexal pathology should be ruled out. Pelvic ultrasound is a reliable tool that will evaluate not only the adnexa, but it will better characterize the location and size of the myomas. The presence or absence of concurrent adnexal pathology may guide the final treatment that the patient receives. Furthermore, the endometrium in this patient older than 35 years with abnormal uterine bleeding should be evaluated prior to surgery.

32.3 **A.** Associated endometritis is noted in patient with fibroids and menorrhagia.

Clinical Pearls

See Table 1-2 for definition of level of evidence and strength of recommendation

- Most women with leiomyoma will be asymptomatic and will not require treatment (Level A).
- Menorrhagia is the most common type of abnormal uterine bleeding associated with leiomyoma (Level B).
- If all other causes of infertility are ruled out, in the presence of leiomyoma, a myomectomy can improve fertility outcome (Level B).
- Hysterectomy is the only surgical procedure that will not allow myomas to form or allow the previously remaining ones to increase in size (Level B).
- Malignancy originating from leiomyoma is very rare (Level A).
- Most common differential diagnosis for pelvic mass is leiomyoma, adenomyosis, pregnancy, and adnexal pathology (Level B).

REFERENCES

1. Parker W, Berek J, Fu YS. Uterine sarcoma in patients operated on for presumed leiomyomas and rapidly growing leiomyomas. *Obstet and Gynecol.* 1994; 83:414-8.
2. Benson CB, Chow JS, Chang-Lee W, Hill JA 3rd, Doubilet PM. Outcome of pregnancies in women with uterine leiomyomas identified by sonography in the first trimester. *J Clin Ultrasound.* 2001;29:261-264.
3. Buttran VC, Reiter RC. Uterine leiomyomata: etiology, symptomatology, and management. *Fertil Steril.* 1981;36:433-435.
4. Farrer-Brown G, Beilby JO, Tarbit MH. The vascular patterns in myomatous uteri. *J Obstet Gynaecol Br Commonw.* 1970;77:967-975.
5. Farrer-Brown G, Beilby JO, Tarbit MH. Venous changes in the endometrium of myomatous uteri. *Obstet Gynecol.* 1971;38:743-751.
6. Katz VL. Benign gynecologic lesions. In Katz VL, Lentz GM, Lobo RA, Gershenson DM, eds. *Comprehensive Gynecology.* 5th ed. Philadelphia, PA: Mosby; 2007:452-557.
7. Li TC, Mortimer R, Cooke ID. Myomectomy: a retrospective study to examine reproductive performance before and after surgery. *Hum Reprod.* 1999;14:1735-1740.
8. Propst AM, Hill JA 3rd. Anatomic factors associated with recurrent pregnancy loss. *Semin Reprod Med.* 2000;18:341-350.
9. Sehgal N, Haskins AL. The mechanism of uterine bleeding in the presence of fibromyomas. *Am Surg.* 1960;26:21-23.
10. Seoud MA, Patterson R, Muasher SJ, Coddington CC 3rd. Effects of myomas or prior myomectomy on in vitro fertilization (IVF) performance. *J Assist Reprod Genet.* 1992;9:217-221.
11. Stewart EA, Nowak RA. Leiomyoma-related bleeding: a classic hypothesis updated for the molecular era. *Hum Reprod Update.* 1996;2:295-306.
12. American College of Ostetricians and Gynecologists. *Surgical Alternatives to Hysterectomy in the Management of Leiomyomas. ACOG Practice Bulletin No. 16.* Washington, DC; May 2000.
13. The Practice Committee of the American Society for Reproductive Medicine. Myomas and reproductive function. *Fertil Steril.* 2006;86(suppl 5):194-199.
14. Wallach EE, Vlahos NF. Uterine myomas: an overview of development, clinical features, and management. *Obstet Gynecol.* 2004;104:393-406.

Case 33

A 42-year-old G2P2 woman, with a recent last menstrual period (LMP), presents complaining of irregular periods for 4 years. She states that her periods are about three to four times a year and very long in duration, up to 21 days. She has gained 50 lb (22.68 kg) in the last 2 years. Four years ago, she was on oral contraceptive pills to regulate her periods. Her last doctor instructed her to take iron daily for her anemia. She is "tired of these heavy periods" and refuses further medical therapy. She wants surgical therapy. Her review of systems is negative for thyroid disease or galactorrhea. She denies any significant past medical, family, or social histories. She had a bilateral tubal ligation 3 years ago.

On examination, her weight is 262 lb (118.85 kg), BP 112/72 mmHg, and pulse 60 bpm. The head and neck examination, including the thyroid gland, is normal. The abdomen is nontender and there are no masses. On pelvic examination, the uterus is noted to be 8- to 10-week size and the adnexa are difficult to assess. A pelvic ultrasound is performed revealing a normal sized uterus, with an endometrial stripe of 10mm and no adenxal masses. A pregnancy test is negative.

➤ What is the most likely diagnosis?

➤ What is the next step?

ANSWERS TO CASE 33:
Surgical Indications for Dysfunctional Uterine Bleeding

Summary: 42-year-old G2 P2 woman has a 4 year history of irregular menses, oligomenorrhea, menorrhagia, obesity, and anemia. She desires surgical therapy.

- **Diagnosis:** Oligomenorrhea or dysfunctional uterine bleeding (DUB)
- **Next step:** Endometrial biopsy

ANALYSIS

Objectives

1. Recognize that DUB is a diagnosis of exclusion.
2. Know the common differential diagnoses that cause DUB.
3. Understand that surgical therapy is indicated only when medical therapy fails and future fertility is no longer desired.
4. Recognize the two surgical therapies for DUB, endometrial ablation, and hysterectomy.

Considerations

This patient has a long history of irregular periods. This is a classic case of anovulation, most likely secondary to her obesity. She weighs 100 lb (45.36 kg) over her ideal body weight. One has to consider an underactive thyroid being a contributor to her obesity. Her age warrants that the next step is to perform an endometrial biopsy. Women older than 35 years should receive an endometrial biopsy (EMB) for any abnormal uterine bleeding. Note that her endometrial stripe is 1 cm. Studies reveal that an EMB using the Pipelle type of device is highly effective in detecting pathology.[1] Her differential diagnosis includes anovulation, hypothyroidism, endometrial polyp, and uterine fibroids. An endometrial polyp or endometrial hyperplasia/neoplasia can be the etiology for an enlarged endometrial stripe. A coagulation defect is unlikely, given the age of the patient. Since DUB is a diagnosis of exclusion, an organic etiology should be ruled out first. After obtaining a negative pregnancy test, check a thyroid-stimulating hormone (TSH), complete blood (cell) count (CBC), and prolactin, even though the patient has a negative past medical history. Premature ovarian failure can be ruled out if the follicle-stimulating hormone (FSH) is less than 40 U/L. An EMB that reveals proliferative endometrium is consistent with anovulation. This patient should be offered medical treatment, first, with hormones. After medical therapy fails or in this case, is refused, surgical therapy is the next option. This patient is a candidate for an endometrial ablation because her uterine size is normal and without evidence of any organic etiology, such as fibroids. The fact that she received a tubal ligation confirms that she does not desire future fertility. Keeping in mind that endometrial ablation has shorter operative time, shorter recovery, and less hospital-associated cost, this procedure should be offered first. Even though hysterectomy is definitive, there is associated morbidity and mortality.[2]

APPROACH TO Dysfunctional Uterine Bleeding

DEFINITIONS

DUB: Excessive uterine bleeding without any demonstrable organic cause.

MENORRHAGIA: Prolonged uterine bleeding longer than 7 days duration or greater than 80 cc.

ENDOMETRIAL ABLATION: Operative destruction, via a hysteroscope, of the endometrium with a variety of different instruments.

OLIGOMENORRHEA: Uterine bleeding that occurs at intervals of longer than 35 days.

MENOMETRORRHAGIA: Prolonged uterine bleeding that occurs at irregular intervals.

POLYMENORRHEA: Uterine bleeding that occurs at intervals every 21 days or fewer.

CLINICAL APPROACH

Heavy menstrual flow can become very disturbing to a woman and can result in disruption of her lifestyle. These changes include absenteeism from work, avoidance of social functions, and restriction to certain physical activities. Over a period of time, women will experience fatigue, anxiety, anemia, and a decrease in quality of life.[3]

Dysfunctional uterine bleeding is defined as noncyclic, menstrual flow, unrelated to organic pathology.[3] It clinically manifests as abnormal volume, timing, and duration of flow. Traditional options for treatment include medical therapy with hormones and surgical therapy, such as endometrial ablation and hysterectomy. The choice of treatment depends on the woman's age and her desire for future fertility.

During a normal menstrual cycle, the endometrium is exposed to the ovarian production of estrogen, in the first half of the cycle and after ovulation, progesterone, in the second half of the cycle. Menses occurs secondary to the estrogen and progesterone withdrawal, to begin another cycle. In DUB, or anovulatory bleeding, a corpus luteum does not form and progesterone is not produced from the ovary. In this clinical scenario, the endometrium continues to be primed with estrogen. As a result, the endometrial lining continues to proliferate. Once the lining is at its maximum thickness, inadvertent shedding of the endometrium will occur in a nonuniform, noncyclic manner. This occurs because the endometrium is very vascular, fragile, and not stable. The end result is prolonged, heavy, uterine bleeding.

A detailed history should be obtained from the patient. It is important to verify what "irregular" means to her. Is the uterine bleeding more than once a month or only monthly, with variable duration? Have the patient quantify her bleeding.

- Number of pads used in a 24-hour period
- Does the bleeding soil her clothes?
- Is her activity restricted?
- Does she stay home from work?
- Passage of clots? If so, what size . . . (ie, penny, nickel, dime, quarter, half-dollar size)

Obtain other relevant history. Certain medications can contribute to abnormal bleeding, such as hormones and psychotropic medications. On the physical examination, look closely for evidence of hirsutism and obesity. Perform a detailed pelvic examination. Examine the external genitalia for lacerations. Insert the speculum and evaluate for lacerations or trauma to the cervix or vagina. Foreign bodies, such as an IUD, can also cause abnormal bleeding. Obtain a Pap smear and cultures. Perform an endometrial biopsy in a woman older than 35 years. Studies show that the endometrial Pipelle is highly effective and accurate in sampling the endometrium.[3] Malignancies can cause abnormal uterine bleeding. This test will usually rule out endometrial hyperplasia and endometrial carcinoma. A TSH and a prolactin should be obtained. If hypothyroidism is diagnosed, then levothyroxine should be prescribed. Once the thyroid hormonal status corrects, usually requiring 3 months, the menorrhagia should improve. Check the pregnancy test. A pelvic ultrasound will evaluate for any organic causes of the uterine bleeding, such as leiomyomas. DUB is a diagnosis of exclusion; other etiologies should be ruled out as a cause of bleeding. Developing a differential diagnosis is important and will differ based on the age of the patient (Table 33–1).

If the TSH, CBC, prolactin, and pelvic ultrasound are normal and the endometrial biopsy is negative for hyperplasia or neoplasia, DUB can be diagnosed. Remember, it is a diagnosis of exclusion.

For women younger than 20 years, a coagulation disorder should be eliminated. All adolescents with prolonged uterine bleeding since menarche need routine screening for coagulation defects. Disorders such as idiopathic thrombocytopenic purpura and von Willebrand disease should be considered. Other disorders that cause platelet dysfunction include leukemia or sepsis. However, the most common diagnosis for DUB in this age group is immaturity of the hypothalamic, pituitary, and gonadal axis. Look for petechiae or bruising on the

Table 33–1 DIFFERENTIAL DIAGNOSES OF DUB

Anovulation
Systemic disease (thyroid)
Pregnancy
Coagulation defects
Infection
Endometrial hyperplasia
Uterine fibroids
Endometrial malignancy

skin during the physical examination. In addition to the earlier-mentioned laboratory tests, also check a prothrombin time and partial thromboplastin time (PTT). An endometrial biopsy (Pipelle) is not necessarily indicated in this age group, unless there is evidence of prolonged unopposed estrogen exposure.

For women, between 20 and 40 years of age, a common disorder is polycystic ovarian syndrome. A triad of symptoms includes obesity, hirsutism, and noncyclic menstrual bleeding (dysfunctional uterine bleeding [DUB]). Hypothyroidism, hyperprolactinemias, and premature ovarian failure should be ruled out. All contribute to irregular menses. On physical examination, note any evidence of acne, hirsutism, and body weight. Perform an endometrial biopsy on women older than 35 years. Check a TSH, FSH, and prolactin. If all are normal, DUB can be diagnosed.

For women between 40 and 51 years of age, anovulatory cycles are common secondary to declining ovarian function. Perform an EMB and ultrasound to rule out fibroids, hyperplasia, and neoplasia. Cancer and hyperplasia incidence is higher in this age group. Check TSH, FSH, and prolactin. If all are normal, DUB is the diagnosis.

Treatment

Treatment options are medical and surgical. The age of the patient will dictate therapy. Medical treatment consists of hormones, such as cyclic progestins, combination oral contraceptives, or nonsteroidal anti-inflammatory drugs (NSAIDs). NSAIDs have been shown to decrease monthly menstrual blood loss and block prostaglandin production. This treatment may be continued up to 6 months. Once medical therapy has failed and the woman does not desire future fertility, surgery can be offered.

Surgical therapy for DUB is twofold: endometrial ablation and hysterectomy. Both are effective treatments for DUB, with hysterectomies being associated with more adverse events.[3]

Endometrial ablation is a minimally invasive technique that was introduced in 1937.[4] It is used to treat heavy menstrual bleeding in women who do not desire future fertility. Its absolute contraindications include pregnancy, uterine size greater than 12 to 14 weeks, active pelvic infection, and evidence of a premalignant or malignant disorder. Older techniques involved the use

Table 33–2 METHODS OF ENDOMETRIAL ABLATION

RESECTOSCOPE
Loop electrode
Rollerball
NONRESECTOSCOPE
Cryoabalation therapy (Her Option)
Heated free fluid (Hydro Therm-Ablator)
Microwave
Radiofrequency electricity (NovaSure)
Thermal balloon (ThermaChoice)

of the resectoscope and now there are newer nonresectoscopic techniques utilizing different energy sources. In the United States, there are several systems approved for use (Table 33–2).

Three instruments are needed to perform an ablation: (1) distention media, (2), operative hysteroscope, (3) ablation instrument. Counselling the patient prior to the procedure is very important. Women should be informed that hypomenorrhea is the usual outcome, even though more than 40% of women can become amenorrheic from the procedure.[5] Priming agents are used before the ablation to thin the endometrium. Danazol and a gonadotropin-releasing hormone (GnRH) analogue (Lupron) are commonly used for 4 to 12 weeks prior to the procedure. Remember, the side effects of Danazol are clitorimegaly, deepening of the voice, acne, and alteration of low-density lipoprotein (LDL) cholesterol.[6] Endometrial thinning can shorten the procedure time and ease the level of difficulty with surgery.

Most studies cite endometrial ablation as an alternative to hysterectomy. Dickersin et al. showed that both endometrial ablation and hysterectomy are effective at 24 months, in improving DUB. However, 32 out of 110 patients who received an endometrial ablation required another operation.[3] Another randomized control trial revealed that 78% of women receiving endometrial ablation were satisfied at 12 months compared to 89% of those receiving a hysterectomy. However, morbidity was higher in the hysterectomy group. Gannon et al.[7] who revealed that endometrial ablation is an alternative to hysterectomy with less operating time, shorter recovery time in the hospital, and cheaper cost compared to hysterectomy, found similar results. No one in this study required a hysterectomy during the follow-up of 12 to 16 months.[8] Endometrial ablation is safe, and Garry et al. showed that out of 600 laser ablations performed, none of the participants experienced any operative morbidity.[6]

Table 33–3 TYPES OF DISTENTION MEDIA

CARBON DIOXIDE GAS	
Electrolyte-rich	**Electrolyte-poor**
Lactated Ringer solution	3% Sorbitol
Normal saline	1.5% Glycine
	5% Mannitol

Complications can occur with endometrial ablation and develop secondary to either the distention media or the operative technique. Table 33–3 shows the different distention media available. Complications with the distention media occur more commonly with the resectoscopic ablations.

Carbon dioxide (CO_2) is a gas used for diagnostic hysteroscopies. If bleeding occurs, CO_2 does not mix well with blood and can disrupt visualization of the endometrial cavity. Watch the flow rate, during the case, to reduce the risk of an air embolus. If the flow is greater than 100 mL/min, the patient is at risk. Sudden desaturation of oxygen, hypotension, or development of cardiac arrhythmias can occur suddenly. Immediately, place the patient in left lateral decubitus position at a 5-degree angle to move the air toward the right ventricle.[9] When liquid media are used, fluid management is critical to avoid complications. Once a deficit of 1 L has been reached, the procedure should be discontinued immediately. The electrolyte-free solutions can get absorbed into the systemic circulation and cause hyponatremia, fluid overload, seizures, brain edema, and rarely death. Hyponatremia is corrected within 24 to 48 hours. Give the patient isotonic solution, normal saline, and infuse 1 to 2 mEq/L/h to correct the sodium level.[9] A diuretic may be given to correct any pulmonary edema, as a result of the fluid overload. Use of the electrolyte-rich media is more likely to cause fluid overload, and not hyponatremia. Other complications described in the literature, during an ablation, include uterine perforation, lacerations of the cervix and vagina, hemorrhage, and thermal injury to the bowel and bladder. If uterine perforation occurs with dilation of the cervix, the perforation is usually in the midline. Lateral perforation can lead to severe bleeding. If this occurs, stop the procedure and perform a laparoscopy to visualize the extent of the damage. Admit the patient and follow serial hematocrits over 24 hours.[9] If hemorrhage develops as a complication, a Foley balloon can be inserted to tamponade the bleeding or a vasopressin can be injected at the site of bleeding to help to decrease the blood loss.[9] These adverse events occur because the ablation extends too deeply into the myometrium and breaches the integrity of surrounding structures.[6]

Hysterectomy, with or without a bilateral salpingo-oophorectomy, is the definitive therapy for DUB. Studies show that for long-term management of bleeding, hysterectomy will be required for DUB in 30% of women.[10] Hysterectomy is the most frequently performed operation in the United States. It is associated with a higher satisfaction rate compared to endometrial ablation, but also its costs are higher.[7] There are complications to consider. Febrile morbidity is the most frequent complication, with abdominal hysterectomies having higher rates compared to vaginal hysterectomies.[2] Others adverse events include thromboembolism; vascular injury; hemorrhage; and damage to the bowel, bladder, and ureteral systems. Accurate knowledge of the anatomy is the key to reducing complication. Ureteral injures occur in 2 to 5 out of 1000 operations.[2] The risk of death is low, keeping in mind that most cases occur as a complication of the surgery.

Comprehension Questions

33.1 A 37-year-old G4P4, with a history of hypothyroidism, stopped taking her medicine last year because she was "feeling fine." Nine months ago, she started having two periods a month. Her laboratory work showed a TSH of 50 U/L and hemoglobin of 11.8 mg/dL. A pelvic ultrasound was normal. What is the most likely diagnosis?

A. Anovulation
B. Hypothyroidism
C. Leukemia
D. Uterine fibroids

33.2 A 17-year-old G0P0 woman presents complaining of heavy bleeding for 10 days every month with her periods, since menarche at the age of 12. Her hemoglobin is 7.5 mg/dL. What is the next step in her workup?

A. Check liver function tests.
B. Draw a TSH.
C. Draw coagulation tests.
D. Order a pelvic ultrasound.

33.3 A 41-year-old G3P3 woman has a resectoscopic endometrial ablation using 1.5% glycine. The ablation lasts for 2 hours and intraoperatively; the nurse states that the fluid deficit is 2500 cc. What is the most likely electrolyte abnormality?

A. Hyponatremia
B. Hypercalcemia
C. Hypoglycemia
D. Hyperkalemia

33.4 A 32-year-old G6P6 woman is having a NovaSure endometrial ablation. You dilate her uterus and insert the hysteroscope and visualize the bowel. What is the most appropriate next step?

A. Proceed with the ablation and repair the uterus after the case.
B. Stop the procedure, perform a laparoscopy, and check serial hematocrits.
C. Repair the uterus first before proceeding with the ablation.
D. Use a different ablation technique.

ANSWERS

33.1 **B.** Hypothyroidism is a systemic etiology for DUB. Once the thyroid gland is regulated with levothyroxine, the menorrhagia will abate in 3 to 6 months.

33.2 **C.** In teenagers, coagulation disorders are the most common etiology for the heavy uterine bleeding. Checking a PT/PTT and von Willebrand factor is the next step to establish a diagnosis.

33.3 **A.** This patient has fluid overload from intravascular absorption of glycine, the distention medium. Hyponatremia is the abnormality that needs to be corrected.

33.4 **B.** Uterine perforation is a complication of this ablation. After visualization of the bowel, the ablation is discontinued and a laparoscopy is performed to judge the extent of injury to the uterus and any other surrounding structures.

Clinical Pearls

See Table 1-2 for definition of level of evidence and strength of recommendation

- Once an organic etiology is ruled out, DUB is the diagnosis for heavy menstrual bleeding (Level B).
- An endometrial biopsy should be performed in all women older than 35 years with heavy uterine bleeding (Level B).
- Differential diagnoses may vary, based on the age of the patient (Level A).
- Surgical therapy for DUB is indicated after medical therapy has failed and future fertility is no longer desired (Level B).
- Endometrial ablation is an alternative to hysterectomy with less morbidity and mortality (Level A).
- Hysterectomy is the most definitive therapy for DUB (Level A).

REFERENCES

1. Goldchmit R, Katz Z, Blickstein I, Caspi B, and Dgani R. The accuracy of endometrial Pipelle sampling with and without sonographic measurement of endometrial thickness. *Obstet Gynecol.* 1993;82:727-730.
2. Peipert JF, Weitzen S, Cruickshank C, Story E, Ethridge D, Lapane K. Risk factors for febrile morbidity after hysterectomy. *Obstet Gynecol.* 2004;103:86-91.
3. Dickersin K, Munro, MG, Clark, M, et al. Hysterectomy compared with endometrial ablation for dysfunctional uterine bleeding. *Obstet Gynecol.* 2007;110:1279-1289.
4. American College of Obstetricians and Gynecologists. Endometrial Ablation. ACOG Practice Bulletin. 2008:1356-1371.
5. Garry R, Shelley-Jones D, Mooney P, et al. Six hundred endometrial laser ablations. *Obstet Gynecol.* 1995;85:24-29.
6. Garry R. Good practice with endometrial ablation. *Obstet Gynecol.* 1995;86:144-151.
7. Gannon MJ, Holt EM, Fairbank J, Fitzgerald M, Milne MA, Crystal AM, et al. A randomised trial comparing endometrial resection and abdominal hysterectomy for the treatment of menorrhagia. *BMJ*. 1991;303:1362-1364.
8. Goldenberg M, Sivan E, Bider D, et al. Endometrial resection vs. abdominal hysterectomy for menorrhagia. *J Reprod Med.* 1996;41:333-336.
9. American College of Obstetricians and Gynecologists. Hysteroscopy. ACOG Practice Bulletin. 2008:350-353.
10. Learman LA, Summitt RL Jr, Varner RE, Richter HE, Lin. F, Ireland CC, et al. Hysterectomy versus expanded medical treatment for abnormal uterine bleeding: clinical outcomes in the medicine or surgery trial. *Obstet Gynecol.* 2004; 103:824-833.
11. American College of Obstetricians and Gynecologists. Anovulatory Bleeding. ACOG Practice Bulletin No. 2008:1049-1056.
12. Pinion SB, Parkin DE, Abramovich DR, Naji A, Alexander. DA, Russell IT, et al. Randomised trial of hysterectomy, endometrial ablation, and transcervical endometrial resection for dysfunctional uterine bleeding. *BMJ*. 1994;309:979-983.
13. Easterday CL, Grimes DA, Riggs JA. Hysterectomy in the United States. *Obstet Gynecol.* 1983;62:203-212.
14. Unger JB, and Meeks GR. Hysterectomy after endometrial ablation. *Am J Obstet Gynecol.* 1996;175:1432-1437.

Case 34

A 33-year-old G4P3013 woman, with a recent last menstrual period, presents to the office complaining of intermittent, lower abdominal pain for 2 years. During the last 6 months, she reports pain with her menstrual cycle and occasional pain during sexual intercourse. When she is not on her menses, she has intermittent pain four to five times a week. She denies any urinary or bowel complaints associated with the pain. For the last 12 months she has been taking oral contraceptives daily, prescribed by her last OB/GYN physician. In addition, she is taking an NSAID two to three times a day for the last 4 months, with minimal relief of her pain. The pain lasts for 1 to 2 hours and is not affected by changes in positions.

Other significant history consists of a mother with endometriosis, diagnosed in her 30s and three prior surgeries, two cesarean sections, and a bilateral tubal ligation. She denies having any medical problems.

On examination, her vitals are temperature, 98.9°F; BP, 110/70 mm Hg; pulse, 90 beats/min. Pertinent findings include abdominal examination, without rebound or guarding; no distention or fluid wave, no tenderness to deep palpation. Pelvic examination reveals normal external genitalia, no cervical motion tenderness, no uterine or left adnexal tenderness, with only mild right adnexal tenderness. An ultrasound of the pelvis is normal.

➤ What is the most likely diagnosis?

➤ What is your next step?

ANSWERS TO CASE 34:
Surgical Indications for Chronic Pelvic Pain

Summary: A 33-year-old multiparous woman presents with chronic pelvic pain, dysmenorrhea, dyspareunia, family history of endometriosis, and no specific etiology of pain clinically or with ultrasound.

- **Most likely diagnosis:** Chronic pelvic pain (possibly endometriosis).
- **Next step:** Laparoscopy.

ANALYSIS

Objectives

1. Know some common differential diagnoses for chronic pelvic pain.
2. Recognize women at risk for developing chronic pelvic pain.
3. Be able to understand that surgical therapy for chronic pelvic pain is indicated once medical management has failed.
4. Identify surgical options available in treating chronic pelvic pain.

Considerations

This patient has a long history of pelvic pain. She has been taking medications, for a minimum of 4 months and a maximum of 1 year, and still experiences pain. She has a pertinent negative history for depression and domestic/sexual abuse. A positive history for either can increase the risk of developing pelvic pain. This persistent pain can also increase the chance of her losing time from work.[1] This patient has both cyclic and noncyclic pain. She has pelvic pain, for greater than 6 months duration, and failed medical therapy. She has an abnormal pelvic examination that shows mild right-sided tenderness, with an ultrasound that reveals normal pelvic organs. Before surgical therapy is offered, sending her to a gastroenterologist should be considered. Studies reveal that irritable bowel syndrome is the most common nongynecologic etiology for chronic pelvic pain.[2] This patient should be offered a laparoscopy as the next step. This will enable a diagnosis to be established. In the presence of an abnormal pelvic examination, studies reveal that up to 80% may have pelvic pathology on laparoscopy.[3] Kresch et al. found that 83% of women with pelvic pain had pathologic findings at laparoscopy.[4] Depending on the diagnosis, treatment can also be offered. In this patient, diagnoses can be multiple. Endometriosis, associated with cyclic pain, is a genetically linked disease and her risk is increased, since her mother also had it. Taking into account that her pain is also noncyclic, one has to rule out other gynecologic causes, such as pelvic adhesions. Her history of three prior surgeries increases her risk for adhesive disease. Since she denies any urinary urgency, or frequency, interstitial cystitis is unlikely. Procedures for midline pain should not be offered in this patient because her pain is not just limited to the midline of the pelvis. If after treatment with laparoscopy and other indicated procedures, via the laparoscope, the patient still has pain, a hysterectomy can be offered as a last resort. Counseling the patient preoperatively is important, remembering that persistent pelvic pain can exist after a hysterectomy.[5,6]

APPROACH TO Chronic Pelvic Pain

DEFINITIONS

PAIN: An unpleasant sensory or emotional experience associated with actual or potential tissue damage.

CHRONIC PELVIC PAIN: Pain in the lower abdomen for greater than 6 months' duration.

ENDOMETRIOSIS: The presence and growth of glands and stroma identical to the lining of the uterus in an aberrant location.

PRIMARY DYSMENORRHEA: Painful, crampy sensation in the lower abdomen that occurs prior to, or during, menses and is not associated with pelvic pathology.

SECONDARY DYSMENORRHEA: Painful, crampy sensation in the lower abdomen that occurs prior to, or during, menses and occurs with pelvic pathology.

PRESACRAL NEURECTOMY: A surgical procedure that consists of excision of the superior hypogastric plexus ("presacral nerve").

PELVIC CONGESTION SYNDROME: Vascular engorgement of the uterus and the vessels of the broad ligament which may lead to pelvic pain.

LAPAROSCOPIC UTERINE NERVE ABLATION (LUNA): A surgical procedure that involves transecting the uterosacral ligaments for the relief of pain.

CLINICAL APPROACH

Chronic pelvic pain complaints can be frustrating and challenging to both the physician and the patient. It can have a profound impact on life. It is defined as a noncyclic, lower abdominal pain for greater than 6 months duration, unrelated to pregnancy.[2] Pain is subjective and may be somatic or visceral. In somatic sensory nerves, perception of the pain is rapid and well localized. In visceral pain, pain is a result of transmission of impulses along the

Table 34–1 COMMON GYNECOLOGIC DIAGNOSES ASSOCIATED CPP

LEVEL A	LEVEL B	LEVEL C
Endometriosis		Adnexal ovarian cysts
Pelvic congestion syndrome	Adhesions	Dysmenorrhea
Pelvic inflammatory disease	Leiomyomas	Chronic endometritis

Level A evidence: good and consistent scientific evidence of causal relationship to CPP; Level B evidence: limited and inconsistent scientific evidence showing causal relationship to CPP; Level C evidence: Causal relationship to CPP per expert opinions

autonomic nervous system that innervates the internal reproductive organs. In general, pelvic pain is poorly localized, and is usually diffuse. The etiologies may be unclear and can range from many disorders, both gynecologic (Table 34–1) and nongynecologic (Table 34–2). An accurate workup is necessary and the appropriate treatment instituted. Treatment is twofold. One is to treat the pain as a diagnosis and the second is to treat the cause of the pain.[7] When medical management fails, surgical therapy is the next step.

It is imperative to obtain a thorough history and physical in patients with chronic pelvic pain. Getting the history can be both, diagnostic and therapeutic for the patient. It shows concern for her well-being, in addition to allowing the patient to tell her story. Have the patient characterize the pain. Pertinent questions for the history include

- Duration of pain
- Location of pain
- Commencement of pain
- Is pain associated with menses or bowel habits?
- What positions (ie, sitting, lying, standing) affect the pain?
- Has the pain affected your quality of life?
- Have you lost time from work?
- Have you taken any over-the-counter medicines for the pain?

Table 34–2 COMMON NONGYNECOLOGIC DISORDERS ASSOCIATED WITH CPP

GASTROINTESTINAL (LEVEL A)	GENITOURINARY (LEVEL A)	MUSCULOSKELETAL (LEVEL B)
Irritable bowel syndrome		
Constipation	Interstitial cystitis	Muscular strains or sprains
Inflammatory bowel disease	Urinary tract infection	Abdominal wall trigger points

The history will identify risk factors associated with pelvic pain. Obtain additional personal, medical, surgical, family, and social histories. Depression and a history of sexual abuse are predictors of pain severity. The association between domestic/sexual abuse and pelvic pain is significant. Sexual abuse is defined as penetration or other direct contact with the patient's unclothed genitals.[8] Patients with a history of sexual abuse have increasing rates of pelvic pain complaints.

Remember that a routine physical examination is very difficult for a patient with chronic pelvic pain. So, be gentle. Examine the patient supine and in the lithotomy positions. On the abdominal examination, have the patient point with one finger to identify the location of the pain. Inspect for abdominal distention, ascites, masses, and bowel sounds. Palpate lightly and deeply. Note any surgical scars and tenderness on the abdomen. On pelvic examination, inspect the external genitalia for any redness, induration, excoriations, ulcerations, and atrophic changes. Use a cotton Q-tip to evaluate for any tenderness or sensation abnormalities at the vestibule. Perform a speculum examination and fully visualize the entire vagina and cervix for any lesions. Obtain a Pap smear and cervical cultures, if necessary. Begin the manual portion of the examination with only one index finger. Palpate both the anterior and vaginal wall to elicit any pain or tenderness. Compress the uterus to evaluate for tenderness. A fixed uterus may indicate scarring in the pelvis. Palpate the rectovaginal septum last during the rectovaginal examination.

Diagnostic tests that may be ordered are based on the history and physical of the patient. All patients should not receive the same diagnostic workup. Establishing a differential diagnosis is important prior to instituting any treatment.

There are different levels of evidence in the medical literature associated with etiologies of chronic pelvic pain.[7]

- Level A: Good and consistent scientific evidence of causal relationship to chronic pelvic pain.
- Level B: Limited or inconsistent scientific evidence of causal relationship to chronic pelvic pain.
- Level C: Causal relationship to chronic pelvic pain based on expert opinions.

Treatment for chronic pelvic pain consists of medical and surgical options. NSAIDs and oral contraceptive pills have been the mainstay of treatment.[5] Tricyclic antidepressants have also been used with success. After a patient has been on medicines and continues to experience pain, it is time to offer surgical intervention. The patient's desire for future fertility will play a role in the type of intervention available.

Laparoscopy should be offered first. It is a simple, cost-efficient, diagnostic tool that can be performed on an outpatient basis. It can be used to establish a diagnosis, treat, or even monitor the course of a specific disease. If the patient has endometriosis, ablative or excisional therapy can be offered through the laparoscope. Adhesiolysis via the laparoscope is another alternative, if the patient has extensive pelvic adhesions.

Complications of laparoscopy include hemorrhage, bowel injuries, uterine perforation, vascular injuries, and infection. Reports of complications in the literature range from 0.2 out of 1000 to 4.6 out of 1000.[9] Cardiac arrest can occur at the time of induction of anesthesia, rapid or excessive insufflation of gas, or extreme Trendelenburg positions.[9]

In patients with midline pain, such as dysmenorrhea, and failed medical management, a presacral neurectomy or a LUNA procedure can be offered. Presacral neurectomy has become less popular over the years. Removing the "presacral nerve" or the superior hypogastric plexus has been shown to relieve pain in 60% to 80% of patients.[10] The operation can be difficult and lengthy. Acute complications include laceration of the middle sacral vein, hemorrhage, hypotension, and small bowel obstruction.

The LUNA is another alternative in relieving midline pain in women desiring future fertility. It was first described in 1899.[11] Through the laparoscope, the uterus is stretched upward and the uterosacral ligaments are coagulated and transected at their insertion into the posterior cervix. The goal is to interrupt the afferent-efferent sympathetic and parasympathetic neuronal pathways.[11] Be careful to identify the ureters to avoid injury. With the uterosacral ligaments supporting the uterus, a side effect of this procedure can be uterine prolapse.

Presacral neurectomy and LUNA, done in conjunction, do not offer any additional pain relief.[12]

For women with persistent pelvic pain who completed of their childbearing and failed medical management, a hysterectomy should be offered. Chronic pelvic pain is the indication for 10% of hysterectomies reviewed.[13] Before offering this final surgical alternative, it is imperative that nongynecologic etiologies for pain have been ruled out. Stovall et al. showed that, out of 99 women with pelvic pain followed 12 months after a hysterectomy (with or without a bilateral salpingo-oophorectomy [BOS]), 22% still had persistent pelvic pain.[5] Hillis et al. showed results consistent with the latter, up to 24 to 40% with persistent pain, 1 year after surgery.[6] If a treatable condition is found and treated before proceeding with surgery, it is possible that the patient's pain may resolve. Once a hysterectomy is decided, the associated morbidity should be discussed with the patient. The risk of bleeding; infection; and damage to bowel, bladder, or vascular structures should be included in the consent form. Thrombotic complications are increased after a hysterectomy. There is an increase in both infectious and febrile morbidity after a hysterectomy. Risk factors for febrile morbidity have been documented in the literature secondary to a hysterectomy.[14] Peipert et al. showed that febrile morbidity was 14% in over 680 charts reviewed. Morbidity can be decreased by the route of hysterectomy. Vaginal cases have less febrile morbidity than abdominal cases. Administering prophylactic antibiotics, 1 hour prior to starting the surgery, decreases febrile risk. In addition, meticulous surgical technique, by minimizing blood loss, also lessens febrile morbidity. With febrile morbidity, there are longer hospital stays and increasing costs to the patient.[14] Reports show that after a hysterectomy, symptoms, and quality of life can be improved. The Women's Health Study, of 1299 women, showed improvement in pain and overall participation in social functions after receiving a hysterectomy.[15] After 1 year, 87% of women reported improvement and after 2 years 88% improved.

Hysterectomy is the final surgical option offered for treatment of chronic pelvic pain. It may give long-term improvement of symptoms.

Comprehension Questions

34.1 A 19-year-old G0P0 woman complains of pain with her menses that started at menarche. Her pain is relieved with monthly NSAIDs. Her pelvic examination and pelvic ultrasound are normal. What is her most likely diagnosis?

A. Primary dysmenorrhea
B. Secondary dysmenorrhea
C. Pelvic inflammatory disease
D. Ruptured right corpus luteal cyst

34.2 A 45-year-old G5P5 woman has a 5-year history of chronic pelvic pain secondary to endometriosis. Her surgical history consists of two laparoscopic laser treatments for her endometriosis. She has been on continuous oral contraceptives and NSAIDs for the last 6 months with continued pain. What is the next step?

A. Total abdominal hysterectomy (TAH) with a bilateral salpingo-oophorectomy (BOS)
B. Repeat laser therapy via the laparoscope
C. Six more months of medical therapy
D. Partial hysterectomy

34.3 A 35-year-old G2P2, thin, woman with a recent last menstrual period received a laparoscopy for persistent pelvic pain. At the initiation of the surgery, she became suddenly hypotensive, with a BP of 70/30 mm Hg and a pulse of 125 beats/min. What is the most likely surgical complication?

A. Cardiac arrest
B. Vascular injury
C. Ureteral injury
D. Bowel laceration

34.4 A 40-year-old G0P0 woman had a LUNA procedure for dysmenorrhea. On postoperative day 1, her H/H was 10.5/32 and a creatinine 1.0. On postoperative day 2, her hemoglobin level was unchanged, but her creatinine increased to 1.8 and she now has back pain. What is the most likely complication of this surgery?

A. Bladder laceration
B. Bowel injury
C. Ureteral injury
D. Kidney puncture

ANSWERS

34.1 **A.** Primary dysmenorrhea is the pain before or during menses with no organic cause that usually begins at menarche. Her normal pelvic ultrasound is absent of any pelvic pathology.

34.2 **A.** This patient has failed medical therapy and previous conservative surgery via the laparoscope. With persistent pelvic pain secondary to her endometriosis, she requires definitive therapy, a TAH/BSO.

34.3 **B.** This patient has a vascular injury secondary to insertion of the Veress needle. As a result of acute hemorrhage, there is sudden hypotension and tachycardia. The laparoscopy is immediately converted to a laparotomy for repair of the injured vessel.

34.4 **C.** The ureter has been compromised in this patient. Early diagnosis is the key. Her rising creatinine is a clue.

Clinical Pearls

See Table 1-2 for definition of level of evidence and strength of recommendation

- Chronic pelvic pain can be caused by gynecologic or nongynecologic disorders.
- Obtaining a detailed history and physical examination is the key in establishing a diagnosis for pelvic pain (Level B).
- After medical therapy has failed, a laparoscopy is offered in order to establish a diagnosis (Level B).
- Surgical therapy is directed based on the patient's desires for future fertility (Level B).
- Presacral neurectomy and the LUNA procedures are performed in patients with midline or central pelvic pain (Level A).
- Ten percent of all hysterectomies are performed for chronic pelvic pain.

REFERENCES

1. Mathias SD, Kuppermann M, Liberman RF, Lipschutz AC, Steege JF. Chronic pelvic pain: prevalance, health-related quality of life, and economic correlates. *Obstet Gynecol.* 1996;87:321-327.
2. Zondervan KT, Yudkin PL, Vessey MP, et al. Chronic pelvic pain in the community—symptoms, investigations, and diagnoses. *Am J Obstet Gynecol.* 2001; 184:1149-1155.
3. Cunanan RG Jr, Courey NG, Lippes J. Laparoscopic findings in patients with pelvic pain. *Am J Obstet Gynecol.* 1983;146(5):589-591.
4. Kresch AJ, Seifer DB, Sachs LB, Barraes I. Laparoscopy in 100 women with chronic pelvic pain. *Obstet Gynecol.* 1984;64(5):672-674.
5. Stovall TG, Ling FW, Crawford DA. Hysterectomy for chronic pelvic pain of presumed uterine etiology. *Obstet Gynecol.* 1990;75(4):676-679.
6. Hillis SD, Marchbanks PA, Peterson HB. The effectiveness of hysterectomy for chronic pelvic pain. *Obstet Gynecol.* 1995;86:941-945.
7. Howard FM. Chronic pelvic pain. *Obstet Gynecol.* 2003;101:594-611.
8. Jamieson DJ, Steege JF. The association of sexual abuse with pelvic pain complaints in a primary care population. *Am J Obstet Gynecol.* 1997;177(6):1408-1412.
9. Cunanan RG, Coury NG, Lippes J. Complications of laparoscopic tubal sterilization. *Obstet Gynecol.* 1980;55:501-506.
10. Lee RB, Stone K, Magelssen D, Belts RP, Benson WL. Presacral neurectomy for chronic pelvic pain. *Obstet Gynecol.* 1986;68:517-521.
11. Lichten EM, Bombard J. Surgical therapy of primary dysmenorrhea with laparoscopic uterine nerve ablation. *J Reprod Med.* 1987;32:37-41.
12. ACOG Practical Bulletin. Chronic Pelvic Pain. No. 51. 2004:1184-1199.
13. Carlson KJ, Nichols DH, Schiff I. Indications for hysterectomy. *NEJM.* 1993;328:856-861.
14. Peipert JF, Weitzen S, Cruickshank C, Story E, Ethridge D, Lapane K. Risk factors for febrile morbidity after hysterectomy. *Obstet Gynecol.* 2004;103(1):86-91.
15. Kjerulff KH, Langenberg PW, Rhodes JC, et al. Effectiveness of hysterectomy. *Obstet Gynecol.* 2000;95:319-326.

Case 35

A 62-year-old G1P1 menopausal woman with a 6-month history of postmenopausal bleeding is undergoing hysteroscopy. She states that, on many occasions, her undergarments are blood tinged. She denies any nausea, vomiting, or abdominal pain. She has been menopausal for 5 years. Her past medical history is significant for type 2 diabetes for 10 years and is controlled with an oral hypoglycemic agent daily. Socially, she runs 3 miles, two times a week. A pelvic examination was noncontributory, without masses. A transvaginal ultrasound reveals a small uterus, with an 8-mm endometrial stripe; normal ovaries. An endometrial biopsy was negative for hyperplasia and carcinoma.

Prior to inserting the hysteroscope, the cervical canal is dilated with the Hegar dilators. She undergoes a dilation and curettage (D&C) with an operative hysteroscopy which reveals an endometrial polyp. The 30-degree hysteroscope is placed through a 10-mm outer sheath and glycine 1.5% is used as the distention medium. Upon entering the uterine cavity, the endocervix, the anterior and posterior walls, and the tubal ostia are all visualized. The endometrium appears pale, and a fundal endometrial polyp is visualized. The polyp extends into the endometrial cavity, while its broad base remains attached to the fundus, closer to the right tubal ostia. Grasping forceps are used in an attempt to provide adequate visualization of the base of the polyp, in its entirety. The loop resectoscope is used to resect the polyp at the base. Forty-five minutes after the start of the procedure, the nurse announces that there is a 900-cc fluid deficit. The polyp is only partially resected. The procedure continues, and the loop electrode is placed anterior to the base of the polyp and the resection continues. After several passes with the resectoscope, there is noted to be an immediate loss in intrauterine pressure to 30 mm Hg.

- ➤ What is the intraoperative diagnosis?
- ➤ What are the risk factors associated with this intraoperative diagnosis?
- ➤ What is the next step in managing this patient?

ANSWERS TO CASE 35: Hysteroscopic Complications

Summary: This is a 62-year-old woman with postmenopausal bleeding for 6 months. An operative hysteroscopy revealed an endometrial polyp as the etiology for her bleeding. During the surgery to resect the polyp, adequate visualization was difficult to obtain in order to resect the polyp. However, the resection began, under poor visualization and a uterine perforation occurred. Of note, at the time of the perforation, there was a fluid deficit approaching 1 L.

➤ **Intraoperative diagnosis (points of injury):** Uterine perforation is a complication of hysteroscopy. The uterus is at the greatest risk of being damaged in two instances: (1) at the time of cervical dilation or entry into the uterus and (2) thermal injury secondary to use of electrical current. Of special note, the uterine wall is very thin near both tubal ostia. Care must be taken when using the loop resectoscope in this area.

➤ **Risk factors associated with intraoperative diagnosis:** An unrecognized injury to the uterine wall may result in trauma to the intra-abdominal organs, or the pelvic vessels. Complications during operative hysteroscopy can occur during one of the following instances: (1) intraoperatively, (2) immediately postoperatively, or (3) as a late complication.

➤ **Next step:** A good surgeon prepares the patient preoperatively for the indicated procedure. All risks, benefits, and possible complications should be discussed during the preoperative counseling session. A discussion has to occur to understand that if a complication occurs, the procedure has to be discontinued. In this patient, the intraoperative diagnosis was a uterine perforation. An immediate loss of intrauterine pressure is noted at the time of perforation secondary to the loop resectoscope, which signals the diagnosis of a uterine perforation. The next step is to discontinue the hysteroscopy and evaluate the extent of damage done to the uterus, via laparoscopy.

ANALYSIS

Objectives

1. Know the different categories of hysteroscopic complications and be able to recognize them.
2. Be familiar with the advantages and disadvantages of each distending medium used during hysteroscopy.

3. Understand that there are legal risks associated with hysteroscopic complications.
4. Know the six most common gynecologic procedures that are associated with a higher incidence of complications.

Considerations

This is a 62-year-old G1P1 woman with postmenopausal bleeding who undergoes an operative hysteroscopy for removal of the endometrial polyp (Figure 35–1). Hysteroscopy is a quick, minimally invasive diagnostic and therapeutic procedure. Hysteroscopic surgery decreases morbidity and adds to a speedy recovery, but this advantage is minimal if complications occur. The experience of the surgeon is a strong predictor of complications. A preoperative workup revealed there to be an organic cause of the bleeding. The differential diagnosis for postmenopausal bleeding is numerous. The most common cause is atrophy of the endometrium. Other diagnoses that cause postmenopausal bleeding include endometrial hyperplasia, endometrial polyp, and endometrial carcinoma. There should be some prerequisites in place to minimize the risk of hysteroscopic complications: (1) There has to be accurate visualization of the uterine cavity and the lesion in its entirety. (2) Bleeding should be kept to a minimal because it impairs vision. (3) Laparoscopy may be used simultaneously, in some instances, to increase the safety of the procedure. (4) Accurate balancing of fluid intake and output must occur.

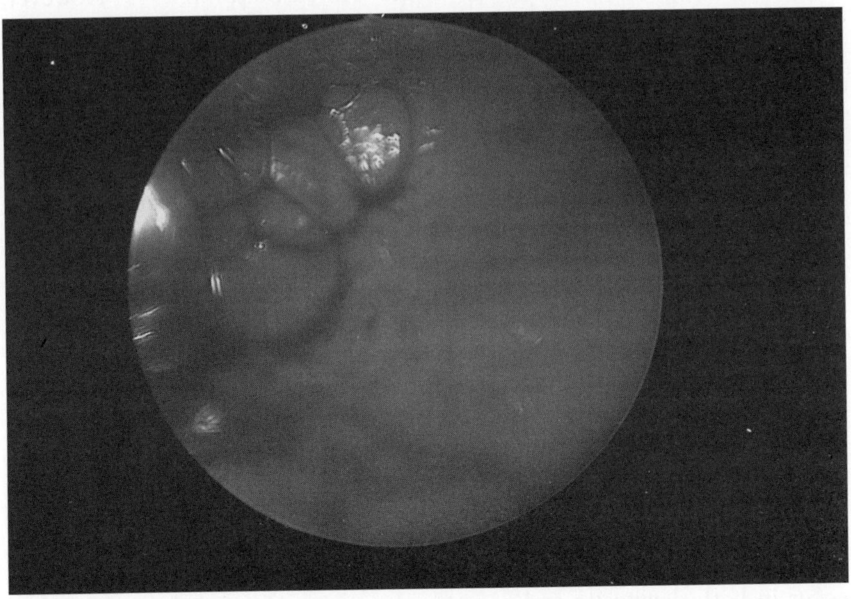

Figure 35–1. Endometrial polyps noted in the uterine cavity.

APPROACH TO Hysteroscopic Complications

DEFINITIONS:

HYSTEROSCOPE: A telescope that transmits light and carries the image to the viewer's eye. It contains the eyepiece, barrel, and lens.

DIAGNOSTIC HYSTEROSCOPY: A hysteroscope that is introduced into the endometrial cavity to detect intrauterine pathology, which aids in diagnosis.

OPERATIVE HYSTEROSCOPY: A hysteroscope, which is placed through an operative sheath that allows the introduction of flexile instruments to perform intrauterine surgery.

SHEATH: A device that is fitted over the telescope, which allows infusion of distention media.

DISTENTION MEDIUM: Fluid used to separate the walls of the uterus in order to perform the intrauterine surgery.

CLINICAL APPROACH

History

Baggish first reported hysteroscopy in the United States in 1979. However, the first hysteroscope was developed in the early nineteenth century. In 1807, a hollow tube was invented to explore the natural human cavity.[1] Today, hysteroscopes are used to aid in gynecologic diagnoses.

Instrumentation

The hysteroscope is placed in an 8- to 10-mm operative sheath, and a retractable hand piece is placed through the hysteroscope to perform electrosurgery within the uterine cavity. A variety of instruments may be used which include the monopolar loop electrodes, grasping forceps, biopsy forceps and scissors, and bipolar instruments, such as the VersaPoint (Gynecare Versapoint™ Bipolar Electrosurgery System). The surgeon should be aware of the type of angulation of the lens; in general, the 0-degree hysteroscope gives a more "straight-on" view, whereas the 30-degree hysteroscope allows for good visualization of the entire uterine cavity (Figure 35-2A and B).

Prior to the start of the procedure, the surgeon must select the type of distention media to be used. The distention medium flows through the operative sheath and it separates the anterior and posterior walls of the uterus. It also creates sufficient intrauterine pressure for the procedure. Complications occur in both diagnostic and operative hysteroscopic procedures. However, the reported complication rates are lowest with diagnostic procedures.[1]

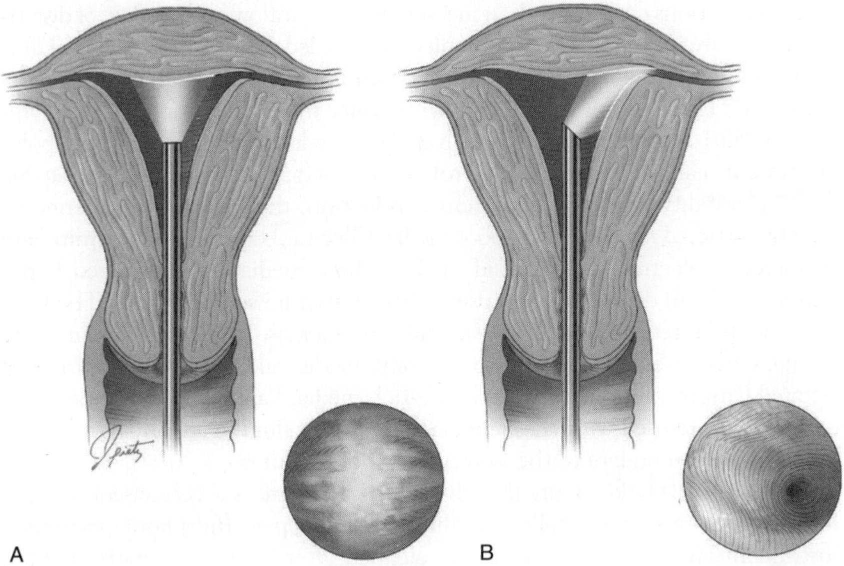

Figure 35–2. Different types of hysteroscopes. The 0-degree hysteroscope (A) gives a "straight-on" view which has a limited field of vision, whereas the 30-degree hysteroscope (B) gives a wider view of the uterine cavity, so long as the operator is aware of the direction of the fore-oblique lens. *(Reproduced, with permission, from Schorge JO, Schaffer JI, Halvorson LM, et al.* Williams Gynecology. *New York: McGraw-Hill, 2008:950.)*

Intraoperative Complications

Uterine perforation is the most common complication reported to be associated with hysteroscopy.[2,3] This complication commonly occurs during dilation of the cervix and if there is a lack of knowledge of the specific location of the uterine position. Perforation can also occur when the cervical os is stenotic and the uterus is small or sharply ante- or retroflexed. The likelihood of a perforation increases when the woman is nulliparous, menopausal, and has a history of a prior cone biopsy, and if undue force is placed while dilating. If cervical stenosis is encountered, there are pharmacologic methods used to aid in ripening.[2] Vaginal misoprostol and laminaria tent can be used.[3] Keep in mind that persons allergic to shellfish should not receive laminaria. Be mindful that, if there is a stenotic cervical os, a false passage can be created with the Hegar dilators, which too increases the risk of uterine rupture. Once the uterus is perforated, the procedure is immediately stopped and evaluation for trauma to intra-abdominal organs and/or pelvic vessels has to occur. After 6 weeks, the operative hysteroscopy may be rescheduled.[2] Cervical mucosal lacerations can also occur from use of the tenaculum. Treatment consists of applying pressure, cautery, or suturing the cervix.

Complications can occur when measurements of inflow and outflow of distention media are inaccurately or incompletely recorded. The type of electrical unit used, such as monopolar or bipolar, will determine the type of distention media to choose. There are two types of low-viscosity fluids: hypotonic (electrolyte-poor media) and isotonic (electrolyte-rich media). In general, monopolar instruments cannot be used in electrolyte rich media such as normal saline due to the possibility to electrical current conduction; thus, these instruments are usually restricted for electrolyte poor media. Glycine, sorbitol, and mannitol are examples of electrolyte-poor fluid media. These media are considered hypo-osmolar and will decrease serum osmolality and serum sodium levels. The fluid overload that results from these media will increase the risk of pulmonary edema, cerebral edema, and death. Isotonic media, such as normal saline and lactated Ringer solutions, are electrolyte-rich media. Laser and bipolar electrical instruments are used with these media. The risk of fluid overload and hyponatremia is less, secondary to the isotonicity of these fluids.

Dextran 70 (Hyskon), another distention medium, is a very viscous, sticky solution that provides excellent visibility, but is a powerful plasma expander. Instruments need to be meticulously cleaned after being used with dextran; residual material can ruin the instrumentation. The major disadvantage is that the maximum volume to be used is 500 cc, because for every 100 cc absorbed, the plasma volume expands 850 cc.[4]

Carbon dioxide gas is the final medium that can be used during hysteroscopy, but should not generally be used with operative hysteroscopy. This medium is immiscible with blood and has a high risk of carbon dioxide embolism with operative procedures. Signs and symptoms of gas emboli include pulmonary hypertension, arrhythmia, hypercarbia, hypoxia, tachypnea, and systemic hypotension.

Immediate Postoperative Complications

All fluids used with operative hysteroscopy can be associated with complications. To avoid the fluid overload, accurate balancing of inflow and outflow of distention media is required. The surgeon and surgical team are responsible for calculating the difference between the amount of fluid infused and the amount of fluid expelled during the surgery. The difference, between the two, is defined as the fluid deficit. The deficit should be less than 1 L. If the deficit is greater than 1.5 L, surgery should generally be terminated immediately.[5] This deficit can become absorbed rapidly and can cause fluid overload syndrome. Absorption or intravasation may occur via several mechanisms: (1) directly into vascular structures during surgical resection, (2) across the walls of the endometrium, and (3) via the fallopian tubes with absorption from the peritoneum.[6] The first clinical sign of fluid overload is the rapid production of dilute urine. Besides addressing the fluid overload, the patient should be assessed for hyponatremia, which likewise should be treated. Correction can occur over the first 24 hours by raising the sodium levels 1 to 2 mEq/L/h.[4] Keep the patient well oxygenated and use diuretics to manage the volume overload.

The best two means to prevent the fluid overload complication are to accurately measure the inflow and outflow of distention media and to control the intrauterine irrigation pressure that distends the uterus. Intrauterine pressures that are safe remain less than 100 mm Hg.

Hemorrhage, defined as greater than 500 cc, can occur during the procedure and immediately postoperatively.[7] Remember, clear vision is required to adequately perform operative hysteroscopy. A few methods, used to control intrauterine bleeding, are irrigation of the uterine cavity, insertion of a Foley catheter balloon, or injection of vasopressin at the bleeding site, or intravenous oxytocin.[4] These methods should not be considered if the hemorrhage is secondary to an intraoperative complication, such as uterine perforation or laceration of the surrounding pelvic vessels. In these circumstances, the operative hysteroscopy should be stopped immediately.

Infection is rare after operative hysteroscopy. Prophylactic antibiotics are not universally employed, and do not prevent infection.[1] Infection is reported with an incidence of less than 2%.[1] If an infection does occur, it may involve the urinary tract or endometrium. Risk factors that increase the likelihood include extensive endomyometrial destruction, multiple insertions with the hysteroscope, and lengthy procedures.[2]

Late Complications

This category of complications can occur months to years after an operative hysteroscopy. It has been reported that late complications are associated with intrauterine fertility surgeries or after an endometrial ablation for abnormal uterine bleeding.[8] Intrauterine synechiae that result from the operative hysteroscopy can inhibit regular menstrual flow. Commonly recognized conditions that can occur late include development of a hematometra, a pregnancy-related endometrial cancer, or post-tubal sterilization syndrome. The majority of these complications occur after an endometrial ablation.

Prompt recognition of complications is a must. Patients may complain of a myriad of complaints, such as increasing pain, bleeding, and persistent nausea and vomiting, postoperatively. Remember, if the procedure was completely uncomplicated, a patient will not call the office repeatedly. A patient who repeatedly calls the office may be experiencing a late complication, which previously had been occult. An astute surgeon has to be prompt in the diagnosis and treatment of associated complications. Legal risks can increase if a surgeon maintains a cavalier attitude, fails to accurately document fluid balance, and fails to respond promptly to possible complaints of a complication.

Indications

Operative hysteroscopy allows for visualization of the endometrial cavity, and it uses a variety of electrical current to treat intrauterine pathology. Unlike diagnostic hysteroscopy that can be performed in an office setting under local anesthesia, operative hysteroscopy is performed in a surgical suite under general or regional anesthesia. There are a variety of angled tip lenses available on the hysteroscope. The two most common are 0- and 30 degree. A 0-degree hysteroscope gives a straightforward, panoramic view of the anterior and posterior walls of the uterus and the tubal ostia. It is very similar to normal vision. A 30-degree hysteroscope allows visualization of the fundus; however, in order to see the tubal ostia, the scope has to be turned to a 90-degree angle to view the tubal ostia.

Symptoms which indicate that a hysteroscopy should be performed are abnormal uterine bleeding, infertility, or postmenopausal bleeding. Contraindications for performing the procedure, include pregnancy, infection, and endometrial carcinoma. Complications related to operative hysteroscopy are directly associated with the type of surgical procedure being performed. The six most common procedures, performed via the hysteroscope, are myomectomy septum resection, adhesiolysis, D&C with hysteroscopy, endometrial ablation, and polypectomy (Figure 35–3).[7] While polypectomy and endometrial ablations have lower rates of complications, myomectomy, adhesiolysis, and resections of a uterine septa are associated with higher complication rates.

Rates of Injury

Complications are more likely to occur with operative rather than diagnostic hysteroscopy.[1] Accurate vision is the first step in order to minimize the complication risk. The time required to perform the procedure is directly

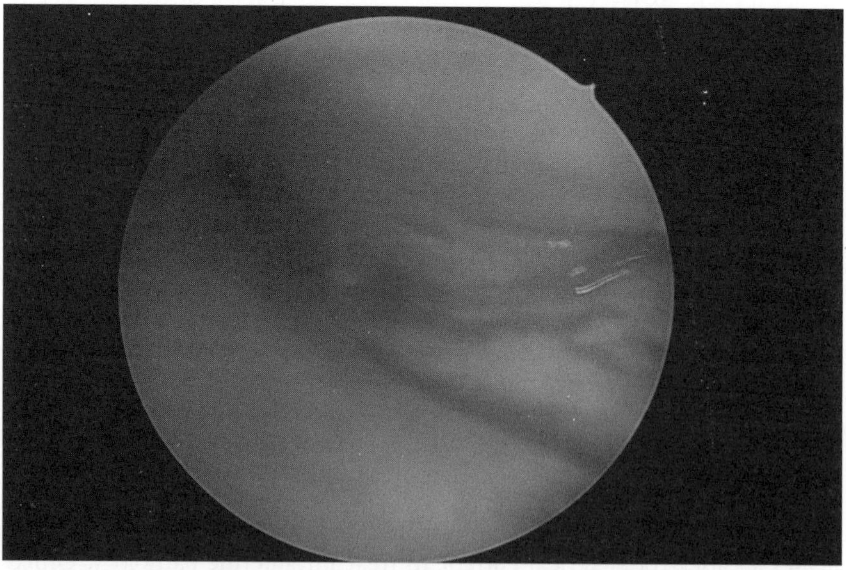

Figure 35–3. A submucous myoma is noted by hysteroscopy. This fibroid can be resected hysteroscopically.

associated with the risk of complications. It was reported that out of 925 patients, myomectomy had the highest percentage of complications (10%), compared to a polypectomy, which has the lowest rate (0.4%).[7] In another study, 38 complications occurred after 13,000 procedures. The complication rate for diagnostic hysteroscopy is 0.4% as compared to 0.95% of operative hysteroscopy.[1]

Comprehension Questions

35.1 A 25-year-old woman is undergoing hysteroscopic resection of submucous uterine fibroids. The surgeon is using 1.5% glycine solution as a distention medium. After 40 minutes of the procedure, the nurse informs the surgeon that there is a 500-mL fluid deficit. What is your next step?

A. Stop the procedure at this time.
B. Continue the procedure and carefully monitor fluid deficit.
C. Switch the fluid media to normal saline.
D. Give the patient furosemide and then continue the procedure.

35.2 The surgeon is using electrosurgery in a hysteroscopic procedure. Normal saline is used as a distention medium. Which of the following is the most accurate statement?

A. Normal saline should not be used with electrosurgery due to the possibility of conduction of electricity.
B. Normal saline may be used with a bipolar cautery device such as VersaPoint.
C. Normal saline has a greater risk of volume overload than dextran solution.
D. Normal saline is not often used as a distention medium due to the danger of hypernatremia, and instead half-normal saline is recommended.

ANSWERS

35.1 **B.** Until the fluid deficit with glycine or sorbitol reaches 1000 mL, the procedure can continue.

35.2 **B.** Normal saline is a commonly used distention medium, and is less likely to lead to fluid overload or DIC as compared to dextran, although these complications can occur. A bipolar device may be used with normal saline, and because the electrical current flows between the electrodes, it is safe to use with saline.

Clinical Pearls

See Table 1-2 for definition of level of evidence and strength of recommendation

- The hysteroscope contains the eyepiece, barrel, and lens (Level B).
- Accurate and clear visualization of the uterine lesions is the key to decreasing the risk of intraoperative complications (Level B).
- Uterine perforation is the most common complication associated with operative hysteroscopy (Level A).
- Pharmacologic agents, such as vaginal misoprostol and laminaria, may be used to ripen the cervical os prior to an operative hysteroscopy. This decreases the risk of uterine perforation (Level B).
- Each distention medium has its own advantages and disadvantages (Level A).
- Accurate balancing of fluid inflow and outflow will decrease the risk of the fluid overload and hyponatremia complication (Level B).
- Procedures which have longer operative times have a higher incidence of complications, such as myomectomy, adhesiolysis, and resection of a uterine septum (Level B).
- Once an intraoperative complication occurs, the hysteroscopy is immediately terminated (Level B).
- Late complications may occur months to years after an operative hysteroscopy (Level B).

REFERENCES

1. Julian TM. Hysteroscopic complications. *J Low Genit Tract Dis*. 2002;6(1):39-47.
2. Bradley LD. Complications in hysteroscopy: prevention, treatment, and legal risk. *Curr Opin Obstet Gynecol*. 2002;14:409-415.
3. Shveiky D, Rojansky N, Revel A, Benshushan A, Laufer N, Shushan A. Complications of hysteroscopic surgery: "beyond the learning curve." *J Minim Invasive Gynecol*. 2007;14:218-222.
4. ACOG Technical Assessment. *Hysteroscopy*. August 2005;4:350-353.
5. Konig M, Meyer A, Aydeniz B, Kurek R, Wallwiener D. Hysteroscopic surgery—complications and their prevention. *Contrib Gynecol Obstet*. 2000;20:161-170.
6. Hsieh MH, Chen TL, Lin YH, Chang CC, Lin CS, Lee YW. Acute pulmonary edema from unrecognized high irrigation pressure in hysteroscopy: a report of two cases. *J Clin Anesth*. 2009;20:614-617.
7. Propst AM, Lieberman RF, Harlow BL, Ginsburg ES. Complications of hysteroscopic surgery: predicting patients at risk. *Obstet Gynecol*. October 2000;96(4):517-520.
8. Cooper JM, Brady RM. Late complications of operative hysteroscopy. *Obstet Gynecol Clin North Am*. June 2000;27(2):367-374.
9. Jansen FW, Vredevoogd CB, Ulzen KV, Hermans J, Trimbos B, Trimbos-Kemper TCM. Complications of hysteroscopy: a prospective, multicenter study. *Obstet Gynecol*. August 2000;96(2):266-270.

Case 36

A 24-year-old nulliparous Caucasian woman presents to your office for her annual well-woman examination. She is a recent college graduate and has a monogamous relationship. Yearly Pap smears began at age 19 and have always been normal. She denies any medical conditions, and her only medication is a combination oral contraceptive pill (OCP). She does not smoke or engage in any illicit drug usage. She does drink alcohol socially.

On examination, you note no irregularities of the cervix or vagina on speculum examination; a Pap smear is performed. Bimanual examination reveals findings suggestive of an adnexal mass on the patient's right side. Palpation of the mass does not provoke pain or discomfort. She denies recent unintentional weight loss or weight gain, early satiety, abdominal bloating, dyspareunia, or vaginal discharge. She states that she has been taking her OCP regularly as directed.

Urine pregnancy test was negative in the office and a confirmatory serum β-human chorionic gonadotropin (β-hCG) level was sent to the laboratory. Transvaginal ultrasound was performed in the office and an 8-cm mass with both solid and cystic characteristics was seen on the right ovary. The mass also had areas that appeared to be calcified within the cystic portion of the mass.

➤ What is the most likely diagnosis?

➤ What is your next step?

➤ What options for management may be utilized?

ANSWERS TO CASE 36:
Ovarian Cystectomy

Summary: This is a 24-year-old nulliparous Caucasian woman having an asymptomatic ovarian mass suggestive of a cystic teratoma. The patient has an unremarkable past medical history and is asymptomatic.

- **Most likely diagnosis:** Benign cystic teratoma (dermoid).
- **Next step:** Operative removal.
- **Management options:** Surgical excision either via laparotomy, laparoscopy, or a combination of these procedures.

ANALYSIS

Objectives

1. List the surgical options available for ovarian cystectomy.
2. Describe the diagnostic features of an ovarian cyst.
3. Describe the potential complications that may arise and the solutions to them during removal of cyst.

Considerations

This is a 24-year-old Caucasian woman who presents for a routine yearly health maintenance visit. During the course of the visit, a right-sided adnexal mass is palpated during bimanual examination. Formal evaluation of the mass confirmed a right-sided ovarian mass consistent with a dermoid cyst. Pregnancy was excluded initially by urine pregnancy test, thus making the mass less likely to be an ectopic pregnancy.

The patient is further screened by questioning for evidence of ovarian cancer. The line of questioning did not provide evidence for suspicion of malignancy. Ultrasound imaging demonstrated characteristics of benign cystic teratoma. The image demonstrated regional diffuse bright echoes with or without posterior acoustic shadowing, shadowing echodensity, and a fluid-fluid level.

Further workup may be employed to differentiate the mass as benign or malignant. Dysgerminoma is a malignant form of germ cell tumor and the serum marker is lactate dehydrogenase 1 (LDH-1) and LDH-2. If this was to be suspected in the patient, it would be prudent to draw a baseline level as a way to measure response to treatment rather than a screening method. Serum markers have not been shown to be an accurate method for screening for ovarian malignancy.

Operative management is the treatment of choice in this patient. The possibility of bilateral involvement of both ovaries must be discussed with the patient. Malignant transformation is present in approximately 2% of teratomas, and thus the possibility of malignancy and the need for a staging procedure must be explained to the patient. Operative technique may be either via laparoscopic or laparotomy approach. Each approach has benefits and downfalls that the patient must be made aware of. Various methods within each modality will be discussed in detail in the following section.

As with any operation, the risk of complications must be addressed and taken into account before operation is attempted.

APPROACH TO Ovarian Cystectomy

DEFINITIONS

TERATOMA: Tissue that recapitulates the three layers of the developing embryo (ectoderm, mesoderm, and endoderm). One or more of the layers may be represented. Mature (benign) or immature (malignant) subtypes further differentiate. Arise from a single germ and have a karyotype of 46,XX.

ROKITANSKY PROTUBERANCE: Area seen on both ultrasound and pathologic specimen where fatty tissue, teeth, and bone protrude into the lumen of the teratoma.

SPILLAGE: Potential complication arising from laparoscopic (minimally from laparotomy) surgery where the contents of the cystic mass may escape from a ruptured cyst into the abdominal cavity.

CLINICAL APPROACH

Benign Cystic Teratomas

Ovarian cysts are a common occurrence in both premenopausal and postmenopausal women. Germ cell tumors account for 20% to 25% of all ovarian tumors. The most common ovarian neoplasm in women younger than 30 years is the dermoid, accounting for 25% of all ovarian neoplasms.

Dermoid cysts, or benign cystic teratomas, are a member of the germ cell tumor family. These tumors primarily arise during the reproductive years but may occur in both the postmenopausal and prepubescent women. These tumors have the ability to produce adult tissue: skin, bone, teeth, hair, and dermal tissue. Generally dermoids are unilateral, but 10% to 15% are bilateral. The gross appearance is a smooth outside wall with a yellowish appearance due to the sebaceous fatty tissue within the cyst. Size may range from 0.5 cm to more than 40 cm in diameter. Approximately 90% will be less than 15 cm in diameter. The cellular composition is derived from all three layers of embryonic origin: ectoderm, mesoderm, and endoderm. Malignancy may be present in 2% of cases.

Most teratomas are discovered incidentally at time of examination or imaging for an unrelated reason. Thus, the most common symptom is an asymptomatic patient. Patients with symptoms usually present with abdominal pain, abdominal mass or swelling, and abnormal uterine bleeding. Abnormal uterine bleeding and its subsequent relief after cyst removal suggest hormone synthesis by the tumor. Histologic evaluation has not shown evidence of endocrine function.

Complications that arise from dermoid cysts include torsion and rupture. Torsion is the presenting symptom in 11% to 20% of cases, depending on the study. Torsion has been seen to be more common during pregnancy. Rupture is relatively uncommon but serious. Chemical peritonitis and adhesion formation may result. Infection and malignant change are other potential complications. The logic and reasoning behind removal of the cyst lies in the potential for complications such as torsion, spontaneous rupture, risk of chemical peritonitis, and malignancy.

Diagnostic Evaluation Debate ensues concerning the proper workup for ovarian masses. O'Connell and associates demonstrated the reliability of transvaginal ultrasonographic diagnosis associated with negative cancer antigen 125 (CA-125), and clinical oncological examination provide a highly certain diagnosis of benign ovarian swelling and hence dermoid cysts.[1] The utilization of tumor markers before operative intervention has been addressed and currently not specific enough to be used as a reliable screening tool, rather usage has been implemented in order to evaluate response to treatment and recurrence. Beyond the scope of this case is proper transvaginal ultrasonographic diagnosis to differentiate a benign cyst from one that may be suspicious for malignancy. The importance of this weighs heavily in regard to the modality of operative removal of the cyst. Suspicion of malignancy would necessitate a proper oncology workup and possibly staging. Benacerraf et al. report a 15% failure rate in the ultrasonographic diagnosis of malignant cysts.[2] Morgante and associates suggest that frozen section at time of removal in patients where suspicion of malignancy is present (> age 40 with uncertain ultrasonographic parameters and high tumor marker levels) is crucial.[3]

Surgical Approach The classic modality utilized in removal of ovarian cysts is via open laparotomy. Laparoscopic approaches have also been utilized with equal success rates. Operative approaches via laparoscopy or vaginal routes without laparoscope efforts have been demonstrated to be viable options. The size of the tumor, perceived mobility of the adnexa, possibility of malignancy, and the skill of the surgeon must be considered when choosing the best method for removal.

Open laparotomy is the traditional method of removal of benign ovarian cysts. In the premenopausal women, removal of the ovarian cysts is performed. In the postmenopausal women, oophorectomy and salpingectomy are standards of care. The method of removal of the cyst in the premenopausal women in this case would be cystectomy. An elliptical incision is made through the cortex of the ovary (see Figure 36–1). The placement of this incision is debatable, with some advocating for it to be as near as possible to the functional part of the ovary while others arguing that it should be placed at the apex of the dome of the cyst. The importance of the initial incision is to allow for symmetric reconstruction of the ovary. Development of a plane is then performed using a blunt instrument (Figure 36–2). Fine-needle electrocautery may also be used to develop the plane. After properly separating the cyst wall from the overlying ovarian cortex, the cyst can be shelled out without rupture. Rupture has been encountered in 4% to 13% of tumor removals via laparotomy even with the most precise techniques. This is generally due to the thin nature of the cyst wall. Packing the pelvis with wet laparotomy pads before attempts at cyst removal has been described as a way to prevent contamination if rupture were to occur. A wet surgical towel encompassing the infundibulopelvic ligament has been utilized at our institution as a means to protect the pelvis if

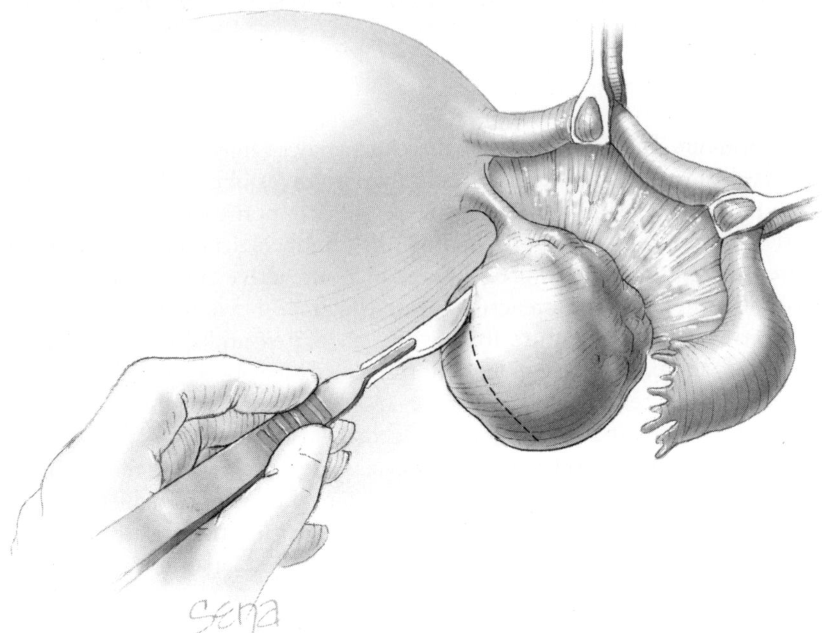

Figure 36–1. An incision is made on the surface of the ovary. *(Reproduced, with permission, from Schorge JO, Schaffer JI, Halvorson LM, et al.* Williams Gynecology. *New York: McGraw-Hill, 2008:925.)*

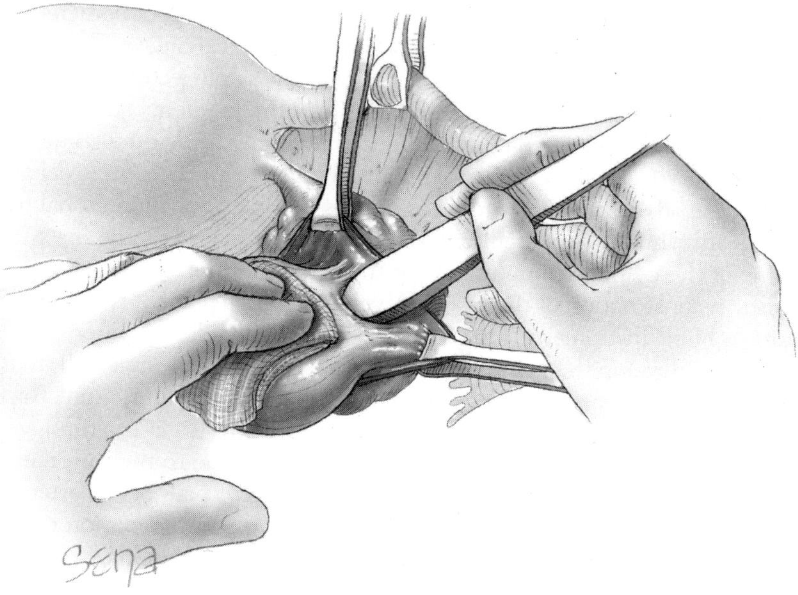

Figure 36–2. The ovarian cyst is bluntly dissected. *(Reproduced, with permission, from Schorge JO, Schaffer JI, Halvorson LM, et al.* Williams Gynecology. *New York: McGraw-Hill, 2008:925.)*

rupture occurs. Reconstruction of the ovary may or may not be utilized after the cyst has been removed. The technique involves obliteration of the dead space in a purse string fashion, using suture of a nonreactive material. The ovarian surface is then reapproximated using a subcortical running suture of a nonreactive suture, interrupted sutures of nonreactive suture, or a running "baseball" stitch using nonreactive suture (Figures 36–3 and 36–4). Care must be taken not to place suture in the ovarian cortex and disturb the normal ovarian structure. Excessive redundant thin cortex may be removed if necessary. Morgante et al. recommend not reconstructing the ovary after cystectomy.[3] They site an increased risk of adhesion formation at the ovary that may impair reproductive function and cause postsurgical pain. If the ovary is reconstructed, they advocate using a barrier method to isolate the ovary to reduce adhesion formation. Further studies are required to compare the efficacy of these systems in reducing adhesion formation after laparoscopy and laparotomy.

Laparoscopy Laparoscopic methods of removal are the more common approach today with the advancement of laparoscopic techniques in the last two decades. The technique is similar to laparotomy in that an elliptical incision is made through the cortex of the ovary. As mentioned before, the placement of the incision should be made in such a manner as to not disturb

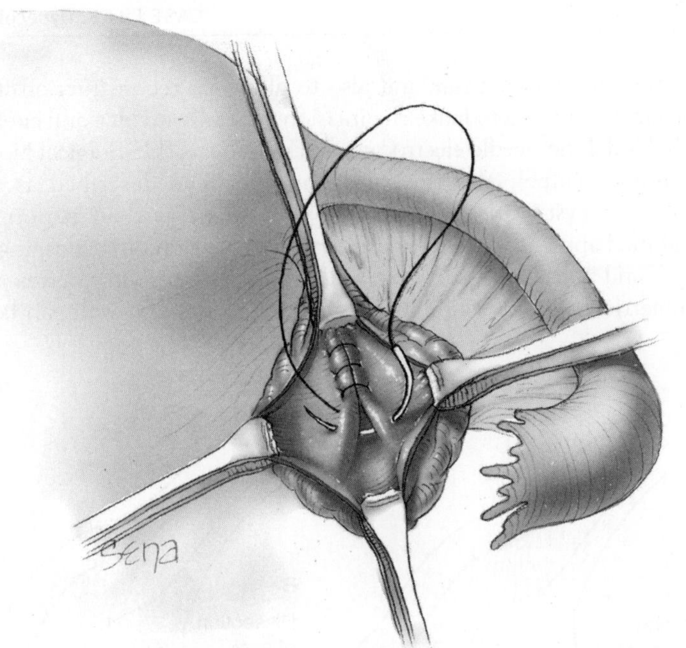

Figure 36–3. The ovary is then repaired using a continuous running closure. *(Reproduced, with permission, from Schorge JO, Schaffer JI, Halvorson LM, et al.* Williams Gynecology. *New York: McGraw-Hill, 2008:926.)*

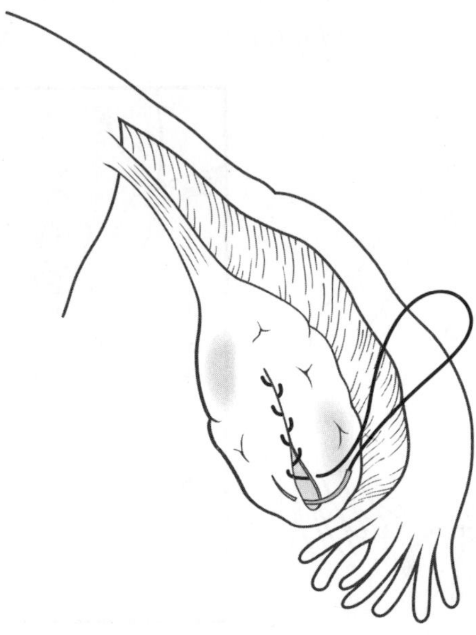

Figure 36–4. The epithelium of the ovary is closed, sometimes using a "baseball stitch" to reduce the amount of suture on the ovarian surface, thus reducing adhesion risk.

the normal ovarian tissue and also to allow for reconstruction if so desired. Instruments utilized to make the incision generally involve and energy source of some kind. Fine-needle electrocautery, EndoShears (US Surgical Norwark, CT), harmonic scalpel, and the laser have all been described as methods to incise the cyst wall. Development of a plane is then performed using a combined approach either by using hydrodissection or by grasping the incised edges and separating the cyst wall from the overlying cortex with gentle symmetric pulling (Figure 36–5). Shelling of the cyst wall can be performed

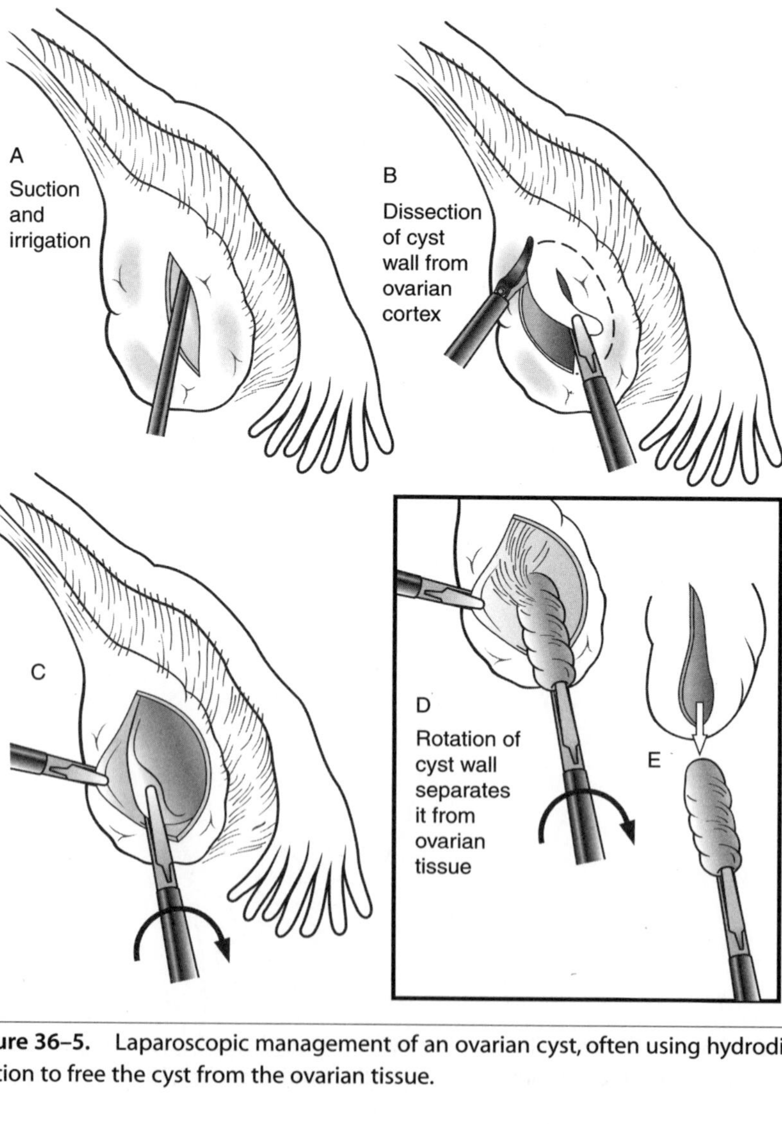

Figure 36–5. Laparoscopic management of an ovarian cyst, often using hydrodissection to free the cyst from the ovarian tissue.

using the laser to focus energy at the adhesions between the cyst wall and the cortex, using a sharp instrument (ie, Endoshears, fine-needle electrocautery), hydrodissection, or with a combination of approaches. Energy source (ie, laser or bipolar cautery) may be used to achieve hemostasis. Ovarian reconstruction generally is not performed as discussed prior, but may be performed at this time. Removal of the cyst may be performed using an impermeable sac (Endobag: Ethicon, Somerville, New Jersey) through the 10-mm umbilical trocar site. If the cyst is too large to remove from this port, various methods have been described to remedy the situation. Decompression of the cyst by removal of cyst contents either via large-bore needle aspiration or by direct removal of tissue using a grasping instrument has been utilized. Enlarging an ancillary trocar incision is another option. Removal of the cyst using laparoscopy and colpotomy, as reported by Teng and associates, is another approach for removal of the large ovarian cyst.

Comparison of Laparotomy versus Laparoscopy

Comparison between laparotomy and laparoscopic procedures has been chronicled by Morgante and associates,[3] Nezhat and associates,[4] and Curtin.[5] When consideration is given to blood loss, hospital stay, patient morbidity, cosmetic results, pain, need for analgesics, level of recovery after a week, and adhesion formation, all these parameters favor laparoscopic intervention. Laparotomy has been demonstrated to have a slight advantage in that it has less operative time to complete.

Spillage rates have been addressed and range from 15% to 100% for laparoscopy compared to 4% to 13% for laparotomy, as reported by Nezhat and associates.[4] Mecke and Savvas addressed the potential complication that arises from spillage and found no serious complications in patients with intraperitoneal contamination.[6] They advocate extensive irrigation of the abdominal cavity with sodium chloride until there is no fatty tissue remaining in the lavage. Nezhat and associates concluded that the risk of chemical peritonitis following laparoscopic removal of dermoid cysts was 0.2%.[4]

Although Dembo and associates reported that malignant ovarian cyst rupture may not affect the prognosis for ovarian cancer, spread of malignancy is still a potential problem for laparoscopic management.[7] Pelvis washings should be performed during both laparoscopic and laparotomy procedures before cystectomy. Postoperative chemotherapy may be used in case of unexpected rupture of a malignant cyst.

Bilateral dermoids occur in approximately 10% to 15% of cases and would be removed. Current treatment involves preservation of the contralateral ovary if it grossly appears normal.

Comprehension Questions

36.1 A 54-year-old postmenopausal woman presents with a complaint of abdominal bloating and pelvic pressure over the last 4 months. Ultrasound shows a 16-cm left ovarian mass with both solid and cystic component. CA-125 levels are normal. What would be the proper management in this patient?

A. Observation
B. Ovarian cystectomy
C. Total abdominal hysterectomy and bilateral salpingo-oophorectomy
D. Operative laparoscopy with drainage of cyst

36.2 A 16-year-old G0 woman presents with acute right-sided continuous pain beginning 2 hours prior to presentation and the finding of a large complex adnexal mass on ultrasound. Her pregnancy test result is negative. She is thought to likely have ovarian torsion. Which of the following is the best initial management plan?

A. Pain medication and observation
B. Immediate exploratory laparotomy
C. Immediate laparoscopy
D. Chemotherapy

36.3 The finding of which tissue influences the grade and prognosis of malignant immature teratomas?

A Neuroepithelium
B. Bone
C. Hair
D. Teeth

ANSWERS

36.1 **C.** Total abdominal hysterectomy along with bilateral salpingo-oophorectomy is the current therapy recommended for women beyond childbearing years. Especially in a woman with clinical symptoms that are related to malignancy (ie, abdominal bloating, early satiety, weight loss or gain, and occasionally abdominal pain), abdominal hysterectomy with removal of tubes and ovaries should be considered. Conservative measures may be employed if frozen section is performed and is benign. Cystic teratomas can undergo malignant degeneration, usually after menopause. This occurs rarely in only 2% of the tumors.

36.2 **C.** Torsion presents with approximately 16% of teratomas and may be the only presenting symptom. In this case, a negative serum pregnancy test would exclude an ectopic pregnancy. Torsion would be very likely in a teenager with an enlarged ovarian cyst, such as a benign cystic teratoma. This is an emergent situation. Surgical management must be employed expediently if preservation of the ovary is the focus. Immediate laparoscopy is indicated in this situation with evaluation of adnexal mass. A unilateral ovarian cystectomy or oophorectomy may be chosen, depending on the ability to reestablish blood flow after untwisting the pedicle, and no evidence of necrosis is present. Mage and associates demonstrated that the majority of patients with torsion can be treated with laparoscopic untwisting of adnexa (and removal of adnexal cyst), and no further intervention is needed.[8]

36.3 **A.** Teratomas are considered either mature or immature, depending on the histologic composition of the tissue. Mature teratomas are benign while immature teratomas are malignant. Immature teratomas account for 20% of the malignant ovarian tumors in women younger than 20 years. They comprise less than 1% of all ovarian cancers. These tumors do not occur in postmenopausal women. The prognosis for patients is related to the grade of the tumor. The grade of the tumor is based on the degree of immaturity. The highest grade (grade 3) tumors have a high proportion of neuroepithelium.

Clinical Pearls

See Table 1-2 for definition of level of evidence and strength of recommendation

- Serious complications are minimal in patients with intraperitoneal spillage of cystic contents and copious abdominal irrigation (Level B).
- Torsion is a potential and common complication of benign cystic teratomas (Level B).
- Malignancy occurs in less than 2% of teratomas (Level B).
- The majority of adnexal torsions from benign neoplasm can be laparoscopically untwisted with conservation of the ovary if surgical intervention is undertaken rapidly (Level B).
- Ultrasound fails to diagnose malignant ovarian cysts 15% of the time (Level B).
- Laparoscopic ovarian cystectomy should be the elective treatment for women with suspected dermoid cysts (Level C).

REFERENCES

1. O'Connell GJ, Ryan E, Murphy KJ, Prefontaine M. Predictive value of CA125 for ovarian carcinoma in patients presenting with pelvic masses. *Obstet Gynecol.* 1987;70:930-932.
2. Benacerraf B, Finkler N, Wojciechowski C, Knapp R. Sonographic accuracy in the diagnosis of ovarian masses. *J Reprod Med.* 1990;35:491-495.
3. Morgante G, Ditto A, la Marca A, et al. Surgical treatment of ovarian dermoid cysts. *Eur J Obstet Gynecol Reprod Biol.* 1998;81:47-50.
4. Nezhat CR, Kalyoncu S, Nezhat H, et al. Laparoscopic management of ovarian dermoid cysts: ten years' experience. *JSLS.* 1999;3:179-184.
5. Curtin J. Management of the adnexal mass. *Gynecol Oncol.* 1994;55:542-546.
6. Mecke H, Savvas V. Laparoscopic surgery of dermoid cysts—intraoperative spillage and complications. *Eur J Obstet Gynecol Reprod Biol.* 2001;96:80-84.
7. Dembo AJ, Davy M, Stenwig AE, Berle EJ, Bush RS, Kjorstad K. Prognostic factors in patients with stage I epithelial ovarian cancer. *Obstet Gynecol.* 1990;75:263-273.
8. Mage G, Canis M, Mandes H, et al. Laparoscopic management of adnexal torsion: a review of 35 cases. *J Reprod Med.* 1989;34:520-524.
9. Benjapibal M, Boriboonhirunsarn D, Suphanit I, Sangkarat S. Benign cystic teratoma of the ovary: a review of 608 patients. *J Med Assoc Thai.* 2000;83:1016-1120.
10. Callen PW. Ovarian sonography. In: *Ultrasonography in Obstetrics and Gynecology.* 4th ed. Philadelphia, PA: Saunders; 2000:878-880.
11. Caruso PA, Marsh MR, Minicowitz S, Karten G. An intense clinicopathologic study of 305 teratomas of the ovary. *Cancer.* 1971;27:343-348.
12. Ferrari MM, Mezzopane R, Bulfoni A, et al. Surgical treatment of ovarian dermoid cysts: a comparison between laparoscopic and vaginal removal. *Eur J Obstet Gynecol Reprod Biol.* 2003;109:88-91.
13. Rock JA, Jones HW III. Surgery for the benign disease of the ovary. In: *Te Linde's Operative Gynecology.* 10th ed. Philadelphia: Lippincott Williams & Wilkins. 2008:629-646.
14. Sah SP, Uprety D, Rani S. Germ cell tumors of the ovary: a clinicopathologic study of 121 cases from Nepal. *J Obstet Gynaecol Res.* 2004;30(4):303-308.
15. Stenchever MA, Droegemueller W, Herbst AL, Mischell DR. Neoplastic diseases of the ovary. In: *Comprehensive. Gynecology.* 4th ed. St. Louis: Mosby; 2001:955-998.
16. Yazbek J, Helmy S, Ben-Nagi J, et al. Value of preoperative ultrasound examination in the selection of women with adnexal masses for laparoscopic surgery. *Ultrasound Obstet Gynecol.* 2007;30:883-888.

Case 37

A 56-year-old G3P3 postmenopausal woman presents to your office with complaints of urinary incontinence for the last 6 months. She reports leakage of large amounts of urine (saturating sanitary pads) after coughing, laughing, or sneezing. She denies dysuria, frequency, or hesitancy. At times, she does have urge symptoms and nocturia. She has no known medical history and is not taking any medications. She denies loss of stool. Her previous primary care physician instructed her on Kegel exercises which she performs daily.

Her physical examination is within normal limits. Specifically, her pelvic examination revealed a parous cervical os and a mobile 7-week-size uterus with no adnexal masses. No cystocele or rectocele is appreciated. Upon Valsalva maneuver, there was no evidence of loss of urine or evidence of urethral hypermobility. Urine culture performed was negative for organisms. Her fasting blood sugar is 97 mg/dL.

- What is the most likely diagnosis?
- What would be your next management step?

ANSWERS TO CASE 37: Urodynamic Testing

Summary: This is a 56-year-old G3P3 woman with urinary incontinence of large volumes of urine with Valsalva, nocturia, and some urgency. Her physical examination demonstrates no evidence of urinary incontinence or pelvic floor relaxation.

- **Most likely diagnosis:** This patient's presentation is most consistent with mixed stress and urge incontinence.
- **Next management step:** Postvoid residual (PVR), voiding diary, and urodynamic testing.

ANALYSIS

Objectives

1. List the indications for urodynamic testing.
2. Be able to interpret some basic urodynamic studies.
3. Describe the steps of basic office urodynamics.
4. Understand how to use urodynamic results to guide management of the patient.

Considerations

The patient presented in this case has an initial complaint that appears to be most consistent with stress incontinence (loss of urine with Valsalva). However, upon further questioning, other factors are evident. The patient reports losing large amounts of urine with each episode, nocturia, and urge symptoms all found with urge incontinence. In addition, her physical examination did not support the diagnosis of stress incontinence. This patient would benefit from a voiding diary to adequately assess fluid intake/output and determine precise timing of incontinence. After the diary is obtained, urodynamic studies should be performed due to her urge symptoms and normal physical examination. **Other indications for urodynamic studies include failed previous treatment (either with medication or surgery), suspected neurogenic component, or suspected voiding disorders. After urodynamic studies are performed, the appropriate management plan can then be made.**

APPROACH TO
Urodynamics

DEFINITIONS

URODYNAMIC STUDIES: Study of the bladder and its pressure-volume relationship.

URODYNAMIC STRESS INCONTINENCE: Involuntary stress incontinence when intravesical pressure exceeds the maximum urethral pressure in absence of detrusor activity.

STRESS URINARY INCONTINENCE: The symptom of involuntary urinary leakage on exertion or effort.

URETHRAL PRESSURE PROFILE: Intraluminal pressure within the urethra while bladder is not active.

URGE URINARY INCONTINENCE: The involuntary loss of urine associated with urgency.

CLINICAL APPROACH

Urodynamics is essentially the study of the bladder and its pressure-volume relationship. Urodynamic studies allow for a better understanding of lower urinary tract disorders and help to guide management plans. Quite often, simple office urodynamic studies can be performed and provide useful information. Sometimes, complex multichannel devices are required. Prior to any urodynamic study, a urine culture should be obtained.

Office Urodynamics

Office urodynamic studies are sometimes referred to as eye cystometry (Figure 37–1). Below is an outline of the steps used in office urodynamics:

1. The patient is instructed to void completely, and then the bladder is catheterized, and a postvoid residual (PVR) is then calculated. The PVR is considered normal if less than 50 cc and abnormal if greater than 200 cc. Measurements between 50 and 200 cc require clinical correlation.
2. Approximately 400 to 500 cc of sterile saline (room or body temperature) is slowly infused into the bladder using a 60-cc Foley tip syringe. The patient is either in standing or semierect position for the examination.

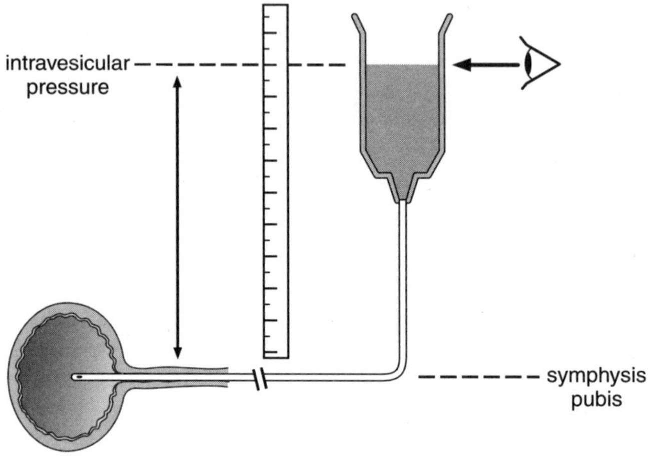

Figure 37–1. Simple cystometry using a water manometer.

3. The syringe is held 10 to 15 cm above the pubic symphysis and closely observed as the bladder is being filled in 60-cc increments. This is continued until the patient is uncomfortable and no longer able to tolerate and the number recorded as the bladder capacity. The normal bladder capacity is at least 350 to 400 cc.
4. If the meniscus in the syringe rises while filling, a detrusor contraction is suspected.

Multichannel Urodynamic Studies

Complex multichannel urodynamic studies measure the pressure within the bladder and intra-abdominal cavity during filling. Because a rise in bladder pressure can be the result of either a bladder contraction or abdominal pressure, complex urodynamic studies allow for the abdominal pressure to be substracted from the bladder pressure, resulting in an indirect determination of the true detrusor pressure. As with office urodynamics, the patient is asked to void and a PVR is obtained. The patient is placed in semierect position and room/body temperature fluid (saline or sterile water) is then instilled at a constant rate. While the bladder is filling, pressure catheters located in the bladder and rectum/or vagina (for abdominal pressure) record the pressure in centimeter H_2O. As the bladder is filling, the patient is asked to perform Valsalva maneuvers to possibly evoke incontinence. The presence of incontinence with the Valsalva confirms either stress continence or intrinsic sphincter deficiency and a leak point pressure can be determined. As the patient coughs or strains, the pressure is transmitted to both the abdominal and bladder pressure catheters, resulting in a net zero detrusor pressure change. However, if the patient has a rise in bladder pressure without an increase in abdominal pressure, the net effect would be an increase in detrusor pressure consistent with a detrusor contraction. During the filling stage, bladder sensation can be assessed along with determination of bladder capacity.

After the bladder has reached its capacity, urethra function can be assessed with a passive urethral pressure profile. The urethral catheter is withdrawn from the bladder at a fixed rate. As the catheter passes through the urethra and its sphincter, an increase in pressure is transmitted to the catheter. Urethral pressure rises to a maximum urethral closure pressure and then returns to zero after catheter leaves the urethra (Figure 37–2).

Office or multichannel urodynamic studies allow the clinician to have a better understanding of bladder function and to develop the optimal management plan. Patients who have a large PVR or decreased bladder sensation often have a neurogenic problem, resulting in their incontinence. Patients with neurogenic bladder problems are best treated with intermittent self-catheterization and referred to urologic specialist. Increased detrusor activity during filling is consistent with urge incontinence and can be managed with numerous medication or even behavioral/biofeedback techniques. Patients who have a loss of urine with Valsalva or cough may have either simple stress incontinence or possibly intrinsic sphincter dysfunction. The finding of an abnormal urethral pressure profile or low leak point pressure implies an intrinsic sphincter problem best managed by a suburethral sling, periurethral bulking agent, or artificial sphincter. When stress incontinence is confirmed, surgery (suburethral sling or urethropexy) is often needed.

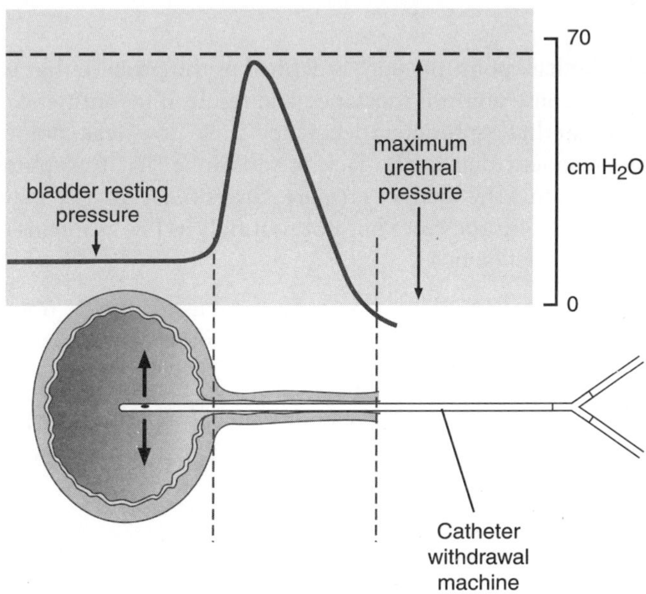

Figure 37–2. Urethral pressure profile.

Comprehension Questions

37.1 Which of the following conditions is most likely to be associated with a low leak point pressure?
A. Bladder hyperreflexia
B. Detrusor instability
C. Intrinsic urethral sphincter dysfunction
D. Stress incontinence

37.2 A 35-year-old woman is noted to have possible urinary retention. Which of the following is a normal postvoid residual?
A. < 25 cc.
B. < 50 cc.
C. < 100 cc.
D. Absolute normal values for PVR have not been established.

37.3 A 39-year-old woman is noted to have bladder hypersensitivity and reduced bladder capacity. Which of the following is the most likely diagnosis?
A. Interstitial cystitis
B. Stress urinary incontinence
C. Neurogenic bladder
D. Diabetes mellitus

ANSWERS

37.1 **C.** The leak point pressure is defined as the pressure that is required to overcome urethral resistance and result in incontinence. Patients with urethral sphincter deficiency have low leak point pressure measurement due to the lack of resistance that the sphincter provides against the bladder pressure. Stress incontinence may occur at low leak point pressures but not routinely as low as intrinsic urethral sphincter deficiency.

37.2 **D.** No absolute value has been established for a normal PVR. However, values greater than 200 mL can be considered abnormal.

37.3 **A.** Incontinent patients who have a history of spinal cord injury often suffer from overflow incontinence. Interstitial cystitis, cystitis, and detrusor instability all have bladder hyperactivity with reduced bladder capacity.

Clinical Pearls

See Table 1-2 for definition of level of evidence and strength of recommendation

- Indications for urodynamic studies include (Level C).
  - Mixed symptomatology
  - Suspected voiding disorder
  - Previous unsuccessful incontinence surgery
  - Neurogenic bladder disorders
  - Clinical examination not consistent with history
  - Patients in whom conservative measures have failed
- Patients with abnormal urethral pressure profiles or low leak point pressures should be referred to a urologist and treated with either a suburethral sling, periurethral bulking agent, or artificial sphincter (Level C).
- No absolute value has been established for a normal postvoid residual (Level C).
- Urodynamic studies are generally reliable among different observers (especially in presence of stress urinary incontinence) (Level A).

REFERENCES

1. Abrams P. Urodynamic techniques. In: Abrams P. ed. *Urodynamics* 3rd ed. Bristol, UK: Springer; 2006:39-46, 99-109.
2. Cardozo L, Staskin D. Cystometry. In: Cardozo L and Staskin D. eds. *Textbook of Female Urology and Urogynaecology*. London, UK: Isis Medical Media Ltd; 2001: 198-204.
3. Cardozo L, Staskin D. Urethral pressure measurements. In: *Textbook of Female Urology and Urogynaecology*. 2001:216-224.
4. Diokno AC, Wells TJ, Brink CA. Urinary incontinence in elderly women: urodynamic evaluation. *J Am Geriatr Soc*. 1987;35:940-946.
5. Fritel X, Fauconnier A, Pigné A. Circumstances of leakage related to low urethral closure pressure. *J Urol*. 2008;180:223-236.
6. Haylen BT, Lee J, Logan V, Husselbee S, Zhou J, Law M. Immediate postvoid residual volumes in women with symptoms of pelvic floor dysfunction. *Obstet Gynecol*. 2008;111:1305-1312.
7. Katz VL, Lentz GM, Lobo RA, Gershenson DM. Urogynecology. In: *Comprehensive Gynecology*. 5th ed. Philadelphia, PA: Mosby; 2007:537-565.
8. Swift SE, Ostegard DR. Evaluation of current urodynamic testing methods in the diagnosis of genuine stress incontinence. *Obstet Gynecol*. 1995;86:85-91.
9. Theofrastous JP, Swift SE. Urodynamic Testing. In: *Ostergard's Urogynecology and Pelvic Floor Dysfunction*. Philadelphia, PA: Lippincott Williams & Wilkins; 2003:115-139.
10. Wall LL, Wiskind AK, Taylor PA. Simple bladder filling with a cough stress test compared with subtracted cystometry for the diagnosis of urinary incontinence. *Am J Obstet Gynecol*. 1994;171:1472-1477.

11. Weber AM. Is urethral pressure profilometry a useful diagnostic test for stress urinary incontinence? *Obstet Gynecol Surv*. 2001;56:720-735.
12. Weber AM. Leak point pressure measurement and stress urinary incontinence. *Curr Womens Health Rep*. 2001;1:45-52.
13. Weir J, Jacques PF. Large-capacity bladder. A urodynamic survey. *Urology*. 1974;4:544-548.
14. Whiteside JL, Hijaz A, Imrey PB, et al. Reliability and agreement of urodynamics interpretations in a female pelvic medicine center. *Obstet Gynecol*. 2006;108:315-323.

Case 38

A 24-year-old G1P0 woman at 26 weeks' gestation presents to your clinic for routine prenatal care. Upon reviewing her laboratory results from her initial visit, she is found to have an abnormal Pap smear. The Pap smear demonstrated low-grade squamous intraepithelial lesion (LSIL). The patient is brought back to clinic for colposcopy which revealed no lesions.

➤ What is your next step of management?

➤ Was the referral for colposcopy warranted?

➤ How does a colposcopic examination in pregnancy differ from that in a nonpregnant patient?

ANSWERS TO CASE 38: Colposcopy

Summary: A 24-year-old G1P0 woman at 26 weeks' gestation with abnormal Pap smear demonstrating LSIL and subsequent normal colposcopy.

- **Next step in management:** Repeat Pap in 6 and 12 months.
- **Referral for colposcopy warranted:** Yes.
- **Colposcopy in pregnancy:** More conservative; goal is to rule out invasive disease with follow-up after delivery; no endocervical curettage (ECC) should be performed during pregnancy.

ANALYSIS

Objectives

1. List the criteria of an adequate colposcopic examination.
2. Describe the different colposcopic features of dysplasia.
3. Describe common pitfalls of colposcopy and how to avoid them.
4. Become familiar with how pregnancy affects colposcopy.

Considerations

This is a 24-year-old pregnant woman at 26 weeks' gestation with cervical dysplasia noted on Pap smear. The finding of cervical dyplasia is not uncommon in pregnancy. Her access to prenatal care may be the first time in which cervical cancer screening is done. The management of cervical dysplasia does not change appreciably in pregnancy. Patients with LSIL and high-grade squamous intraepithelial lesion (HSIL) still require a colposcopy for further evaluation. The method in which a colposcopy is performed is not any different from that in a nonpregnant state, except that an ECC is contraindicated in pregnancy. Colposcopic examination during pregnancy can be challenging due to the increased vasculature and hormonal changes to the cervix. Acetic acid and Lugol solution can both be applied to the cervix with no risk to the pregnancy. Biopsies should only be performed in areas of suspected advanced disease. All minor colposcopic changes should await further evaluation after pregnancy. The goal in pregnancy is to rule out invasive carcinoma. Treatment of dysplasia can take place after the pregnancy is completed. In addition, it is not too uncommon for the dysplastic cells to regress/slough off after delivery. For this patient, no lesions were seen on colposcopy and she can be reevaluated in 6 months.

APPROACH TO Colposcopy

DEFINITIONS

TRANSFORMATION ZONE: The area located between the original squamous epithelium and columnar epithelium.

ACETOWHITE EPITHELIUM: Areas of high nuclear activity which appear white. The more dense/pearl the epithelium appears, the higher the grade lesion.

PUNCTATION: Focal area with capillaries appearing like dots. The coarser the punctation, the higher the grade lesion.

MOSAIC: Focal appearance in which the capillaries appear to surround abnormal areas as tiles. A higher-grade lesion will be found to have a coarser, wider, and more irregular mosaic.

ATYPICAL VESSELS: Focal area in which vessels appear horizontal with irregular caliber and branching (appearing like commas, cork screw, etc.). The finding of atypical vessels is suggestive of invasive cancer.

CLINICAL APPROACH

Prenatal care provides many opportunities to screen for important conditions which could affect both the mother and fetus. One important screening test is the Pap smear. Cervical dysplasia occurs in 1% of childbearing women who are screened annually, and 2% to 8% of all pregnant women will have an abnormal Pap smear. The incidence of cervical neoplasia (including carcinoma in situ [CIS] and invasive carcinoma) in the pregnant population is estimated to be 1.5 to 12/100,000 pregnancies. Although patients with cervical neoplasia often are asymptomatic, common signs/symptoms of invasive cancer are often attributed to pregnancy changes when a patient is pregnant. Fortunately, if cervical cancer is detected, it is often in the preinvasive or early invasive stage.

The management of cervical dysplasia in pregnancy is similar to, but less aggressive than in nonpregnant women. In general, the management is conservative with the ultimate goal of ruling out an invasive malignancy. Treatment for cervical intraepithelial neoplasia (CIN) is generally delayed due to the potential serious complications with therapy, minimal risk of disease progression, high rate of spontaneous disease resolution, and high rate of incomplete excision. In this case, a pregnant patient with LSIL should be evaluated with a colposcopy. Her colposcopy can be performed in a similar fashion to a nonpregnant patient, except for the fact that an ECC should not be done and cervical biopsy performed only if invasive disease is suspected. In the presence of this patient's normal colposcopy, a repeat Pap can be performed postpartum.

Studies have suggested a higher CIN regression rate than that of a non pregnant patient.[1-3] The regression rate is likely increased due to several factors. The local inflammatory reaction and increased shedding and turnover of the cervical epithelium stimulated by cervical trauma (dilation) may improve regression rates. In addition, the extensive metaplasia and cell turnover in the cervix during pregnancy may also contribute to the higher rate of regression. Studies are conflicting as to whether a vaginal delivery yields higher regression compared to a cesarean delivery. Although some studies have suggested a higher rate of regression after a vaginal delivery, the mode of delivery should be made based on obstetrical indications.

Colposcopy

Colposcopy is a method of visually examining the cervix, vagina, and vulva for intraepithelial neoplasia and early invasive carcinoma. It uses an external white light source under magnification to highlight abnormal changes of the tissue (Figure 38–1). Changes in the relationship between the epithelium and stroma with exposure to external light allow the colposcopist to identify potential lesions. As light passes through the colorless epithelium, it is either absorbed or reflected by the underlying stroma (which appears red). The thickness and optical density of the epithelium along with vascularity of the underlying stroma determine the amount of reflected light seen under magnification. When acetic acid is applied to the cervix, surface cells undergo cytoplasmic dehydration. This dimunition of cytoplasm results in more reflected light that appears white on colposcope. When the nuclear to cytoplasm ratio is high (dysplasia/cancer), more reflected light is noted, thus producing the acetowhite change (Figure 38–2). When acetic acid is applied to the columnar epithelium, most of the light is absorbed and little is reflected due to the high mucin content rendering the endocervix highly transparent. Thus, the endocervix appears dark pink to red in color with grapelike appearance (Figures 38–3 and 38–4 for examples of LSIL and HSIL). Punctation, mosaicism, and atypical vessels are seen as stromal vessels have traversed the stroma and lie close to the epithelium. (Figure 38–5 shows mosaic epithelium consistent with HSIL.) When vessel changes occur within the acetowhite epithelium, an underlying neoplastic process should be suspected. Atypical vessels are highly suggestive of advanced neoplasia as new vessels are formed under the influence of tumor angiogenic factor. Iodine can also be applied to the cervix to highlight changes in the epithelium. Normal squamous cells will stain brown due to the abundant glycogen content in the cytoplasm. The cytoplasmic glycogen absorbs the iodine, resulting in brown color. Cells with limited cytoplasmic glycogen (neoplasia, estrogen-deficient states, and inflammation) will not stain as darkly.

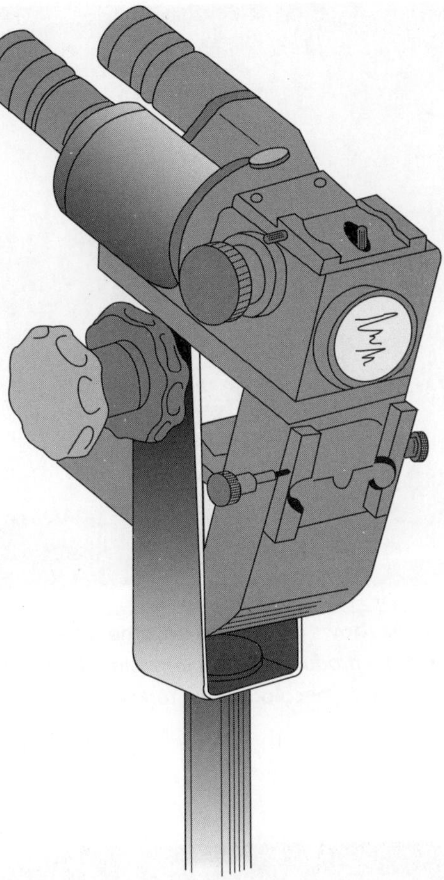

Figure 38–1. Colposcope reveals a binocular magnifying device used to magnify the image of the cervix. *(Reproduced, with permission, from DeCherney AH, Nathan L, Goodwin TM, et al.* Current Diagnosis & Treatment: Obstetrics & Gynecology, *10th ed. New York: McGraw-Hill 2007:534.)*

The majority of neoplasia occurs in the transformation zone of the cervix. This area lies between the original squamocolumnar junction and the new squamocolumnar junction. For a colposcopy to be considered **adequate, two criteria must be met:** (1) the entire transformation zone must be visualized and, (2) if a lesion is present, it must be seen completely. The original squamocolumnar junction is often difficult to visualize due to the metaplasia which has occurred. Therefore, visualization of the new squamocolumnar junction in its entirety is considered a satisfactory colposcopy. When the colposcopy is considered inadequate, a diagnostic cone biopsy is recommended. Other indications for a diagnostic cone are positive endocervical curettings, Pap/colpo discrepancy, and suspected microinvasive disease.

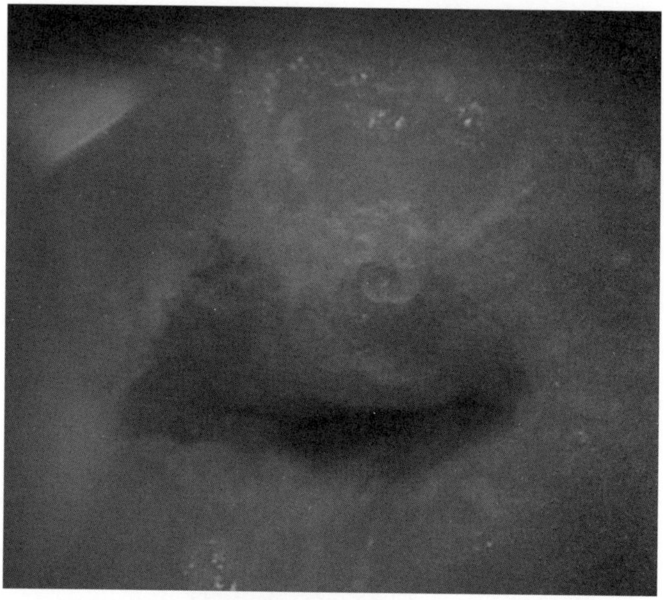

Figure 38–2. The cervix shows changes to become white in color due to the addition of 5% acetic acid. *(Reproduced, with permission, from Schorge JO, Schaffer JI, Halvorson LM, et al.* Williams Gynecology. *New York: McGraw-Hill, 2008:631.)*

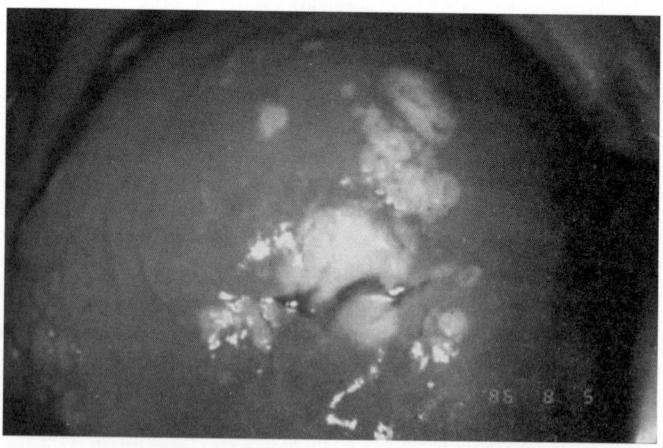

Figure 38–3. Low-grade squamous intraepithelial neoplasia after adding 5% acetic acid. *(Reproduced, with permission, from Schorge JO, Schaffer JI, Halvorson LM, et al.* Williams Gynecology. *New York: McGraw-Hill, 2008:926.)*

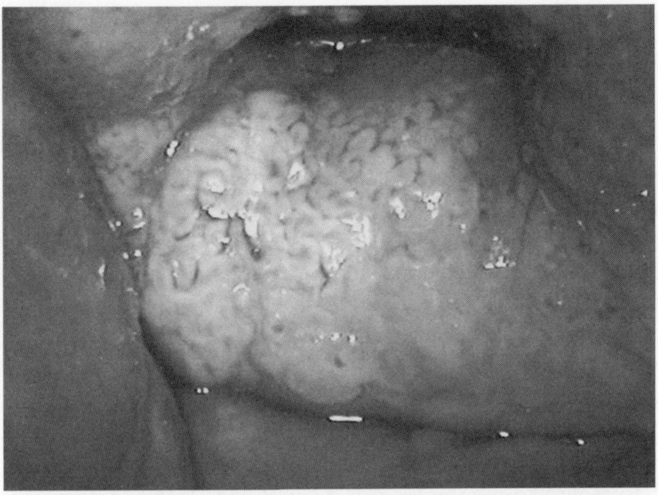

Figure 38–4. High-grade squamous intraepithelial neoplasia after adding 5% acetic acid. *(Reproduced, with permission, from Schorge JO, Schaffer JI, Halvorson LM, et al.* Williams Gynecology. *New York: McGraw-Hill, 2008:632.)*

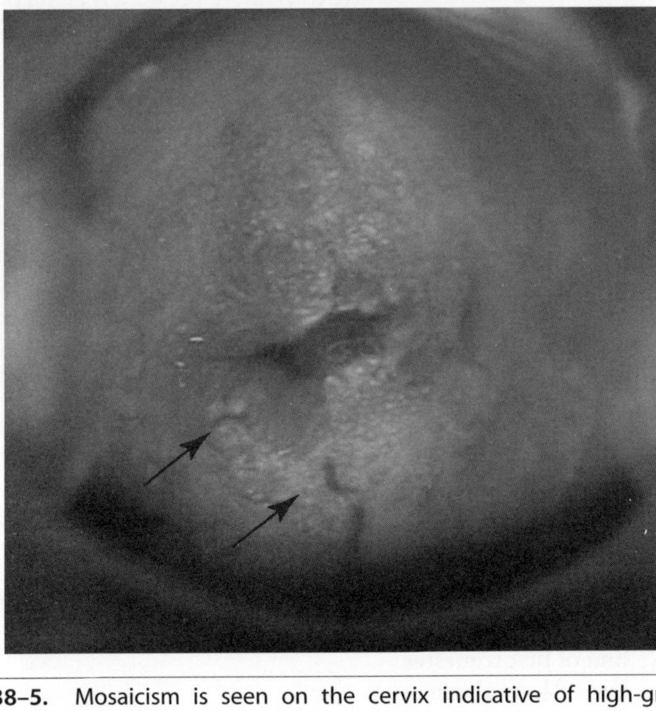

Figure 38–5. Mosaicism is seen on the cervix indicative of high-grade CIN. *(Reproduced, with permission, from Schorge JO, Schaffer JI, Halvorson LM, et al.* Williams Gynecology. *New York: McGraw-Hill, 2008:632.)*

When trying to interpret the colposcopic lesions and predict histology, various colposcopic findings need to be assessed. High-grade lesions are often found to have dull gray or oyster white color with the application of acetic acid. In addition, the acetowhite changes occur rapidly after the application of acetic acid and persist longer than that of lower-grade lesions. High-grade lesions also have irregular surface contours and well-demarcated borders. The finding of atypical vessels within the well-demarcated lesion is also suspicious for advance neoplasia. Several grading systems (Reid Index) have been developed to provide a structured approach for systematically assessing the severity of cervical neoplasia. Despite the use of grading systems, current research suggests a poor correlation between the colposcopic impression and subsequent histology. The sensitivity of colposcopy for CIN 3 has been reported to be between 54% and 85%. Findings from the ALTS (ASCUS-LSIL Triage Study) trial also revealed poor intraobserver agreement in the assessment of colposcopy. Recent studies have also determined that timing of the colposcopy (in regard to menses) is not a significant factor. The sensitivity may also be affected by the thickness of the epithelium covering the lesions (the thinner the epithelium over the lesion, the less abnormal and less likely to be biopsied). To increase sensitivity, studies have shown that random biopsies may increase the detection by 37.4% and another 5.5% with an ECC. At present, with more sensitive screening tests, more pressure is being put on the colposcopist to identify early lesions not previously known to exist. New studies are underway to improve colposcopic detection.

A colposcopy performed during pregnancy requires an understanding of the normal gestational physiologic changes of the cervix. It is important to make sure that the pathologist is aware of the pregnancy state as the physiology of pregnancy alters cellular morphology. Because of increased pelvic congestion, vaginal wall protrusion and redundancy may affect visualization at the time of colposcopy. Other challenges to colposcopy when pregnant include increased friability from eversion of endocervix, an enlarged cervix, cervical distortion form fetal head, early effacement, and poor visualization from mucus plug. Because of eversion of endocervix, after 20 weeks' gestation, almost all colposcopies will be adequate. Acetowhite and vessel changes are similar to those of the nonpregnant state.

Comprehension Questions

38.1 When does eversion of the endocervix take place in a primigravid patient?

A. End of first trimester
B. End of second trimester
C. End of third trimester
D. After delivery

38.2 Which of the following is true?
   A. Lugol solution is more sensitive than acetic acid.
   B. Lugol solution stains areas of dysplasia.
   C. Vaginal atrophy would cause Lugol solution to not stain.
   D. Lugol solution stains area of cervical trauma darker.

38.3 The performance of an ECC with colposcopy (in a nonpregnant patient) increases the sensitivity by what percentage?
   A. 1%
   B. 5%
   C. 10%
   D. Has not been shown to increase sensitivity

ANSWERS

38.1 **A.** Endocervical eversion occurs after the first trimester during a patient's first pregnancy as compared to the last trimester in multigravid patient.

38.2 **C.** Lugol solution nonstaining lesions can be caused by inflammation, atrophy, trauma, in addition to dyplasia, making it less sensitive than acetic acid.

38.3 **B.** Studies have shown that adding an ECC with colposcopy increases the sensivity by approximately 5% and should be considered on all nonpregnant colposcopies.

Clinical Pearls

See Table 1-2 for definition of level of evidence and strength of recommendation

- Colposcopy has poor sensitivity in detecting early lesions but sensitivity can be improved by adding an ECC and random biopsy (Level A).
- The colposcopic finding of atypical vessels is the most consistent colposcopic finding of invasive neoplasia (Level A).
- Colposcopy is performed in a similar fashion during pregnancy as non pregnant but with primary goal to rule out invasive disease (Level B).
- In order for a colposcopy to be adequate, the transformation zone (new squamocolumnar junction) and lesion need to be seen entirely (Level C).

REFERENCES

1. Hunter MI, Monk BJ, Tewar KS. Cervical neoplasia in pregnancy. Part 1: screening and management of preinvasive disease. *Am J Obstet Gynecol.* 2008;199:3-9.
2. Baliga BS. Colposcopic terminology and colposcopic appearances of the cervix. *Principles and Practice of Coloposcopy.* New York, NY: McGraw Hill; 2004:53-59.
3. Broderick D, Matityahu D, Didhdhai M, Alter S. Histologic and colposcopic correlates of ASCUS Pap smears in pregnancy. *J Low Genit Tract Dis.* 2002;6:116-119.
4. American College of Obstetricians and Gynecologists. *Management of Abnormal Cervical Cytology and Histology. ACOG Practice Bulletin*, 66. Washington DC; 2005.
5. Baliga BS. Colposcopy in pregnancy. *Principles and Practice of Coloposcopy.* New York, NY: McGraw Hill; 2004:138-143.
6. Cantor SB, Cárdenas-Turanzas M, Cox DD, et al. Accuracy of colposcopy in the diagnostic setting compared with the screennig setting. *Obstet Gynecol.* 2007;111:7-14.
7. Carcopino X, Akkawi R, Conroy R, Prendiville W. Specific timing for colposcopy: Is it worthwhile? *Obstet Gynecol.* 2008;111:373-377.
8. Cox JT. More questions about the accuracy of colposcopy: What does this mean for cervical cancer prevention? *Obstet Gynecol.* 2008;111:1266-1267.
9. Everson JA, Stika CS, Lurain JR. Postpartum evolution of cervical squamous intraepithelial lesions with respect to the route of delivery. *J Low Genit Tract Dis.* 2002;6:212-217.
10. Ferris DG, Litaker MS. Colposcopy quality control by remote review of digitized colposcopic images. *Am J Obstet Gynec.* 2004;191:1934-1941.
11. Ferris DG, Litaker MS. Prediction of cervical histologic results using an abbreviated Reid colposcopic index during ALTS. *Am J Obstet Gynecol.* 2006;194:704-710.
12. Jeronimo J, Schiffman M. Colposcopy at a crossroads. *Am J Obstet Gynecol.* 2006;195:349-353.
13. Katz VL, Lentz GM, Lobo RA, Gershenson DM. Intraepithelial neoplasia of the lower genital tract (cervix, vulva). In: Katz VL, Lentz GM, Lobo RA, Gershenson DM. eds. *Comprehensive Gynecology.* 5th ed. Philadelphia, PA: Mosby; 2007:743-757.
14. Massad LS, Jeronimo J, Schiffman M. Interobserver agreement in the assessment of components of colposcopic grading. *Obstet Gynecol.* 2008;111:1279-1284.
15. Muller CY, Smith HO. Cervical neoplasia complicating pregnancy. *Obstet Gynecol Clin North Am.* 2005;32:533-546.
16. Yang B, Pretorius RG, Belinson JL, Zhang X, Burchette R, Qiao Y. False negative colposcopy is associated with thinner cervical intraepithelial neoplasia 2 and 3. *Gynecol Oncol.* 2008;111:332-336.
17. Walker JL, Wang SS, Schiffman M. Predicting absolute risk of CIN3 during postcolposcopic follow-up: results from the ASCUS LSIL Triage Study (ALTS) group. *Am J Obstet Gynecol.* 2006;195:341-348.
18. Wright TC, Massad LS, Dunton CJ, Spitzer M, Wilkinson EJ, Solomon D. 2006 consensus guidelines for the management of women with cervical intraepithelial neoplasia or adenocarcinoma in situ. *J Low Genital Tract Dis.* 2007;11:223-239.

Case 39

A 23-year-old nulliparous woman presents to your clinic for follow-up of her abnormal Pap smear. She was previously found to have LSIL on Pap smear, with a finding of CIN 1 on cervical biopsy during her colposcopy. She was managed conservatively and a repeat Pap was performed 6 months later. This Pap also demonstrated LSIL and CIN 2 at the time of colposcopy. She denies postcoital spotting, irregular bleeding, and vaginal discharge. Her sexually transmitted disease (STD) screen was negative.

- ➤ What is your management plan?
- ➤ Would checking human papillomavirus (HPV) subtypes be helpful in her management at this point?
- ➤ Was performing a colposcopy with the first Pap smear demonstrating LSIL warranted?

ANSWERS TO CASE 39: Treatment of Cervical Dysplasia

Summary: A 23-year-old G0P0 woman with persistent cervical dysplasia (CIN 2) on colposcopy after 6 months of observation.

- **Management plan:** Treatment with either excision or ablation.
- **HPV testing:** No, the majority (83%) of patients with CIN 1 lesions have high-risk subtypes of HPV and testing would add little to the management.
- **Colposcopy for LSIL:** Yes, studies have shown a 15% to 30% risk of CIN 2/3 at initial colposcopy after an LSIL Pap.

ANALYSIS

Objectives

1. Become familiar with the management of CIN 1.
2. Learn the technique of both cryotherapy and loop electrosurgical excisional procedure (LEEP).
3. Become familiar with outcomes of both cryotherapy and LEEP.
4. Understand the obstetrical implications after both a cryotherapy and LEEP.

Considerations

The patient is a 23-year-old nulliparous woman with persistent cervical dysplasia. She initially had LSIL on Pap and CIN 1 on colposcopic-directed biopsy. Given the high rate of regression from CIN 1, the patient was appropriately observed with repeat cytology at a 6-month interval. Her follow-up Pap revealed LSIL and she underwent a repeat colposcopy with CIN 2 on biopsy.

At this point, observation is no longer an option and treatment should be undertaken. Cervical dysplasia can be treated with cryotherapy or conization. Given her nulliparity, cryotherapy or a LEEP conization would be the most appropriate management options.

APPROACH TO Treating CIN

DEFINITIONS

CERVICAL INTRAEPITHELIAL NEOPLASIA (CIN): Premalignant histologic changes found in cervical epithelium. It is graded as CIN 1 through CIN 3.

LOOP ELECTROSURGICAL EXCISIONAL PROCEDURE (LEEP): A conization of the cervix using a thin electric wire loop.

LOW-GRADE SQUAMOUS INTRAEPITHELIAL LESION (LSIL): A cytologic diagnosis which has changes consistent with CIN 1.

HIGH-GRADE SQUAMOUS INTRAEPITHELIAL LESION (HSIL): A cytologic diagnosis which has cellular changes consistent with CIN 2 and CIN 3.

CLINICAL APPROACH

Worldwide, cervical cancer remains one of the leading causes of death in women in the world. Fortunately, in developed countries where cervical cancer screening programs are in place, the incidence has decreased dramatically. Screening programs allow the practitioner the opportunity to detect and effectively treat precancerous lesions, cervical intraepithelial neoplasia, before the development of invasive cervical cancer. A survey performed by the College of American Pathologists demonstrated that cervical intraepithelial lesions are a common problem and that the rate of the abnormal cytology continues to rise (1 million women/year with CIN 1). Appropriate management of cervical intraepithelial neoplasia is important for both the prevention of invasive cervical cancer and avoidance of overtreating the lesion.

Patients found to have LSIL on Pap should be referred for colposcopy due to the fact that 15% to 30% of the time CIN 2/3 is identified histologically.[1,2] When colposcopy confirms CIN 1 or less, the patient should be counseled about management options of expectant management or treatment. She should be counseled about the 13% risk of progression to CIN 2/3 at 2-year follow-up and 57% rate of spontaneous regression (91% at 36 months in women aged 13 to 23 years old).[3] In a younger patient who has never been pregnant and is found to have CIN 1, expectant management is a very reasonable initial management plan. When managed expectantly, cervical cytology should be obtained every 6 months twice before returning to annual cytology. If cervical dysplasia persists on subsequent cytology, treatment with either ablation or excision is indicated. HPV subtype testing has no role in the management of CIN 1 because it is found in 83% of all CIN 1 lesions.

Treatment

In general, there are two categories of treatment for CIN: ablative and excisional procedures. Studies have shown a similar rate of CIN and HPV clearance with both excisional and ablative procedures. Ablative procedures can be performed by either cryotherapy or laser vaporization. Both procedures are well tolerated by the patient and are effective (both from a recurrence and cost-effectiveness standpoint). However, ablations should not be performed in patients with endocervical dysplasia and, prior to any ablative procedure, an endocervical curettage (ECC) should be done to rule out dysplasia of the endocervix. LEEP is the most common form of excisional procedure. Cold knife and laser conization are other excisional procedures less commonly used. An advantage of excisional procedures is their ability to evaluate the specimen histology. A major limitation of ablative procedures is the lack of histology for further evaluation. It has been reported that 2% to 3% of patients thought to only have CIN 2/3 were found to have adenocarcinoma in situ (AIS) or invasive cancer on excised specimens.[4] With this knowledge, many practitioners prefer excision to ablation for management of CIN 2/3.

Cryotherapy utilizes either carbon dioxide or nitrous oxide to freeze the epithelium of the cervix. It can be easily performed in the office without anesthesia (when used on cervix). Water-soluble gel is often applied to the probe to enhance contact with the cervix. A two-freeze technique is often used to achieve an ice ball extension 4 to 5 mm beyond the edge of the lesion. Freeze sessions often require 5 minutes each. An ECC should be performed prior to the ablation to rule out endocervical disease. The most common complication after cryotherapy is a profuse water vaginal discharge, although cervical stenosis has also been observed.

A LEEP procedure (see Figure 39–1) can be done as an outpatient, in the OR or in the office setting (with appropriate selected patient). A cervical block using lidocaine and epinephrine is usually sufficient for anesthesia. Depending on the size of the lesion, various size loops are available based on the size of the loop (0.5, 1, 1.5, and 2 cm). A pure cutting or blended (blend 1) current is then used to excise the specimen with 50- to 60-W cutting power. Care should be taken to cause "charring" of the margins by using the appropriate current and not performing the procedure too slowly or quickly (dragging the loop). If endocervical involvement is suspected or a high-grade lesion is present, additional tissue may be excised from the endocervical canal using a small loop (5 mm). This is commonly called a "top hat." Using a smaller loop in just the endocervical canal is thought to conserve cervical stroma and minimize risk of adverse pregnancy outcomes in the future. When using the smaller loop, the cutting power should be reduced to 30 to 40 W. The surgical bed can then be cauterized with a roller ball. Monsel solution can be applied with a cotton-tipped applicator if bleeding persists.

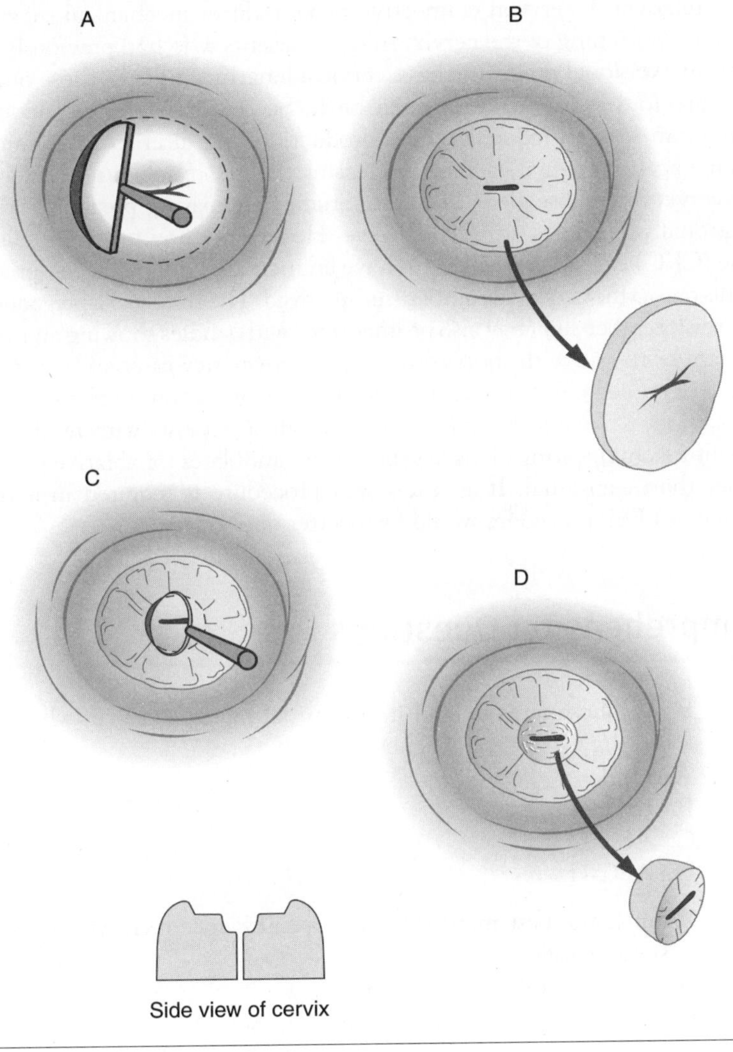

Figure 39–1. LEEP with "top hat."

Complications

Adverse pregnancy outcomes such as cervical stenosis, incompetent cervix, preterm labor, preterm premature rupture of membranes (PPROM), and low birth weight have been associated with excisional procedures, however, not with ablative procedures. An exact percentage risk has not been established. Abnormal pregnancy outcomes are thought to result from two mechanisms.

First, removal of cervical connective tissue reduces mechanical support and possible shortening of the cervix. In fact, patients who had previously undergone an excisional procedure have cervical lengths similar to those of women with previous spontaneous preterm birth. Second, removal of endocervical glands can lead to reduced mucus production and alter local immunologic defense against vaginal bacteria, increasing the risk of subclinical infection of the cervix and subsequent PPROM. Studies comparing pregnancy risks for excisional procedures are inconclusive. However, many feel that cold knife cone (CKC) excisions are likely to have an increased risk of adverse pregnancy events due to the larger volume of tissue removed. The timing of a pregnancy after an excision procedure may also be important with studies showing an increased preterm birth rate with short conization-to-pregnancy interval (< 3 months). Ablative procedures do not appear to have the same obstetrical complications as excision. Knowing this information, younger patients with mild dysplasia and future childbearing plans may be better candidates for ablative procedures rather than excisional. If an excisional procedure is required in a younger patient, a LEEP procedure would be a better option than CKC.

Comprehension Questions

39.1 HPV subtyping is helpful in the initial management of which of the following cytological diagnosis?

A. HSIL
B. LSIL
C. ASC-US
D. ASC-H

39.2 What is the best management of a LEEP specimen with CIN 3 and positive margins?

A. Repeat cytology in 6 months
B. Immediate repeat LEEP (within 72 hours)
C. Delayed repeat LEEP (6 weeks after initial LEEP)
D. Repeat colposcopy

39.3 Prior to performing an ablative procedure, what test should be done?

A. HPV subtyping
B. Cervical assays for gonorrhea/chlamydia
C. Endocervical curettage
D. Vaginal culture for bacterial vaginosis

ANSWERS

39.1 **C.** HPV subtyping is primarily used in the triage of ASC-US. Patients with CIN already have such a prevalence of HPV that knowing the subtype would not impact your management. Patients with ASC-US can be managed either by repeat cytology, immediate colposcopy, or HPV subtyping. If high-risk HPV subtypes are identified, the patient is referred to for colposcopic examination. If the high-risk subtype is negative, cytology should be repeated in 1 year.

39.2 **A.** A specimen with positive margins can be followed with repeat cytology at 6 months. Rarely would you consider repeating the excisional procedure. Incomplete removal of CIN 3 has been reported to occur in 5% to 16% of excisional procedures. It is thought that the inflammatory response from tissue healing and the cauterization of the cut surface of the conization bed help prevent persistent disease.

39.3 **C.** An ECC should be performed on all patients prior to an ablative procedure since tissue is not obtained for histology. Performing the ECC detects possible underlying dysplasia previously not known and that may alter management.

Clinical Pearls

See Table 1-2 for definition of level of evidence and strength of recommendation

- Patients with LSIL should be referred to colposcopy because of the 15% to 30% risk of CIN 2/3 (Level A).
- Ablative and excisional procedures have equal rates of clearance of dysplasia and HPV (Level A).
- HPV typing is primarily useful with ASC-US cytology (Level A).
- All excisional procedures are associated with an increased chance of adverse obstetrical outcomes (CKC possibly the highest) (Level B).
- An ECC should be obtained prior to all ablative procedures (Level C).

REFERENCES

1. Law KS, Chang TC, Hsueh S, et al. High prevalence of high grade squamous intraepithelial lesions and microinvasive carcinoma in women with a cytologic diagnosis of low grade squamous intraepithelial lesions. *J Reprod Med.* 2001;46:61.
2. Lonky NM, Sadeghi M, Tsadik GW, Petitti D. The clinical significance of the poor correlation of cervical dysplasia and cervical malignancy with referral cytologic results. *Am J Obstet Gynecol.* 1999;181:560-566.
3. Ostor AG. Natural history of cervical intraepithelial neoplasia: a critical review. *Int J Gynecol Pathol.* 1993;12:186-192.

4. Ferenczy A, Choukroun D, Arseneau J. Loop electrosurgical excision procedure for squamous intraepithelial lesions of the cervix: advantages and potential pitfalls. *Obstet Gynecol.* 1996;87:332-337.
5. American College of Obstetricians and Gynecologists. *Management of Abnormal Cervical Cytology and Histology.* ACOG *Practice Bulletin*, 66. Washington DC; 2005.
6. Baggish MS, Karram MM. Cervical surgery: conization of cervix. In: Baggish MS, Karram MM. ed. *Atlas of Pelvic Anatomy and Gynecologic Surgery.* 2nd ed. Philadelphia, PA: Elsevier Saunders; 2006:497-501.
7. Crane JM, Delaney T, Hutchens D. Transvaginal ultrasound in the prediction of preterm birth after treatment for cervical intraepithelial neoplasia. *Obstet Gynecol.* 2006;107:37-44.
8. Fanning J, Padratzik J. Cold knife conization vs. LEEP. Are they the same procedure? *J Reprod Med.* 2002;47:33-35.
9. Greenspan DL, Faubion M, Coonrod DV, Hart KW, Mathieson K. Compliance after loop electrosurgical excision procedure or cold knife cone biopsy. *Obstet Gynecol.* 2007;110:675-680.
10. Himes KP, Simhan HN. Time from cervical conization to pregnancy and preterm birth. *Obstet Gynecol.* 2007;109:314-319.
11. Jakus S, Edmonds P, Dunton C, King S. Margin status and excision of cervical intraepithelial neoplasia: a review. *Obstet Gynecol.* 2000;55:520-527.
12. Jancar N, Rakar S, Poljak M, Fujs K, Kocjan BJ, Vrtacnik-Bokal E. Efficiency of three surgical procedures in eliminating high-risk human papillomavirus infection in women with precancerous cervical lesions. *Eur J Gynaecol Oncol.* 2006;27:239-242.
13. Kalliali I, Nieminen P, Dyba T, Pukkala E, Anttila A. Cancer free survival after CIN treatment: comparisons of treatment methods and histology. *Gynecol Oncol.* 2007;105:228-233.
14. Katz VL, Lentz GM, Lobo RA, Gershenson DM. Intraepithelial neoplasia of the lower genital tract (cervix and vulva). In: Katz VL, Lentz GM, Lobo RA, Gershenson DM. *Comprehensive Gynecology.* 5th ed. Philadelphia, PA: Mosby; 2007:754-755.
15. Kyrgiou M, Koliopoulos G, Martin-Hirsch P, Arbyn M, Prendiville W, Parakevaidis E. Obstetric outcomes after conservative treatment for intraepithelial or early invasive cervical lesions: systematic review and meta-analysis. *Lancet.* 2006;367:489-498.
16. Luciani S, Gonzales M, Munoz S, Jeronimo J, Robles S. Effectiveness of cryotherapy treatment for cervical intraepithelial neoplasia. *Inter J Gynecol Obstet.* 2008;101:172-177.
17. Mathevet P, Chemali E, Roy M, Dargent D. Long-term outcome of a randomized study comparing the three techniques of conization: cold knife, laser, and LEEP. *Eur J Obstet Gynecol.* 2003;106:214-218.
18. Persad VL, Peirotic MA, Guijon FB. Management of cervical neoplasia: a 13-year experience with cryotherapy and laser. *J Low Genit Tract Dis.* 2001;5:199-203.
19. Schiffman M, Solomon D. Findings to date from the ASCUS-LSIL triage study (ALTS). *Arch Pathol Lab Med.* 2003;127:946-949.
20. Stenchever M, Droegemueller W, Herbst A, Mishell D. *Intraepithelial Neoplasia of the Cervix. Comprehensive Gynecology.* 4th ed. St. Louis, MO: Mosby 2001:877-879.
21. The ASCUS-LSIL Triage Study (ALTS) Group. A randomized trial on the management of low-grade squamous intraepithelial lesion cytology interpretations. *Am J Obstet Gynecol.* 2003;188:1393-1400.
22. Wright TC, Massad S, Dunton CJ, Spitzer M, Wilkinson EJ, Solomon D. 2006 consensus guidelines for the management of women with cervical intraepithelial neoplasia or adenocarcinoma in situ. *J Low Genit Tract Dis.* 2007;11:223-239.

Case 40

A 30-year-old African American G1P1001 woman presents for her annual well-woman examination. The patient denies any complaints at this time. She is happily married, and she and her husband desire to conceive another child in the next year. A complete history and physical examination is performed and a Pap smear is obtained. The patient has been receiving annual Pap smears since 21 years of age and denies any history of abnormal Pap smears.

The results of the Pap smear show HSIL. The patient returns to the office and undergoes colposcopy. There is one acetowhite focal lesion present at the squamocolumnar junction extending from the 5 to 7 o'clock position of the exocervix. The colposcopic impression is adequate, with moderate-to-severe dysplasia. A punch biopsy of the lesion is taken and an ECC is performed. The results of the biopsy show carcinoma in situ, *can't rule out microinvasion*, while the ECC is negative. Options were discussed with the patient and she desires conservative management.

- ➤ What is your next step?
- ➤ What are the indications for diagnostic excisional procedure?
- ➤ What are potential complications of this procedure?

ANSWERS TO CASE 40: Cold Knife Cone

Summary: This is a 30-year-old G1P1001 woman with a history of carcinoma in situ (CIS) of the cervix diagnosed by colposcopically directed biopsy. The patient desires future fertility; therefore, she would like to be managed conservatively.

- ➤ **Next step:** Diagnostic and therapeutic cold knife conization (CKC) of the cervix to rule out microinvasion.
- ➤ **Indications for diagnostic excisional procedure:** Inadequate colposcopy, two-grade Pap-colposcopy discrepancy, suspicion of microinvasion, endocervical involvement, adenocarcinoma in situ, treatment of persistent or recurrent CIN after failure of LEEP or ablation.
- ➤ **Potential complications:** Early and late postoperative bleeding, infection, cervical stenosis, cervical incompetence, infertility.

ANALYSIS

Objectives

1. List the indications for a CKC.
2. Describe the technique of CKC.
3. Describe the long-term follow-up after CKC.
4. List the short- and long-term complications of CKC and effects on future childbearing.

Considerations

This is a 30-year-old G1P1001 African American woman with a newly diagnosed CIS of the cervix. The patient desires future fertility and wishes to conceive another child in the next year. After counseling, the patient agrees to conservative management in the form of CKC. Patients with high-grade cervical lesions can be managed conservatively until childbearing wishes are done. For this patient, the excision is not only performed for possible treatment but more importantly to rule out microinvasive disease.

In general, high-grade lesions of the cervix are managed with one of the excisional procedures (LEEP, CKC, or laser conization). It has been shown that 2% to 3% of patients with high-grade dysplasia actually demonstrate unrecognized CIS or even invasive cancer. A pathologist cannot make a final diagnosis of microinvasive cervical cancer on punch biopsy or ECC. It is essential that the pathologist examines a large, well-oriented tissue specimen that is in one piece. In addition, it is important for the margins to be clearly seen to ensure diagnosis and possible treatment. Excisional techniques include LEEP, CKC, and CO_2 laser. An advantage of a CKC is that the specimen has very clear well-defined margins. When excision is performed by the LEEP or laser, coagulation artifact along the margin may be present in 3.3% to 51% of cases.

APPROACH TO Cold Knife Conization

DEFINITIONS

CONIZATION: A large biopsy of the central cervix for the diagnosis or treatment of cervical dysplasia.

COLD KNIFE CONIZATION: A conization of the cervix performed with a scalpel.

MICROINVASIVE CERVICAL CANCER: A small cervical carcinoma detected by microscope only (stage IA cervical cancer).

CLINICAL APPROACH

Indications

There are four clinical scenarios in which diagnostic excisional procedure should be performed. These include:

1. An inadequate colposcopy (entire lesion or squamocolumnar junction [SCJ] not visualized)
2. Suspicion of microinvasion
3. Greater than or equal to two-grade discrepancy between Pap smear and colposcopy/biopsy
4. Endocervical involvement (ECC +)

Either a LEEP or CKC may be performed to obtain a cone biopsy specimen, but keep in mind that coagulation artifact from some LEEP specimens may make interpretation of the surgical margins difficult. A CKC is also the preferred treatment of adenocarcinoma in situ and treatment of persistent or recurrent CIN after failure of LEEP or ablation.

Technique

The traditional CKC (Figures 40–1 and 40–2) has been used for many years in the treatment of CIN. In the past, hot cautery was used to perform the conization of an inflamed, hypertrophic, chronically infected cervix. However, for the excision of CIN, a standard surgical scalpel was more appropriate. Thus, the term "cold knife" was introduced to differentiate these two procedures.

A CKC is generally performed in the OR under anesthesia. The patient is placed supine in the dorsal lithotomy position. After examination under anesthesia, the patient is prepped and draped in sterile fashion. A weighted speculum is placed in the vagina. Lugol solution is placed on the cervix to delineate the

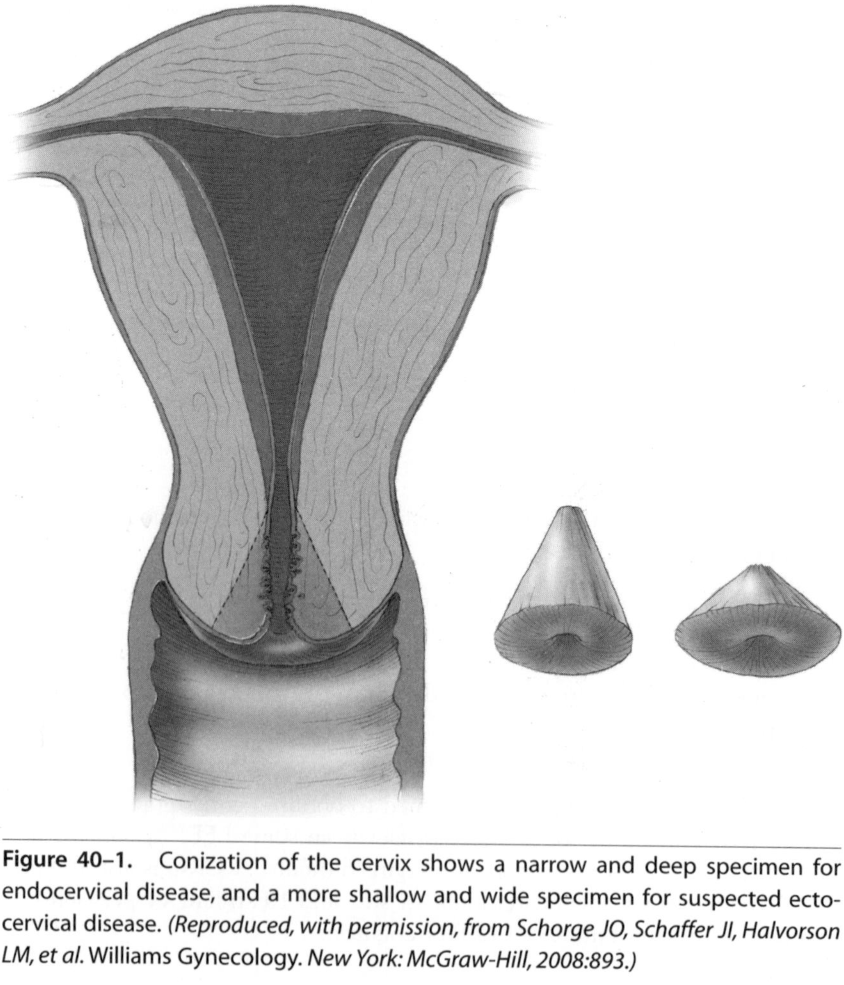

Figure 40–1. Conization of the cervix shows a narrow and deep specimen for endocervical disease, and a more shallow and wide specimen for suspected ectocervical disease. *(Reproduced, with permission, from Schorge JO, Schaffer JI, Halvorson LM, et al.* Williams Gynecology. *New York: McGraw-Hill, 2008:893.)*

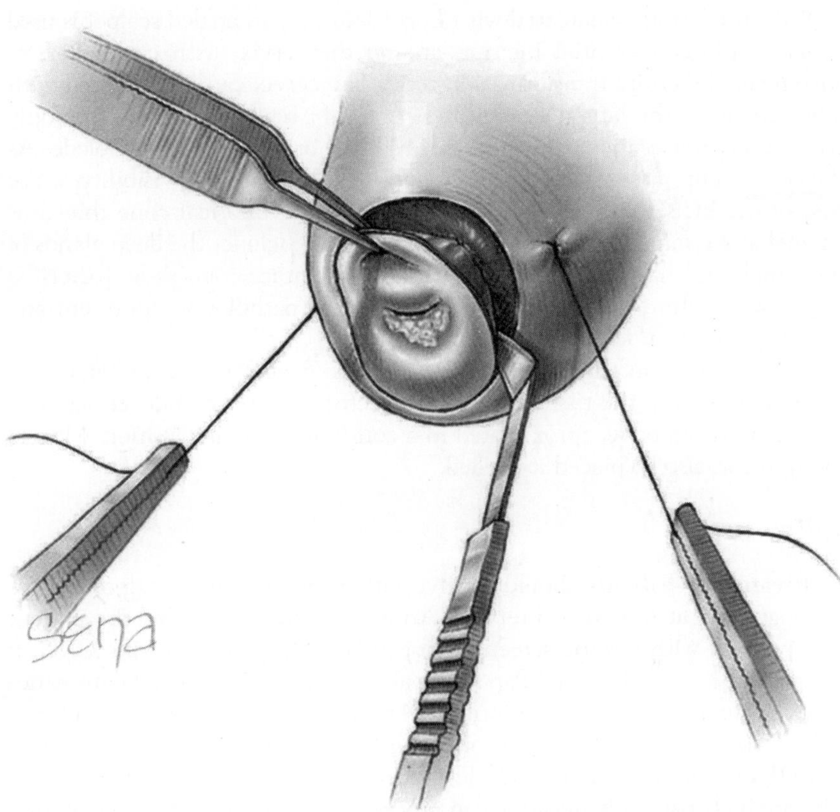

Figure 40–2. Conization of the cervix. Sutures are placed at 3 and 9 o'clock positions of the cervix for hemostasis and also stabilization of the cervix. An angled blade is used to incise the cervix to give a cone biopsy. *(Reproduced, with permission, from Schorge JO, Schaffer JI, Halvorson LM, et al.* Williams Gynecology. *New York: McGraw-Hill, 2008:892.)*

margins of the transformation zone and identify the areas of dysplasia. The cervix is then injected with a vasoconstrictive agent to help decrease blood loss. Approximately 1.5 cc of a mixture of a local anesthetic (lidocaine) with 1:100,000 epinephrine is injected directly into four quadrants of the cervix, that is, 2, 4, 8, and 10 o'clock. A total of 9 to 10 cc is injected and should cause "ballooning" and blanching of the cervix. Because acute hypertension may be caused by this drug, inform the anesthesiologist of its use before injection. Lateral hemostatic sutures (stay sutures), consisting of 2-0 Vicryl or 2-0 Chromic may then be placed at the 3 and 9 o'clock positions of the cervix to ligate the cervical branches of the uterine artery and as a way to apply traction to the cervix. Studies have subsequently shown no benefit to deep lateral sutures in helping reduce blood loss.[1,2]

With the lesion demarcated with Lugol solution, an angled scalpel is used to make a circumferential incision around the cervix, with care taken to encompass the entire transformation zone. The cervix can be stabilized with a tenaculum or the lateral stay sutures. A no. 11 scalpel blade is commonly used; other choices include a larger no. 10 blade or a smaller no. 15 blade. As the cone is cut, it is retracted to the opposite side to provide visibility at the base of the incision. The preferred specimen is a cylindrical cone that runs parallel and symmetric to the endocervical canal, includes the deep glands of the canal, and has its apex in the canal. The intact cone should then be tagged with suture at 12 or 6 o'clock so that the pathologist can orient any positive margins or foci of invasive cancer.

The surgeon can then use electrocautery to coagulate the cervical cone bed. Alternatively, the tissue between the ectocervical and endocervical surgical margin can be reapproximated in a continuous locking fashion. Monsel solution can also be placed if needed.

Follow-up

Posttreatment, patients should receive either cytology with colposcopy or cytology only at 6-month intervals. After two negative results, the patient may proceed with routine screening, for at least 20 years following CKC. If the patient has an abnormal Pap smear at any time, a colposcopy with endocervical curettage must be performed. An alternative posttreatment plan is HPV testing at 6 to 12 months following treatment. Patients who are high-risk HPV positive at testing should proceed with colposcopy/ECC. Patients who are high-risk HPV negative can proceed with routine testing, for at least 20 years following CKC.

CKC is usually considered the definitive treatment of CIN if the cone has encompassed the entire extent of the epithelial change; in other words, the epithelium is clear of disease at the surgical margins. One study evaluated the long-term outcome of patients with CIN 3/CIS after CKC with involved margins.[3] Of the 969 patients with positive margins, 390 patients were followed expectantly for a mean of 19 (range 6-30) years. Results showed a 22% incidence of persistent or recurrent disease in these patients, with 1.3% developing microinvasive cancer and 1% patients with a stage IB lesion. On the other hand, after incomplete excision of CIN 3, most patients did not develop persistent or recurrent disease. This is probably because of the effect of diathermy on the cut cervix after removal of the cone and the inflammatory response associated with wound healing. Dysplastic or malignant epithelium within the inner zone of necrosis and an outer zone of white cell infiltration appears to be eradicated after CKC. Only lesions outside these zones can persist, regress, or progress. The findings suggested that expectant management is reasonable for patients with CIN 3 and positive margins after CKC, provided that careful follow-up is available, particularly during the first year.

Of note, a recent retrospective study showed that compared with office LEEP procedures, CKC patients were significantly more compliant with follow-up appointments.[4] The authors concluded that because LEEP is a less invasive in-office procedure, it may convey to patients the idea that their condition is less severe.

Complications

Cold knife conization is associated with a relatively high complication rate. Short- and long-term complications include early and late postoperative hemorrhage, infection, cervical stenosis, and cervical incompetence. Perioperative and postoperative hemorrhage, the most common complication, generally occurs in 10% to 20% of cases. Hemorrhage is described as early if it occurs within the first 24 hours of surgery. Late hemorrhage typically occurs 10 to 21 days after surgery when the sutures dissolve. Intracervical vasopressors and topical thrombotic agents (Monsel solution) are shown to significantly decrease estimated blood loss, but lateral hemostatic sutures have not been shown to have this effect. There are conflicting results regarding the superior method for obtaining hemostasis of the cervical cone bed. Some studies advocate that electrocautery is more effective in decreasing estimated blood loss, while others insist a continuous suture is the most hemostatic way to close the cone bed.

Cold knife conization, as are all excisional techniques, is associated with a roughly doubled rate of preterm labor (PTL) and delivery.[5] The size of the cone is directly related to the risk of preterm labor. CKC also increases the risk of preterm premature rupture of membranes (PPROM). Two mechanisms have been proposed to account for a higher rate of preterm birth and PPROM after conization. One reason seems to be the disruption of cervical glands and reduced secretion of mucus after removal of cervical tissue. This might result in an impaired defense mechanism against microbial colonization in the cervix, which could facilitate ascending infections and lead to a higher rate of PROM. Another possibility is when part of the connective tissue of the cervix is removed with CKC; this leads to cervical fragility during pregnancy. There is a different collagen composition of the original cervical tissue compared to that of the cervical scar.

Cervical stenosis occurs in about 3% of patients. This is more common in patients who are not having regular menstrual periods. This condition may result in infertility, hematometra, and dysmenorrhea. Data also indicate a slight increase in the incidence of symptomatic cervical tears during vaginal delivery, requiring surgical repair because of postpartum bleeding.

Young women with need for conization should be informed about potential complications in subsequent pregnancies. In addition, closer surveillance, including measurement of the cervical length, might be useful, and information about a prior conization should be available for the obstetrician.

Comprehension Questions

40.1 A 28-year-old G3P3003 woman presents to the office for preoperative evaluation for planned CKC. She asks the physician what risks are associated with this procedure. Which of the following is the most common complication from CKC?

A. Preterm labor
B. Cervical stenosis
C. Postoperative hemorrhage
D. Cervical incompetence
E. Infection

40.2 A 26-year-old G2P2002 woman who underwent CKC for CIN 3 is found to have a positive margin on pathologic evaluation of the specimen. What is the best next step?

A. Repeat CKC immediately.
B. Repeat CKC in 6 weeks, after healing takes place.
C. Perform a Pap smear and colposcopy in 6 weeks after healing takes place.
D. Perform a Pap smear and colposcopy in 6 months.

40.3 A 33-year-old G3P0202 woman at 9 weeks' gestation presents for an initial OB appointment. The patient gives a history of CKC at 23 years of age with no abnormal Pap smears since that time. Her obstetric history is significant for preterm labor and delivery at 32 weeks' gestational age and again at 34 weeks. Which of the following is the best next step in management?

A. Placement of abdominal cerclage
B. Placement of a cervical cerclage using the McDonald technique
C. Measurement of cervical length by sonogram
D. Recommendation of strict bed rest

ANSWERS

40.1 **C.** Early (within 24 hours of surgery) and late (24 hours or more after surgery) postoperative hemorrhage complicates 10% to 20% of cases of CKC. All of the other choices are complications of CKC, but these occur less often. Two options for controlling hemorrhage include placement of a vaginal pack or closure of the cervical bed with a continuous locking suture.

40.2 **D.** Re-exision is not necessary for patients with a positive margin following CKC. Seventy-eight percent or more of patients with involved margins are free of disease at follow-up. The diathermy effect and inflammatory response seems to eradicate the remaining dysplastic cells. These patients should proceed with routine follow-up at 6 months with Pap smear and/or colposcopy or high-risk HPV testing.

40.3 **C.** Following CKC, patients are at increased risk of PTL and PROM. Given this patient's history of two preterm deliveries, cervical incompetence due to previous CKC is a possibility. The next best step in management would be sonographic measurement of her cervical length. Patients with a cervical length of shorter than 2.5 cm are at a higher risk of PTL. An elective McDonald cerclage may be an option for this patient, but it is not the immediate next step; in addition, cerclage placement is preferable at about 12 to 14 weeks' gestational age. Bed rest and abdominal cerclage are not indicated in this situation.

Clinical Pearls

See Table 1-2 for definition of level of evidence and strength of recommendation

- Excisional techniques are recommended in high-grade lesions because excision provides histological confirmation that invasive cancer is not present (Level A).
- For patients with positive margins following CKC for the treatment of CIN 2 or 3, re-excision is not necessary. Patients should be followed at 6-month intervals with cytology and/or colposcopy or high-risk HPV testing (Level B).
- All of the excisional procedures to treat CIN present similar pregnancy-related morbidity, without apparent neonatal morbidity (Level B).

REFERENCES

1. Kamat AA, Kramer P, Soisson AP. Superiority of electrocautery over the suture method for achieving cervical cone bed hemostasis. *Obstet Gynecol.* 2003;102;726-730.
2. Dane C, Dane B, Cetin A, Erginbas M. Haemostasis after cold knife conization: a randomized prospective trial comparing cerclage suture versus electrocauterization. *Aust N Z J Obstet Gynaecol.* 2008;48:343-347.
3. Reich O, Lahousen M, Pickel H, et al. Cervical intraepithelial neoplasia III: long-term outcome after cold-knife conization with involved margins. *Obstet Gynecol.* 2002;99:193-196.
4. Wright TC Jr, Massad LS, Dunton CJ, et al. 2206 American Society for Colposcopy and Cervical Pathology-Sponsored Concensus Conference. 2006 consensus guidelines for the management of women with abnormal cervical cancer screening tests. *Am J Obstet Gynecol.* 2007;197:346-355.

5. Klaritsch P, Reich O, Giuliani A, et al. Delivery outcome after cold-knife conization of the uterine cervix. *Gynecol Oncol*. 2006;103:604-607.
6. Greenspan D, Faubion M, Coonrod D, et al. Compliance after loop electrosurgical excision procedure or cold knife cone biopsy. *Obstet Gynecol*. 2007;110:675-680.
7. Kyrgiou G, Martin-Hirsch P, Arbyn M, et al. Obstetric outcomes after conservative treatment for intraepithelial or early invasive cervical lesions: systematic review and meta-analysis. *Lancet*. 2006;367:489-498.
8. Mathevet P, Chemali E, Roy M, et al. Long-term outcome of a randomized study comparing three techniques of conization: cold knife, laser, and LEEP. *Eur J Obstet Gynecol Reprod Bio*. 2003;106:214-218.
9. Reich O, Pickel H, Lahousen M, et al. Cervical intraepithelial neoplasia III: long-term outcome after cold-knife conization with clear margins. *Obstet Gynecol*. 2001;97:428-430.
10. Rock J, Jones H. Cervical cancer precursors and their management. In: Rock J, Jones H. ed. *Te Linde's Operative Gynecology*. 10th ed. Philadelphia, PA: Lippincott Williams & Wilkins; 2008:1208-1225.

SECTION III

Listing of Cases

- Listing by Case Number
- Listing by Disorder (Alphabetical)

Listing by Case Number

Listing by Disorder (Alphabetical)

INDEX

Page numbers followed by *f* or *t* indicate figures or tables, respectively.